Surgical Principles of Minimally Invasive Procedures

H. Jaap Bonjer
Editor

Surgical Principles of Minimally Invasive Procedures

Manual of the European Association of Endoscopic Surgery (EAES)

Springer

Editor
H. Jaap Bonjer
Department of Surgery
VU University Medical Center Amsterdam
Amsterdam
The Netherlands

ISBN 978-3-319-43194-9 ISBN 978-3-319-43196-3 (eBook)
DOI 10.1007/978-3-319-43196-3

Library of Congress Control Number: 2016960774

Printed on acid-free paper

This Springer imprint is published by Springer Nature
The registered company is Springer International Publishing AG
The registered company address is: Gewerbestrasse 11, 6330 Cham, Switzerland

Preface

Surgical Principles of Minimally Invasive Procedures guides surgeons and surgical residents in managing patients who undergo minimally invasive surgery. Surgeons with vast experience in minimally invasive surgery liberally share their own considerations, thoughts, and lessons learned in this Manual of the European Association of Endoscopic Surgery (EAES). Selection of patients including discussion of contraindications for minimally invasive surgery and caveats is followed by detailed description on preparation for surgery, operation room setup, and patient positioning. The authors of *Surgical Principles of Minimally Invasive Procedures* have dissected the surgical procedures in operative steps and address risks, troubleshooting, and when to convert to open surgery. Each chapter offers advice on postoperative care and early recognition and management of complications.

This manual is a product of teamwork and I wish to acknowledge and thank all the listed contributors. Selman Uranues and Roberto Bergamaschi, initiators of the manual, and Stavros Antoniou, Alfred Cuschieri, Luigi Boni, Filip Muysoms, Michael Rhodes, Andras Vereczkei, and Ramon Vilallonga, members of the EAES Journal and Publication Committee, who served as editorial committee, are recognized for their significant contributions.

Kevin Fahrman, graphic designer at Foreside Photography, and his team have created excellent illustrations of patient positioning, trocar placement, and surgical scenarios. Guy-Bernard Cadière has graciously permitted access to a wide array of high-quality surgical illustrations, and Miguel Cuesta has provided valuable support in editing and processing the artwork.

The EAES is committed to enhancing the quality of surgical care by sharing knowledge and providing educational resources. Future EAES manuals will focus on minimally invasive pediatric surgery and thoracic surgery.

Amsterdam, The Netherlands H. Jaap Bonjer

Contents

Part I General Principles

1 **Ergonomics for Minimal Access Surgery** ... 3
Abe Fingerhut and George B. Hanna

2 **Safety in the Operating Theatre** ... 9
Linda S.G.L. Wauben, Jenny Dankelman, and Johan F. Lange

3 **Access to the Abdominal and Thoracic Cavity** ... 15
H. Jaap Bonjer and Jan Wolter A. Oosterhuis

Part II Abdominal Wall

4 **Totally Extraperitoneal Endoscopic Inguinal Hernia Repair (TEP)** ... 21
Marc J. Miserez

5 **Inguinal and Femoral Hernia Trans-Abdominal Pre-peritoneal Patch Plasty (TAPP)** ... 27
Jan F. Kukleta

6 **Laparoscopic Ventral Hernia Repair** ... 33
Salvador Morales-Conde, María Socas, and Isaias Alarcón

Part III Oesophagus

7 **Motility Disorders** ... 41
Giovanni Zaninotto and Mario Costantini

8 **Gastroesophageal Reflux Disease (GERD) and Hiatal Hernia** ... 47
Rudolph Pointner

9 **Minimally Invasive Esophageal Resection** ... 53
Donald L. van der Peet and Miguel A. Cuesta

Part IV Stomach

10 **Laparoscopic Gastrectomy** ... 61
Wiley Chung and Teodor P. Grantcharov

11 **Laparoscopic Repair of Perforated Peptic Ulcer** ... 71
Jonathan B. Yuval and Amir Szold

Part V Bariatric Surgery

12 **Selection of Bariatric Procedures** 77
G.-B. Cadière, Jacques Himpens, and Ramon Vilallonga

13 **Gastric Banding** 87
Frank A. Granderath and Andreas Kirschniak

14 **Gastric Bypass** 93
Mario Morino and Gitana Scozzari

15 **Sleeve Gastrectomy** 101
Konstantinos Albanopoulos and Joanna Papailiou

16 **Laparoscopic Biliopancreatic Diversion with Duodenal Switch** 107
Catalin Copaescu

17 **Revisional Procedures for Failed Bariatric Operations** 115
Jacques Himpens and Ramon Vilallonga

Part VI Liver

18 **Laparoscopic Liver Resection** 125
Giulio Belli, Corrado Fantini, Alberto D'Agostino, Luigi Cioffi, Gianluca Russo, Andrea Belli, and Paolo Limongelli

19 **Non-resection: Radiofrequency Ablation, Cryo, Microwave** 131
Roberto Santambrogio, Matteo Barabino, and Enrico Opocher

Part VII Galbladder and Biliary Ducts

20 **Cholecystectomy** 139
Jack J. Jakimowicz and Johannes F. Smulders

21 **Surgical Management of Ductal Calculi** 145
Alessandro M. Paganini, Silvia Quaresima, Andrea Balla, and Emanuele Lezoche

Part VIII Pancreas

22 **Laparoscopic Surgery of Pancreatic Body and Tail** 155
Laureano Fernández-Cruz

23 **Laparoscopic Pancreaticoduodenectomy** 161
Igor E. Khatkov, Victor V. Tsvirkun, Roman E. Izrailov, and Pavel S. Tyutyunnik

24 **Treatment of Severe Complicated Pancreatitis** 167
Alfred Cuschieri

Part IX Spleen

25 **Laparoscopic Surgery of the Spleen** 175
Eduardo M. Targarona Soler

Part X Small Intestine

26 **Adhesiolysis for Bowel Obstruction** 183
Wilhelmus J.H.J. Meijerink

Part XI Colon and Appendix

27 **Diagnostic Laparoscopy in Suspected Appendicitis and Laparoscopic Appendectomy** ... 189
Agneta Montgomery

28 **Laparoscopic Right Colectomy** ... 197
Luigi Boni, Giulia David, and Elisa Cassinotti

29 **Left Colectomy and Sigmoidectomy** ... 201
A.M. Lacy and M. Fernández-Hevia

30 **Total Colectomy** ... 207
Willem A. Bemelman

Part XII Rectum

31 **Laparoscopic Resection of the Rectum** ... 215
Timothy A. Rockall and Bruce F. Levy

32 **Laparoscopic Rectopexy with or without Resection for Full Thickness Rectal Prolapse** ... 225
Syed Abbas and Roberto Bergamaschi

33 **Transanal Endoscopic Microsurgery** ... 231
Mario Morino and Marco E. Allaix

34 **TransAnal Minimally Invasive Surgery (TAMIS)** ... 237
A.M. Lacy and M. Fernández-Hevia

Part XIII Thyroid and Parathyroid

35 **Thyroid and Parathyroid (MIVAT and MIVAP)** ... 245
Paolo Miccoli and Gabriele Materazzi

Part XIV Adrenal

36 **Laparoscopic Transperitoneal Adrenalectomy** ... 253
Luigi Boni, Stefano Rausei, Matteo Di Giuseppe, Elisa Cassinotti, and Gianlorenzo Dionigi

37 **Retroperitoneal Adrenalectomy** ... 259
H. Jaap Bonjer and M. Walz

Part XV Innovative Minimally Invasive Techniques

38 **NOTES and Hybrid NOTES Procedures in Clinical Practice** ... 267
K.H. Fuchs, W. Breithaupt, G. Varga, and T. Schulz

39 **Single Incision Laparoscopy** ... 275
Helmut G. Weiss, Jan Schirnhofer, Eberhard Brunner, Katharina Pimpl, Christof Mittermair, Christian Obrist, and Michael Weiss

40 **Robotic Surgery** ... 285
Ivo A.M.J. Broeders

Index ... 291

Contributors

Isaias Alarcón Unit of Innovation in Minimally Invasive Surgery, University Hospital "Virgen del Rocío", Sevilla, Spain

Konstantinos Albanopoulos, MD, PhD Department of Propaedeutic Surgery, Medical School, University of Athens, Athens, Greece

Marco E. Allaix, MD, PhD Department of Surgical Sciences, University of Torino, Torino, Italy

Stavros A. Antoniou, MD, PhD, FEBS Department of General Surgery, University Hospital of Heraklion, Heraklion, Crete, Greece

Center for Minimally Invasive Surgery, Neuwerk Hospital, Mönchengladbach, Germany

Matteo Barabino, MD Chirurgia Epato-bilio-pancreatica e Digestiva, A.O. San Paolo, Università degli Studi di Milano, Milan, Italy

Andrea Belli, MD Department of Abdominal Oncology, Division of Surgical Oncology, Istituto Nazionale Tumori Fondazione G. Pascale – Istituto Di Ricovero e Cura a Carattere Scientifico, Naples, Italy

Giulio Belli, MD Department of General and Hepato-Pancreato-Biliary Surgery, S.M. Loreto Nuovo Hospital, Naples, Italy

Willem A. Bemelman, PhD Academic Medical Center, University of Amsterdam, Amsterdam, The Netherlands

Roberto Bergamaschi, MD, PhD Division of Colon & Rectal Surgery, State University of New York, Stony Brook, NY, USA

Luigi Boni, MD, FACS Minimally Invasive Surgery Research Center, University of Insubria, Azienda Ospedaliero Universitaria, Fondazione Macchi, Varese, Italy

H. Jaap Bonjer, MD, PhD, FRCSC Department of Surgery, VU University Medical Center, Amsterdam, The Netherlands

W. Breithaupt Department of Surgery, Agaplesion Markus-Krankenhaus, Frankfurt, Germany

Ivo A.M.J. Broeders Department of Surgery, Meander Medical Centre, Amersfoort, The Netherlands

Eberhard Brunner, MD General Surgery Department, Saint John of God Hospital, Salzburg, Austria

G-B Cadiere, MD, PhD European School of Laparoscopic Surgery, Centre Hospitalier Universitaire Saint-Pierre, Brussels, Belgium

Elisa Cassinotti, MD Minimally Invasive Surgery Research Center, University of Insubria, Azienda Ospedaliero Universitaria, Fondazione Macchi, Varese, Italy

Wiley Chung Department of General Surgery, St. Michael's Hospital, Toronto, ON, Canada

Luigi Cioffi, MD Department of General and Hepato-Pancreato-Biliary Surgery, S.M. Loreto Nuovo Hospital, Naples, Italy

Catalin Copaescu, MD, PhD Minimal Invasive & Bariatric Surgery Department, Delta Hospital, Bucharest, Romania

Mario Costantini, MD Department of Surgery, Gastroenterology and Oncology, University of Padova, School of Medicine, Padova, Italy

Miguel A. Cuesta, MD Department of Surgery, VU University Medical Center, Amsterdam, The Netherlands

Alfred Cuschieri, MD, ChM, DSc, FRSE, FRCS, FACS Department of Surgery and Molecular Oncology, Ninewells Hospital and Medical School, Dundee, Scotland

Alberto D'Agostino, MD Department of General and Hepato-Pancreato-Biliary Surgery, S.M. Loreto Nuovo Hospital, Naples, Italy

Jenny Dankelman, PhD Department of BioMechanical Engineering, Delft University of Technology, Delft, The Netherlands

Giulia David, MD Minimally Invasive Surgery Center, Department of Surgical and Morphological Sciences, University of Insubria, Varese, Italy

Charlotte Deijen Department of Surgery, VU University Medical Center, Amsterdam, The Netherlands

Matteo Di Giuseppe, MD Minimally Invasive Surgery Research Center, University of Insubria, Azienda Ospedaliero Universitaria, Fondazione Macchi, Varese, Italy

Gianlorenzo Dionigi, MD, FACS Minimally Invasive Surgery Research Center, University of Insubria, Azienda Ospedaliero Universitaria, Fondazione Macchi, Varese, Italy

Corrado Fantini, MD Department of General and Hepato-Pancreato-Biliary Surgery, S.M. Loreto Nuovo Hospital, Naples, Italy

Laureano Fernández-Cruz Professor of Surgery, University of Barcelona, Department of Surgery, Hospital Clinic i Provincial de Barcelona, Villarroel 170, escalera 6, 4ª planta, 08036 Barcelona, Spain

M. Fernández-Hevia Department of Surgery, Hospital Clinic de Barcelona, Barcelona, Spain

Abe Fingerhut, MD, FACS, FRCPS(g), FRCS(hon) Ed Poissy, France

Caterina Foppa, MD Division of Colon and Rectal Surgery, State University of New York, Stony Brook, NY, USA

K.H. Fuchs, PhD Department of Surgery, Agaplesion Markus-Krankenhaus, Frankfurt, Germany

Frank A. Granderath, PhD Department of General and Visceral Surgery, Hospital Neuwerk "Maria von den Aposteln", Mönchengladbach, Germany

Teodor P. Grantcharov, MD, PhD, FACS Department of General Surgery, St. Michael's Hospital, Toronto, ON, Canada

George Hanna Department of Surgery, Imperial College, London, UK

Jacques Himpens, MD, PhD Obesity Department, AZ Sint Blasius, Brussels, Belgium

Papailiou Ioanna, MD, MSc, PhD 1st Department of Propaedeutic Surgery, Medical School, University of Athens, AG.PARASKEVI, Athens, Greece

Roman E. Izrailov, MD, PhD Moscow Clinical Scientific Center, Moscow, Russia
Moscow State University of Medicine and Dentistry, Moscow, Russia

Jack J. Jakimowicz, MD, PhD, FRCS, Ed. Department of Research and Education, Catharina Hospital, Technical University of Delft, Eindhoven, The Netherlands

Igor E. Khatkov, MD, PhD Moscow Clinical Scientific Center, Moscow, Russia
Moscow State University of Medicine and Dentistry, Moscow, Russia

Andreas Kirschniak Department for General, Visceral and Transplant Surgery, University Hospital Tübingen, Tübingen, Germany

Jan F. Kukleta, MD, FMCH Zurich, Switzerland

A.M. Lacy Department of Surgery, Hospital Clinic de Barcelona, Barcelona, Spain

Johan F. Lange, PhD, MD Department of Surgery, Erasmus University Medical Center, Rotterdam, The Netherlands

Bruce F. Levy, MBChB, MRCS Minimal Access Therapy Training Unit, Post Graduate Medical School, University of Surrey, Guildford, Surrey, UK

Emanuele Lezoche, MD, FACS Chirurgia Generale, Specialita' Chirurgiche e Trapianti d'Organo "Paride Stefanini", Policlinico Umberto I, Rome, Italy

Giovanni Lezoche, MD Department of General Surgery, Ospedali Riuniti, Universita' Politecnica Delle Marche, Ancona, Italy

Paolo Limongelli, MD, PhD Department of General and Hepato-Pancreato-Biliary Surgery, S.M. Loreto Nuovo Hospital, Naples, Italy

Gabriele Materazzi, MD Dipartimento di Chirurgia, Rome, Italy

Wilhelmus J.H.J. Meijerink, MD, PhD Department of Gastro-Intestinal and Advanced Laparoscopy, VU University Medical Center, Amsterdam, The Netherlands

Paolo Miccoli, MD Department of Surgery, University of Pisa, Pisa, Italy

Marc J. Miserez, MD, PhD Department of Abdominal Surgery, University Hospital Gasthuisberg, Katholieke Universiteit Leuven, Leuven, Belgium

Christof Mittermair, MD General Surgery Department, Saint John of God Hospital, Salzburg, Austria

Agneta Montgomery, MD, PhD Department of Surgery, Skåne University Hospital, Malmö, Sweden

Salvador Morales-Conde Unit of Innovation in Minimally Invasive Surgery, University Hospital "Virgen del Rocío", Sevilla, Spain

Mario Morino, MD Digestive, Colorectal and Minimal Invasive Surgery, University of Torino, Torino, Italy

Filip Muysoms Department of Surgery, Maria Middelares, Ghent, Belgium

Christian Obrist, MD General Surgery Department, Saint John of God Hospital, Salzburg, Austria

Jan Wolter A. Oosterhuis, MD, PhD Department of Surgery, VU University Medical Center, Amsterdam, The Netherlands

Enrico Opocher, MD Chirurgia Epato-bilio-pancreatica e Digestiva, A.O. San Paolo, Università degli Studi di Milano, Milan, Italy

Alessandro M. Paganini, MD, PhD, FACS Chirurgia Generale, Specialita' Chirurgiche e Trapianti D'Organo "Paride Stefanini", Policlinico Umberto I, Rome, Italy

Joanna Papailiou Department of Propaedeutic Surgery, Medical School, University of Athens, Athens, Greece

Katharina Pimpl, MD General Surgery Department, Saint John of God Hospital, Salzburg, Austria

Rudolph Pointner, PhD Department of Surgery, A.ö. Krankenhaus Zell am See, Zell am See, Austria

Stefano Rausei, MD Minimally Invasive Surgery Research Center, University of Insubria, Azienda Ospedaliero Universitaria, Fondazione Macchi, Varese, Italy

Michael Rhodes Stepping Hill Hospital, Stockport, Manchester, UK

Timothy A. Rockall, MB BS, FRCS, MD Minimal Access Therapy Training Unit, Post Graduate Medical School, University of Surrey, Guildford, Surrey, UK

Gianluca Russo, MD Department of General and Hepato-Pancreato-Biliary Surgery, S.M. Loreto Nuovo Hospital, Naples, Italy

Roberto Santambrogio, MD Chirurgia Epato-Bilio-Pancreatica e Digestiva, San Paolo Hospital, University of Milan, Milan, Italy

Jan Schirnhofer, MD General Surgery Department, Saint John of God Hospital, Salzburg, Austria

T. Schulz Department of Surgery, Agaplesion Markus-Krankenhaus, Frankfurt, Germany

Gitana Scozzari, MD Digestive, Colorectal and Minimal Invasive Surgery, University of Torino, Torino, Italy

Johannes F. Smulders, MD Department of Research and Education, Catharina Hospital, Eindhoven, The Netherlands

María Socas Unit of Innovation in Minimally Invasive Surgery, University Hospital "Virgen del Rocío", Sevilla, Spain

Amir Szold, MD Assia Medical Group, Assuta Medical Center, Tel Aviv, Israel

Edyuardo M. Targarona Soler, MD, PhD Department of Surgery, Hospital de Sant Pau, Barcelona, Spain

Victor V. Tsvirkun, MD, PhD Moscow Clinical Scientific Center, Moscow, Russia

Moscow State University of Medicine and Dentistry, Moscow, Russia

Pavel S. Tyutyunnik, MD Moscow Clinical Scientific Center, Moscow, Russia

Moscow State University of Medicine and Dentistry, Moscow, Russia

Donald L. van der Peet Department of Surgery, VU University Medical Center, Amsterdam, The Netherlands

Susanne van der Velde, MD, PhD Oncologic and GE surgeon, VUMC, Amsterdam, The Netherlands

G. Varga Department of Surgery, Agaplesion Markus-Krankenhaus, Frankfurt, Germany

Andras Vereczkei Department of Surgery, Medical School, University of Pécs, Pecs, Hungary

Ramon Vilallonga, MD, PhD Endocrine-Metabolic and Bariatric Surgery Unit, Robotic Surgery, EAC-BS Center of Excellence, Vall d'Hebron Hospital, Barcelona, Spain

Universitat Autònoma de Barcelona, Barcelona, Spain

M. Walz Department of Surgery, Center of Minimally invasive Surgery, Kliniken Essen-Mitte, Amsterdam, The Netherlands

Linda S.G.L. Wauben, PhD, MSc Department of BioMechanical Engineering, Delft University of Technology, Delft, The Netherlands

Helmut G. Weiss, MD, MSc, FEBS General Surgery Department, Saint John of God Hospital, Salzburg, Austria

Michael Weiss, CM General Surgery Department, Saint John of God Hospital, Salzburg, Austria

Jonathan B. Yuval, MD Department of Surgery, Hadassah-Hebrew University Medical Center, Jerusalem, Israel

Giovanni Zaninotto, MD, FACS Department of Academic Surgery, St Mary's Hospital, Imperial College, London, UK

Part I

General Principles

Ergonomics for Minimal Access Surgery 1

Abe Fingerhut and George B. Hanna

1.1 Introduction

"Ergonomics" can be defined as the scientific study of people at work, applying biological and engineering information to the operating room layout and personnel (including the patient) in a system approach taking into account the anatomic, physiologic, and psychological variabilities of the people who work within the given environment. The goal of ergonomics is to enhance effectiveness and efficiency in the man–machine interaction while reducing surgeon discomfort, fatigue and errors, and, ultimately, increasing patient safety.

In contrast to conventional "open" surgery, the surgeon performs laparoscopic operations with instruments fixed by a fulcrum point via the trocar inserted into the body wall of the cavity of interest. Loss of depth perception (in two-dimensional screens), impaired peripheral vision, decoupling of the visual and motor axes and the need to unceasingly adapt to ever evolving high technology applications are among the challenges with which surgeons interact with the given environment.

1.1.1 Constraints in Endoscopic Surgery

Endoscopic surgery creates a set of mechanical and visual restrictions on the execution of surgical tasks, which can degrade the performance (Table 1.1).

1. Mechanical restrictions (handling of tissues)
   - Standard endoscopic instruments have 4° of freedom of movement: in and out, rotation, side to side and up and down
   - Direct tactile feedback (hand to tissue) is lost and the indirect tactile feedback (through the instrument) is markedly diminished due to the length of instruments and the friction between the instruments and the ports.
   - Long thin instruments have a poor mechanical advantage; the length of endoscopic instruments exaggerates hand tremors especially in a magnified endoscopic field.
2. Visual limitations
   - Standard monitors reproduce two dimensional (2-D) images, with only 2-D depth (pictorial) cues of the operative field.
   - Conventional operating room layouts lead to: (a) crowding of free standing equipment often precluding optimal placement of the viewing monitor, (b) monitor being often far removed from the surgeon.
   - Absence of shadow and depth cues
   - Reduced field of peripheral vision

1.2 Layout of Operating Room

Ergonomics in the operating room concern the patient, the surgeon and anesthesiologist with their respective teams, the operating room staff (nurses and floor assistants), the operation table, the apparatuses necessary to run the operation and their wire/cable connections, and last the image display (monitor).

1.2.1 Patient

The patient is usually positioned supine, but occasionally, in one of the lateral positions or in ventral decubitus. The patient arms must not interfere with adequate vision or surgeon stance: this often requires that arms be tucked alongside, at least unilaterally. Patient's legs may be spread apart, the "French" position, thighs slightly extended over the pelvis so that instruments do not clash with the thigh in low elevation angle situations. Last the patient should be adequately and securely fixed to the operation table to prevent sliding, or limb fall, without undue compression of sensitive

A. Fingerhut, MD, FACS, FRCPS(g), FRCS Ed (✉)
Department of Surgical Research, University Hospital, Graz, Austria
e-mail: abefingerhut@aol.com

G.B. Hanna, MD, MBChB, PhD, FRCSEd, MErgS
Department of Surgery, Imperial College, London, UK

H.J. Bonjer (ed.), *Surgical Principles of Minimally Invasive Procedures*, DOI 10.1007/978-3-319-43196-3_1

compartments or superficial nerves during extreme table tilting or inclination.

Foot pedals must be easily found and effortlessly triggered, without disturbing the surgeon's equilibrium.

1.2.2 Operating Teams

The postures surgeons hold during laparoscopic surgery are more static than during open surgery, most likely related to increased concentration and fine instrument movements. Surgeons must remember to breathe, relax, intermittently loosen hand muscle strain, and move about, particularly during the more difficult, long, and complex parts of procedures.

Table 1.1 Constraints in endoscopic surgery

Mechanical restrictions
1. Limited number of degrees of freedom
2. Diminished tactile feedback
3. Small and long endoscopic instruments
4. Problems of tissue retrieval
5. Fulcrum effect
Visual limitations
1. Loss of normal binocular vision
2. Decoupling of motor and sensory spaces (monitor location)
3. Coaxial alignment of lens system and light fibres
4. Reduced size of endoscopic field of view
5. Disturbed endoscope-instrument-tissue relationship (port location)
6. Angle between the optical axis of endoscope and instruments' plane
7. Reverse alignment of the endoscope and instruments
8. Limitations of the quality of endoscopic image

1.2.3 Operating Table

The operating table must be robust but versatile, allowing inclinations in the horizontal and longitudinal planes as well as left and right tilts. Whereas in open surgery, the surgeon adjusts his stance and hands to the situation, this is more difficult in laparoscopic surgery where the relations between table height, position, and angle of vision of the target change according to table tilt and inclination.

The ideal operating table therefore should allow to obtain low tabletop vertical heights (64–77 cm above floor level), even with the obese patient, and to obtain both Trendelenburg and reverse Trendelenburg positions as well as sidewise rotations. The ideal table height is such that the handles of the instruments are at elbow height, with the table height 0–10 cm lower than the elbows. This corresponds to elbow flexion between 90° and 120° (Fig. 1.1).

1.2.4 Equipment and Cables

All laparoscopic apparatuses in the operating room are potential hazards to traffic as well as to ergonomic and safe movements within the operation room environment. Trolleys occupy floor space, are heavy and time consuming to move

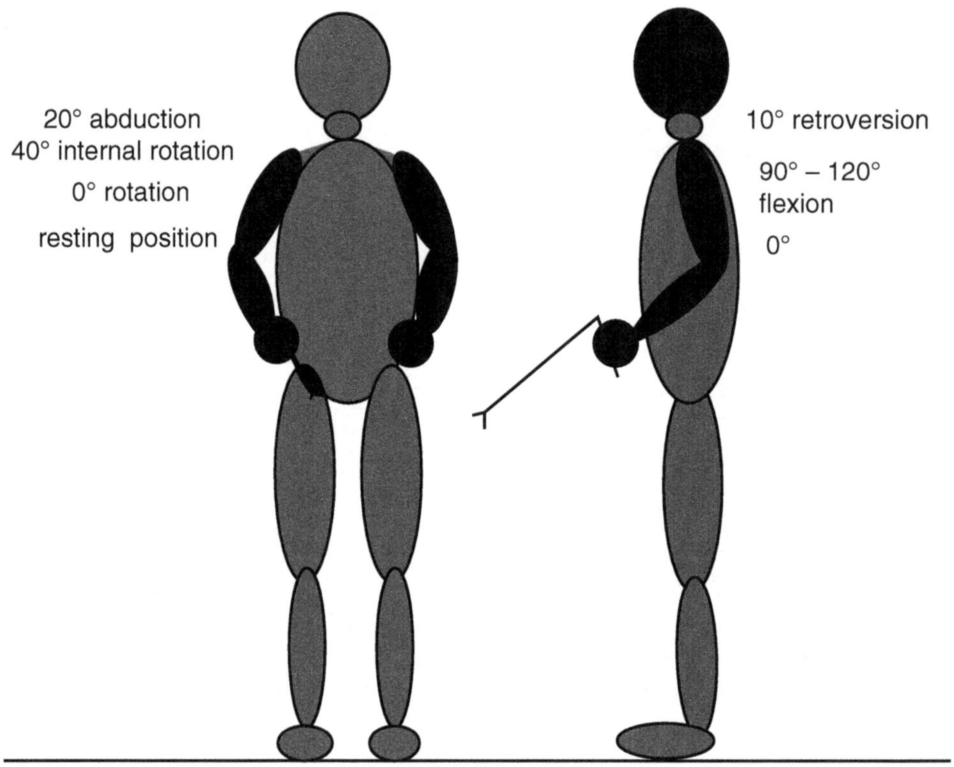

Fig. 1.1 Optimal body positioning for endoscopic surgery

about and place in the adequate position. Attached cables, wiring and tubes are potential hazards on the floor and decrease the efficiency of instrument handling, positioning, and exchanges in the operating field.

Ceiling mounting for all apparatuses and video display systems, along with cameras, light sources, surgical smoke evacuators, coagulation devices, virtually eliminates tripping hazards in the OR and enhance the circulation in the OR.

1.2.5 Image Displays

The position of the screen of the monitor influences the posture of the surgeon and the assistant. Ergonomic studies have shown that the fatigue and musculoskeletal disorders are reduced by optimal posture and head position during tasks making use of video-displays: the ideal posture is neutral without torsion of the back and neck, the head is slightly flexed at an angle of 15°–30° to the horizontal.

Surgical performance is best when the image display is placed in front of the surgeon at the working hand level, the so-called "gaze-down" viewing (which corresponds to the head being flexed 15°–30°). This is ideally achieved by placing a flat liquid crystal display (LCD) immediately above the patient's abdomen and adjacent to the access ports. Some surgeons prefer the screen slightly (15°) below eye level rather than the gaze-down position.

The flat screen is preferred to the standard cathode-ray tube (CRT) from a physical comfort and psychological comfort point of view. The optimal distance between the eyes of the operator and the (flat) screen has been determined to be 600 mm, but the ideal distance depends also on the size of the screen.

Alignment between the eyes and working hands of the surgeon, the target and the screen provides better knot-quality and performance scores, improves execution time, shortens operation or task times, especially intracavity suturing and knotting, and reduces error scores. Suturing is easier and more effective in the vertical than in the horizontal plane with isoplanar visual display (Fig. 1.2).

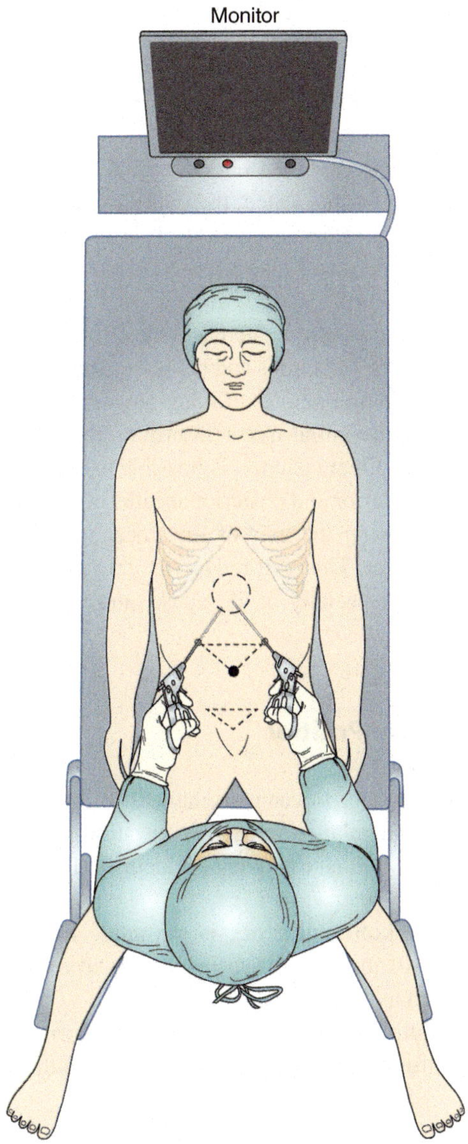

Fig. 1.2 Alignment of surgeon's eyes, endoscope, object and screen

Surgeons may be tempted to use off-axis placement of the optical device and working instruments, also called "sectorization" (optical device placed on one side of the working instruments) when the operating surgeon's hand and/or instruments and those of the assistant get in each other's way. Most of these clashing position related problems can be overcome with adapted trocar position of the optical port, table tilt and inclination, rather than off axis working.

If required or preferred (e.g. incisional hernia repair during which the surgeon often changes from one side of the patient to the other), working with both hands on the non-dominant hand side of the optical device increases performances and decreases muscle work and fatigue (compared with the dominant side). Working with the instruments opposite the optical port should be avoided as it creates mirror image for instruments' movement.

1.2.6 Theater Lighting

Operating room lights are often turned off in order to increase contrast of the operative image and avoid glaring of operating room lights on the image display system. However, working in relative darkness can negatively impact the choice of instruments and increase the risk of collision hazards. Sufficient lighting is needed for proper instrument selection and safe handling of needles.

1.3 Ergonomics of the Operative Field

1.3.1 Trocar Insertion

The ergonomic aspects related to trocars concern their design, insertion, their position, their retrieval and the necessity of closure or not. An ideal trocar system incorporates a low insertion force, secure retention, and a minimal tissue defect. Of the systems tested, the hybrid type trocar and the radially dilating trocar seem best experimentally, but it is unknown whether these characteristics lead to improvement in patient outcomes.

Working against torque increases the effort needed to perform the simplest of actions and decreases the precision with which the surgeon operates. Taking advantage of the open technique for the initial trocar insertion, but also for those inserted under direct vision, it is possible to stagger the incisions on the anterior and posterior sheaths of all non-midline incisions, allowing the axis of the trocar to point directly toward the target. This will reduce the torque necessary for maneuvering, especially in the obese, and reduce the need for closure.

1.3.2 Trocar Position

The goal of proper trocar placement is to ensure adequate vision and triangulation, adapting elevation and manipulation angles to optimal ergonomic principles (Fig. 1.3):

1. The "elevation angle" αE, is the angle formed by the direction of the shaft of an instrument in relation to the horizontal axis of the patient.
2. The "manipulation angle", α_m is the angle formed between two instruments converging and working in the operative field.

The "azimuth angle" is the angle formed between the optical (scope) shaft and an instrument.

The Dundee school has shown that maximal efficacy in suturing and suture quality was obtained when: a) the manipulation angle (α_m) is between 45° and 75° (ideal being 60°), b) the elevation angle, (α_E) is between 30° and 60°, c) azimuth angles are equal, and d) the optical axis-to-target view (OATV) angle, defined as the angle between the optical axis of the endoscope and the plane of the target, approaches 90°.

When a 30° manipulation angle is used (imposed for instance by the body build or anatomy of the patient), the elevation angle should also be 30°. When the manipulation angle is 60°, a 60° elevation angle should be used. Obviously when the target area is small, the elevation angle is easily determined by the position of the trocar and the depth of the target. When the target area is large, there is little the surgeon

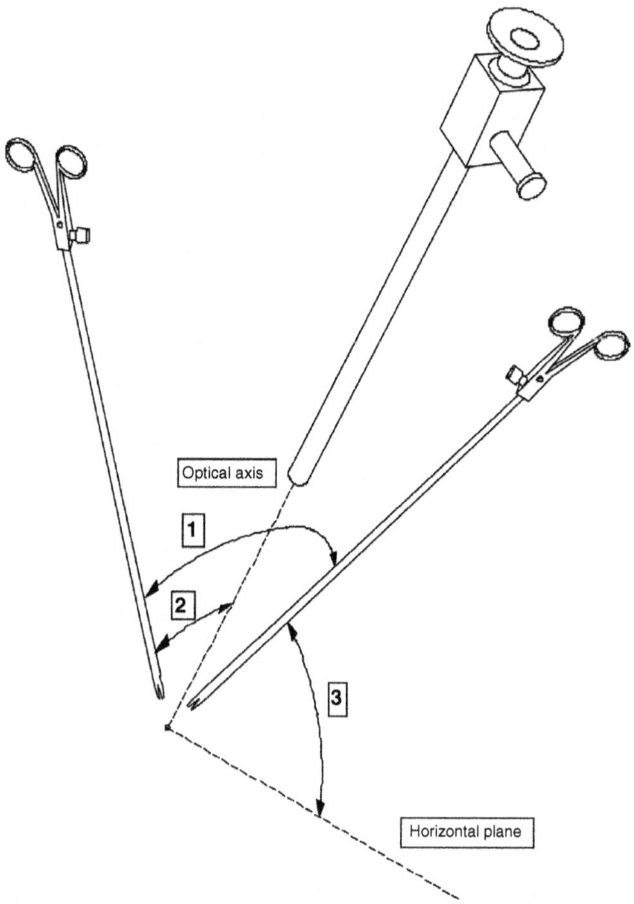

Fig. 1.3 Optimal ergonomy: *1* manipulation angle, *2* azimuth angle and *3* elevation angle

can do to change this angle, so different trocars are necessary. Elevation angles can be fairly easily modified, however, by simply increasing (decreasing) the tilt (Trendelenburg or anti Trendelenburg) of the table, rather than by elevating or lowering the elbow.

1.3.3 Field of Vision

Endoscopes can be of forward viewing (0°) or forward oblique direction of view (30°, 45°). Endoscopes of different directions of view have no significant effect on the execution time or the quality of task performance when the optical axis of the endoscope subtends the same OATV angle. In practice, however, forward-oblique endoscopes are preferable because it is more likely to obtain an OATV angle approaching 90° (Fig. 1.4). However, the visual field changes when the forward oblique endoscope is rotated around its axis relative to the camera whereas the operative field of forward-viewing endoscope is unaltered. Perspectives change by rotation of the forward-oblique endoscopes to provide, for instance visualization of the abdominal wall to control the

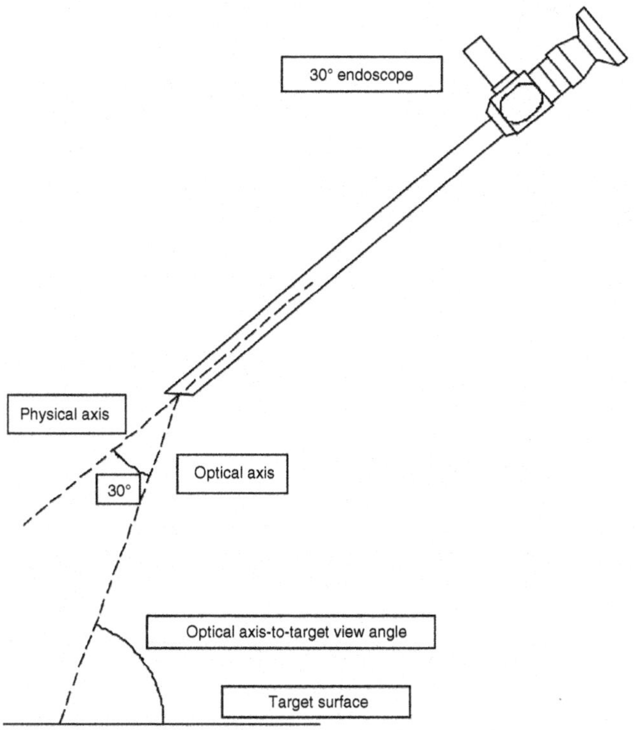

Fig. 1.4 Optical axis to target view

entry of trocars or for the execution of advanced laparoscopic procedures, such as incisional hernia repair.

Variations in the build of patients necessitate a careful selection of the location of the optical port in the individual patient to obtain both an optimum OATV angle and the correct target-to-endoscope distance for a specific endoscopic operation.

The scope must be placed so as to render the field of vision adapted to the task to be accomplished (exploration, suture, stapling, resection). Sometimes the position of the scope has to be changed from one trocar to another, or else, another trocar has to be inserted to improve the field of vision.

Constant attention must be exercised not to lose sight of an instrument tip while performing tasks such as suturing and knot-tying. Safety precautions dictate that all instruments not in use, especially energy-driven devices, be withdrawn. Zooming out and in with the endoscope to locate instrument tips can, however, be time-intensive.

The angle between the optical axis of the endoscope and the instrument plane (OAIP) should ideally be between 0° and +15°, such as that the instruments appear to enter the field of vision (approach angle) from the same direction as the surgeon sees them from the outside, and such that the instruments are seen from above. This means that the principle trocar setup (that is the optical port and the main working ports) have to be planned. Taking into account that the ideal placement of the optical port would be in the direct alignment between the two main working ports, this would not be practical because the working space on the outside (hands of operator and cameraman) as well as on the inside would be reduced and would hinder the manipulations. However, two factors intervene to obtain the ideal OAIP: one is the placement of the trocars used for the optical endoscope and the working instruments, the so-called triangulation setup; the other is related to the angle of tilt of the table. The angle of tilt of the table plays a double role: first, a tilt is necessary in certain operations in order that the viscera fall away by gravity, the second is to allow enough space on the outside so that the hands holding the scope and the hands manipulating the instruments do not come into contact with each other.

The correct position of the scope and the instruments are interrelated. It is possible to work with the scope tip either above (cephalad) or below (caudad) with respect to the interline between the two working trocars. Placed cephalad, the instruments are seen on the monitor display as coming in from below while when the tip of the scope is placed caudad, the instruments are seen to come into vision on the screen from above. Obviously, these images are related to the position of the tip of optical device more than the actual port placement.

There are few studies that have actually looked at the ideal trocar placement as related to specific operations, or anatomic landmarks, other than based on personal experience rather than an objective rationale for selected locations. Standardization of trocar placement in laparoscopic Roux-en-Y gastric bypass and gastroesophageal reflux disease repair has been reported.

1.3.4 Instruments and Tissue Handling

The passage through the trocar determines a fulcrum point for the instrument leading to two unnatural effects that have to be dealt with: the mirror effect and the scaling effect.

The mirror effect is related to the fixed point created by the trocar along the shaft of the instrument: movements inside the body cavity are seen to move in the opposite direction that of the surgeons' hands.

The scaling effect depends on the ratio between the intracorporeal and extracorporeal (I/E) lengths of instruments. When I/E is equal or close to one, the course of the hands at one extremity of the instrument imposes the same cursive length at the other extremity (although in opposite directions (the "mirror effect")). When I/E is less than unity, the intracorporeal movements are scaled down (i.e. hands on the outer extremity of the instrument must travel a less distance than the cursive length of the tip of the instrument). On the other hand when the I/E is greater than unity, the intracorporeal movements are scaled up (i.e. hands on the outer extremity of the instrument must travel little before the cursive length of the tip of the instrument becomes greater).

The ideal length of the shaft of the instruments has hardly been mentioned in the literature. Most instrument shafts are 360 mm in length, but these vary anywhere between 310 and 400 mm. Longer shafts are available for use in the obese, but such shafts may diminish surgeons' performance. The longer the working rod of laparoscopic instruments the more complex internal mechanical linkages that decrease the efficient transmission of force from the surgeon's hand to the instrument tip. A typical disposable laparoscopic grasper transmits the force of the surgeon's hand from the handle to the tip with a ratio of only 1:3, in contrast to a 3:1 ratio with a hemostat. The surgeon must therefore work about six times as hard to accomplish the same grasping task with the laparoscopic instrument compared with a typical grasper used in open surgery.

Of concern is the mental and physical fatigue that can arise from changing instruments, reinserting them through the trocar, and then repositioning them within the abdomen. Such instrument exchanges are laborious and distracting to the surgeon, and time-consuming, hence the need to place a premium on minimizing exchanges and using multifunction instruments. The latter, however, when poorly designed, can be even more difficult to use.

The tasks of suturing (knotting), retraction, cutting, grasping, hemostasis, as well as extraction of the specimen (when necessary) are all influenced by ergonomics.

Intraabdominal manual sewing and knotting skills are often needed for advanced laparoscopic procedures, such as confection of a gastric wrap around the lower esophagus and hiatal crural closure, Heller myotomy, the edges of the myotomy, incisional and inguinal hernia repair, just to name a few. Although patient body build and the degree of difficulty of dissection or encountered pathology influence laparoscopic task performance, the ease and effectiveness of instrument movement is mainly governed by the ergonomics, closely dependent on correct trocar placement.

Intracorporeal knotting represents one of the most difficult tasks to learn in minimal access surgery. It not only requires advanced and well-rehearsed motor skills but also requires dexterity and special spatial cognition qualities. Undue duration of knotting, strenuous efforts to insert the needle, maneuver instruments and suture material, and attain adequate knotting strength can be responsible for further mental and physical stress as well as unsafe maneuvers, sutures or knots. Again, we underscore the need for optimal, ergonomic trocar placement.

Conclusion

Ergonomics are an all important component to safe laparoscopic surgery. A standardized approach to trocar placement, taking into account patient habitus and body build, the foreseeable potential pathological and anatomical modifications, as well as the characteristics of the surgeon (height, body build) and the possibilities of the operating room, table, and instruments is necessary to optimize ergonomics and render laparoscopic surgery a safe practice.

Bibliography

1. Berguer R, Smith WD, Davis S. An ergonomic study on the optimum operating table height for laparoscopic surgery. Surg Endosc. 2002;16:416–21.
2. De Visser H, Heijnsdijk EAM, Herder JL, Pistecky PV. Forces and displacements in colon surgery. Surg Endosc. 2002;16:1426–30.
3. Emam TA, Hanna GB, Kimber C, Dunkley P, Cuschieri A. Effect of intracorporeal extracorporeal instrument length ratio on endoscopic task performance and surgeon movements. Arch Surg. 2000;135:62–5.
4. Emam TA, Hanna G, Cuschieri A. Ergonomic principles of task alignment, visual display, and direction of execution of laparoscopic bowel suturing. Surg Endosc. 2002;16:267–71.
5. Fingerhut A, Hanna GB, Veyrie N, Ferzli G, Millat B, Alexakis N, Leandros E. Optimal trocar placement for ergonomic intracorporeal sewing and knotting in laparoscopic hiatal surgery. Am J Surg. 2010;200:519–28.
6. Ferzli GS, Fingerhut A. Trocar placement for laparoscopic abdominal procedures: a simple standardized method. J Am Coll Surg. 2004;198:163–73.
7. Hanna G, Shimi S, Cushieri A. Task performance in endoscopic surgery is influenced by location of the image display. Ann Surg. 1998;227:481–4.
8. Hanna GB, Shimi S, Cuschieri A. Optimal port locations for endoscopic intracorporeal knotting. Surg Endosc. 1997;11:397–401.
9. Hanna GB, Shimi S, Cuschieri A. Influence of direction of view, target-to-endoscope distance and manipulation angle on endoscopic knot tying. Br J Surg. 1997;84:1460–4.
10. Patil PV, Hanna GB, Cushieri A. Effect of the angle between the optical axis of the endosopic and the instruments' plane on monitor image and surgical performance. Surg Endosc. 2004;18:111–4.
11. Shukla PJ, Maharaj R, Fingerhut A. Ergonomics and technical aspects of minimal access surgery in acute surgery. Eur J Trauma Emerg Surg. 2010;36:3–9.
12. Suppe AN, Kulkarni GV, Supe PA. Ergonomics in laparoscopic surgery. J Min Access Surg. 2010;6:31–6.
13. van Det MJ, Meijerink WJ, Hoff C, Totte ER, Pierie JP. Optimal ergonomics for laparoscopic surgery in minimally invasive surgery suites: a review and guidelines. Surg Endosc. 2009;23:1279–85.

2 Safety in the Operating Theatre

Linda S.G.L. Wauben, Jenny Dankelman, and Johan F. Lange

Human performance is not without error, at best the risk is 'as low as reasonable possible' (ALARP) [1]. As a consequence, errors occur. The most common site for adverse events in hospitals is the operating theatre (OT) [2, 3]. Studies have shown that 30–50 % of errors can be prevented [2, 3]. Although patients and their different condition, pathology and anatomy play and important role, many errors occur due to e.g., the complex non-standardized OT environment, the many people having to work together, the workload, the urgency and uncertainty of decisions, and the large variety of (non-ergonomic) instruments and instrumentation [2, 3, 4, 5]. In other words, the latent conditions in the system can easily lead to active operator errors, which are to be expected and are inevitable [2, 3, 4]. Adopting a system approach (opposed to a persons approach) could reduce the occurrence of preventable patient safety incidents by learning from errors, improving quality of equipment and technology, training of professionals (both technical and non-technical skills), and implementation and compliance to protocols and checklists [2, 3, 4–7]. Furthermore, it could be used to identify which technology needs to be developed or adapted to further improve patient safety.

There are many models describing the system approach and its different interrelated components surrounding the patient and influencing patient safety [3–5, 8]. The components Task, Individual, Team, Physical Work Environment, Organization & Management, and Political & Regulatory were used as a framework for describing safety in the OT in this chapter (see Fig. 2.1).

Linda S.G.L. Wauben, PhD, MSc (✉)
Department of BioMechanical Engineering,
Delft University of Technology, Delft, The Netherlands

Research Centre Innovations in Care,
Rotterdam University of Applied Sciences,
Rotterdam, The Netherlands
e-mail: l.s.g.l.wauben@hr.nl

J. Dankelman, PhD
Department of BioMechanical Engineering,
Delft University of Technology, Delft, The Netherlands
e-mail: l.s.g.l.wauben@tudelft.nl

J.F. Lange, PhD, MD
Department of Surgery, Erasmus University Medical Center,
Rotterdam, The Netherlands

2.1 Task

Task performance can be supported by the use of checks. The most common ones are checklists. Checklists reduce the reliance on memory; they reduce the mental workload for the primary skill based task, saving capacity for the secondary rule and knowledge based tasks [3, 4, 6]. Several paper, electronic, and computer-based checklists can be used for several stages of a surgical procedure [3, 4, 6, 8]:

Pre-operative equipment checklists to check the availability and the safety status of OR devices, anaesthesia equipment, and laparoscopic instruments and apparatus [4, 6].

Pre-operative briefings to check and double-check important patient and procedure related factors before surgery to improve the safety attitude and to improve situation awareness. Some examples are the Surgical Safety Checklist, the SURPASS (SURgical PAtient Safety System), and TOP *plus* [3].

Intra-operative collaborative cross-checks (or double-checks, or the two-challenge rule). Cross-checks are performed by at least two people who examine each others' actions and observable behaviour to assess its validity and accuracy (e.g. critical view of safety during laparoscopic cholecystectomy) [3, 6]. Cross-checks detect erroneous actions, reduce perceptual errors, and improve coordination [3, 9]. Cross-checking also stimulates residents to recognize and respond faster to error prone situations and to 'speak up' [3].

Procedure-specific checklist to perform (and assess) subsequent clinical actions during a surgical procedure.

Post-operative debriefings to discuss and evaluate, with the entire OT team, the surgical procedure performed and dis-

H.J. Bonjer (ed.), *Surgical Principles of Minimally Invasive Procedures*, DOI 10.1007/978-3-319-43196-3_2

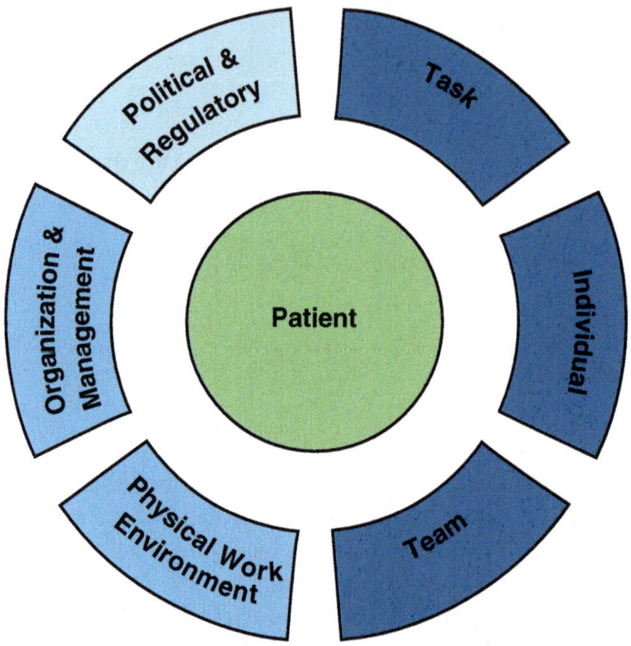

Fig. 2.1 Six interrelated components of the system approach surrounding the patient and influencing patient safety (Based on [3–5, 8])

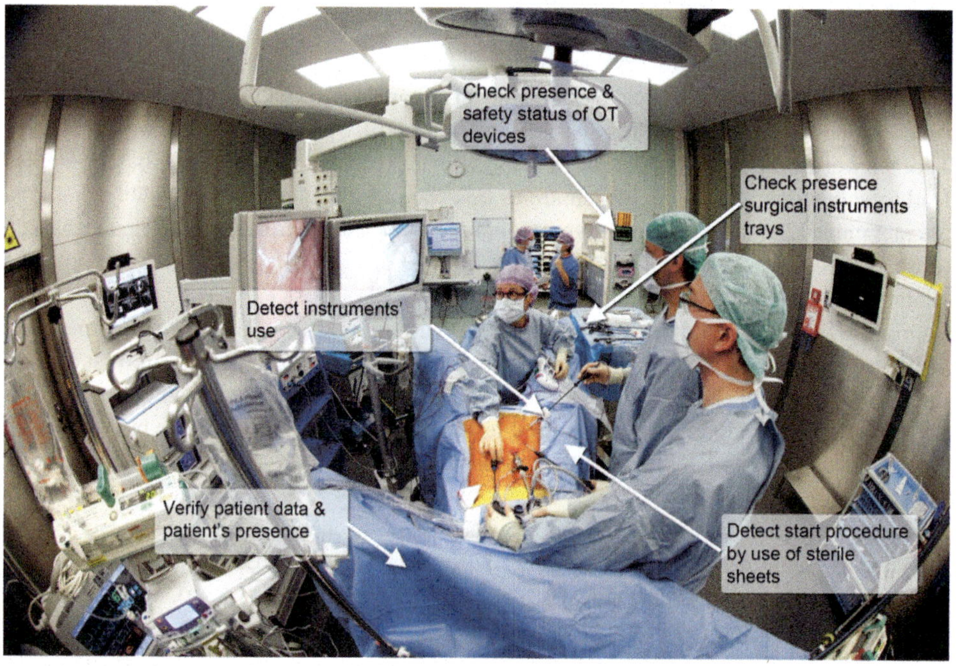

Fig. 2.2 Using technology to automatically check and detect devices, patients and instruments and instrument use in the operating theatre

cuss possible near misses and recommendations for the future to learn from errors made. Checklists, such as the Surgical Safety Checklist, the SURPASS and TOP*plus* include these team debriefings [3].

Checklist can also be used to check important steps during the entire surgical trajectory. Furthermore, smart technology can be used to support healthcare staff during these checks, by e.g., RFID tracking to automatically check the presence and safety status of OT devices, and the location and presence of patients (see Fig. 2.2).

2.2 Individual

Surgeons and OT staff have to be competent and must have adequate knowledge and skills to perform a successful surgical procedure. Performing minimally invasive surgery requires a more complex set of skills (skill based, rule based, and knowledge based behaviour) than open surgery due to e.g., non-ergonomic instruments, limited freedom to manipulate, and limited indirect view on the operative field [3]. Although these skills and behaviour can be trained 'on the job', they are best to be trained 'before the job' in order to prevent patient harm. Individual technical skills can be taught by means of e.g., box trainers, Virtual Reality Simulators, and Augmented Reality trainers [3, 4, 10]. Simulated *common* scenarios can be used to train skill- and rule based behaviour and simulated *crises* scenarios can be used to train all types of behaviours, including knowledge based behaviour [3]. Besides preventing patient harm, training technical skills using simulation also has the advantage that it can provide objective feedback on the individual's technical performance (personal assessment) [3].

Surgical performance and technical skills can be assessed by means of supervision and feedback, and by means of more objective methods, such as: retrospective chart review, procedure-specific checklists, global rating scales, objective structured assessment of technical skills (OSATS), motion analyses, virtual reality simulators or video assessment [3].

2.3 Team

Seventy to 75 % of errors in OT are attributed to the non-technical skills of the OT team (communication, teamwork, leadership, decision-making, situation awareness) [3, 11]. OT team members have discrepant perceptions of teamwork and team members are sometimes discouraged to speak up because of traditional hierarchical structures, authority, social barriers, or differences in professional training and responsibility [3].

There is emerging evidence that team interventions that include both technical as well as non-technical skills support safe surgery [3, 12, 13]. Training aspects of team interventions, such as basic Human Factors Training, Medical Team Training or Crew Resource Management include: no denial/avoidance of the fallibility of human performance, acknowledge errors are made, no blame and shame for the actor of error (legal and ethical issues), situation awareness and vigilance (controlling external distractions, anticipating future events, using all team members for input), leadership and management (assertiveness, inviting input, horizontal authority, flat hierarchy), teamwork and cooperation, problem solving and decision making, and communication [3, 4, 7, 14]. Advantages of trained teams are tension free cross-checks (instead of directly addressing each other, which can be seen as offensive), naturally following guidelines and protocols as 'team dialogue' (now these documents are often not used or known), converting traditional vertical hierarchy into functional flat hierarchy, alternating leader-follower roles, and improve the working atmosphere.

Training individual technical skills as well as non-technical team skills can be done by means of interdisciplinary simulation in an operational environment, for instance e.g. the 'simulated operating theatre' [3]. Here, both common and rare crises scenarios can be trained. Especially for crises scenarios, this simulated environment provides a safe environment, without endangering the patient's safety [3]. However, training of these technical skills can also be done by means of cross-checks or team checks during both simulations as well as during actual surgical procedures [3].

Non-technical skills can be evaluated by means of several methods and techniques, e.g., Surgical Non Technical performance (NOTECHS), Anaesthetists Non-Technical Skills assessments (ANTS), Non-technical Skills for Surgeons (NOTSS), Scrub Practitioners' List of Intra-operative Non-Technical Skills (SPLINTS), Situation Awareness Rating Technique (SART), Situation Awareness Global Assessment Technique (SAGAT), Observational Teamwork Assessment for Surgery (OTAS), and Judgment Analysis [3, 7].

2.4 Physical Work Environment

The OT environment is not standardized and has changed drastically over the last decade, from OTs designed for open procedures only, to specially designed OTs for minimally invasive surgery and/or robotic surgery [3]. More and more technology is incorporated, which is not adapted to the users. This (unergonomic) working environment leads to health risks for both OT staff and patients and leads to inefficient processes. Besides following ergonomics guidelines to e.g. set-up the OT (Chap. 1) other environmental work conditions should be taken into account to reduce complexity and improve control of the OT environment [3, 4].

Both ambient temperature and air condition are important to prevent bacteria growth, patient's hypothermia, discomfort amongst team members, and airborne infection risk of all people in OT. The ambient temperature is kept low (20–23 °C) and high ventilation rate of the plenum or laminar airflow systems are set to reduce contamination. Furthermore, sterile areas, such as the operative table and sterile instrument table, should be placed in this airflow. In order to maintain an optimal airflow, staff movements, door movements and placing obstacles in front of the ventilation vents should be reduced to limit infections.

Staff and patients are exposed to many sounds in OT produced by apparatus and people [15]. Noise (unwanted sounds) affect both patients and OT staff. Particularly, non-predictable and non-controllable sounds and background conversation interfere with the performance of complex tasks, and have an instant and continuing effect. Additionally, noise impairs (critical) conversation. A solution to mask ambient OT noise is to play background music. Music can reduce patients' anxiety, pain levels, and sedative requirements, but can also distract (novice) surgeons performing new tasks [15].

One of the basic necessities to perform safe surgery is good vision of the operative field and related to that the quality and intensity of lighting [16]. Surgical lights should be focused on the operative field taking into account blocking of the light beam by OR staff. The nominal luminance produced by the ambient lights should be approximately 1000 lux, bright enough for the circulating OT staff and anaesthesia staff to perform their tasks. During the endoscopic part of minimally invasive procedures, the surgical lights are often switch off and the ambient lights switched to green light to enhance viewing on the flat screens.

2.5 Organization and Management

Hospitals have to become a learning organization [14]. This requires an organizational safety culture to change the attitude towards errors of both individuals as well as organizations [3, 4]. Staff should be actively engaged and encouraged to report patient safety errors [3, 14, 17]. Currently, incidents are underreported caused by fear of blame, time pressure, resource constraints, perception that reporting is unnecessary, and lack of clear definition [3, 14]. Therefore, reporting should not be used for punitive purposes and reporting errors should be facilitated by providing easy-to-use standardized electronic reporting systems or e.g. video- and audio recordings and new technology should be developed for automatic monitoring [3, 4, 14]. Furthermore, safety and safety significant events and issues have to be given the highest priority and must be constantly assessed by means of self-analysis of the organization [3, 4]. Errors should be analysed and solutions to problems should be planned, using combinations of different risk-assessment methods and incident analyses (e.g., retrospective chart review, event audit, observation, root cause analysis) [3, 4, 17]. Staff should also receive feedback information and recommendations based on these error analyses so they can train and learn from operational experience, leading to a proactive approach of error prevention [3,14, 17].

2.6 Political and Regulatory

In the OT, many protocols and guidelines are used to perform surgery, facilitate training, support clinical decision-making, and support maintaining professional standards in daily practice [2, 18]. These protocols are established by international and national surgical associations and are influenced by demands of e.g., healthcare inspectorates and insurance companies. Following protocols and guidelines also improves communication between team members by clarifying tasks and direction needed to perform safe surgery and increases task-efficiency (less operating time). Protocols also form the basis for information and communication technology for e.g., the electronic medical record and digital operative notes. Developing and implementing methods for (automatic) monitoring to check whether protocols and guidelines are followed properly will further improve patient safety in the OT.

Conclusions

Improving safety in the OT requires changes on different system levels and includes factors related to task performance, individual capability and training, teamwork, the physical work environment, learning capabilities of the organization and management, and political and regulatory demands on (inter)national level. Future interventions should take into account all these system levels, however, focusing first on teams and team skills, smart technology to support the OT team and 'training before the job'.

References

1. Cuschieri A. Human reliability assessment in surgery: a new approach for improving surgical performance and clinical outcome. Ann R Coll Surg Engl. 2000;82:83–7.
2. Kohn LT, Corrigan JM, Donaldson MS. To Err is human: building a safer health system. Washington, DC: National Academy Press; 2000.
3. Wauben LS, Lange JF, Goossens RH. Learning from aviation to improve safety in the operating room: a systematic literature review. J Healthcare Eng. 2012;3:373–90.
4. Dankelman J, Grimbergen CA. Systems approach to reduce errors in surgery. Surg Endosc. 2005;19:1017–21.
5. Vincent C, Moorthy K, Sarker SK, Chang A, Darzi AW. Systems approaches to surgical quality and safety: from concept to measurement. Ann Surg. 2004;239:475–82.
6. Verdaasdonk EG, Stassen LP, Widhiasmara PP, Dankelman J. Requirements for the design and implementation of checklists for surgical processes. Surg Endosc. 2009;23:715–26.
7. Sevdalis N, Davis R, Koutantji M, Undre S, Darzi A, Vincent CA. Reliability of a revised NOTECHS scale for use in surgical teams. Am J Surg. 2008;196:184–90.
8. Vicente K. The Human Factor. New York: Taylor & Francis Group; 2006.
8. de Vries EN, Prins HA, Crolla RM, den Outer AJ, van Andel G, van Helden SH, Schlack WS, van Putten MA, Gouma DJ, Dijkgraaf MG, Smorenburg SM, Boermeester MA. Effect of a comprehensive surgical safety system on patient outcomes. N Engl J Med. 2010;363:1928–37.
9. Diamond T, Mole DJ. Anatomical orientation and cross-checking-the key to safer laparoscopic cholecystectomy. Br J Surg. 2005;92:663–4.
10. Brinkman WM, Tjiam IM, Buzink SN. Assessment of basic laparoscopic skills on virtual reality simulator or box trainer. Surg Endosc. 2013;27:3584–90.
11. Cuschieri A. Nature of human error. Implications for surgical practice. Ann Surg. 2006;244:642–8.
12. Buljac-Samardzic M, Dekker-van Doorn CM, van Wijngaarden J, van Wijk K. Interventions to improve team effectiveness: a systematic review. Health Policy. 2009;94:183–95.
13. Mazzocco K, Petitti DB, Fong KT, Bonacum D, Brookey J, Graham S, Lasky RE, Sexton JB, Thomas EJ. Surgical team behaviors and patient outcomes. Am J Surg. 2009;197:678–85.

14. Benn J, Koutantji M, Wallace L, Spurgeon P, Rejman M, Healey A, Vincent C. Feedback from incident reporting: information and action to improve patient safety. Qual Saf Health Care. 2009;18:11–21.
15. Moorthy K, Munz Y, Undre S, Darzi A. Objective evaluation of the effect of noise on the performance of a complex laparoscopic task. Surgery. 2004;136:25–30.
16. Matern U, Koneczny S. Safety, hazards and ergonomics in the operating room. Surg Endosc. 2007;21:1965–9.
17. Fabri PJ, Zayas-Castro JL. Human error, not communication and systems, underlies surgical complications. Surgery. 2008;144:557–63.
18. Korolija D, Sauerland S, Wood-Dauphinée S, Abbou CC, Eypasch E, García Caballero M, Lumsden MA, Millat B, Monson JRT, Nilsson G, Pointner R, Schwenk W, Shamiyeh A, Szold A, Targarona E, Ure B, Neugebauer EAM. EAES guidelines for endoscopic surgery. Berlin/Heidelberg/Germany: Springer; 2006.

3 Access to the Abdominal and Thoracic Cavity

H. Jaap Bonjer and Jan Wolter A. Oosterhuis

3.1 Access to the Abdominal Cavity

Safe establishment of a pneumoperitoneum is of paramount importance in minimally invasive surgery [1]. Gas insufflation of the abdominal cavity is necessary to create sufficient working space by suppressing the viscera and elevating the abdominal wall. Variously shaped retractors inserted through a small incision and connected to a lifting device have been employed to elevate the anterior abdominal wall and avoid use of gas. However, this technique, gasless laparoscopy, does provide inferior exposure compared to a pneumoperitoneum, and, therefore, has been largely abandoned.

Carbon dioxide is the most frequently used gas for insufflation because it is not combustible, readily absorbable and low in cost. However, carbon dioxide insufflation does cause acidosis in the exposed tissues and is associated with suppression of macrophage function. Surprisingly, humidification of the insufflated carbondioxide and warming the gas to body temperature are rarely used in spite of the damaging effect of cold and dry gas on the peritoneum that has been observed at electron microscopy.

The insufflation pressure needs to be calibrated according to the required exposure and kept as low as possible to limit the reduction of venous return and microcirculation. High insufflation pressures can be due to incomplete muscular relaxation while low pressures combined with high insufflation flow indicate leakage along or through trocars, open stopcock or detachment of the insufflator tubing. It is recommended to lower the insufflation pressure at the end of the procedure to identify any bleeding from venules.

H.J. Bonjer, MD, PhD, FRCSC (✉) • J.W.A. Oosterhuis, MD, PhD
Department of Surgery, VU University Medical Center, Amsterdam, The Netherlands
e-mail: j.bonjer@vumc.nl; jwa.oosterhuis@vumc.nl

3.2 Closed, Hybrid and Open Techniques

A pneumoperitoneum can be established in a closed, semi-closed and open fashion. The choice of first entry is important to place the laparoscope at a site which will provide a good laparoscopic view for the laparoscopic procedure and to avoid adhesions due to previous surgery. The umbilicus is preferred for acquiring access to the peritoneal cavity given its central position in the abdomen and because the abdominal wall is thinnest at the umbilicus. In case of a former midline incision including the umbilicus, it is advisable to choose an entry site more laterally and withstand the temptation to re-use the scar for cosmetic reasons.

The closed method employs the use of the spring loaded Veres needle (Fig. 3.1). This needle is inserted blindly into the peritoneal cavity while the abdominal wall is elevated manually or by graspers placed on the skin to increase the distance between the abdominal wall and the viscera and vessels. The tactile sensation of two 'pops' due to penetration of fascia and peritoneum aids the surgeon to determine the position of the tip of the Veres needle. Once the Veres needle is considered to be in the intraperitoneal cavity, saline can be injected and aspirated through the Veres needle to confirm proper positioning. Filling the Veres needle with saline to the top of its orifice followed by elevating the abdominal wall which should result in a lowering meniscus is another method to assure correct placement. Gas insufflation is started at low flow when the surgeon is confident that the tip of the Veres needle is in the right place. The Veres needle is removed when the set insufflation pressure has been reached. Subsequently the first trocar is inserted while the abdomen is elevated. Rotating the trocar back and forth is important to limit the force exerted on the trocar during insertion. In addition, the shaft of the trocar can be grasped between the index finger and the middle finger of the other hand to avoid sudden uncontrolled advancement of the trocar.

The hybrid method entails insertion of the laparoscope in a trocar with a transparent blunt or semi-blunt tip to provide

H.J. Bonjer (ed.), *Surgical Principles of Minimally Invasive Procedures*, DOI 10.1007/978-3-319-43196-3_3

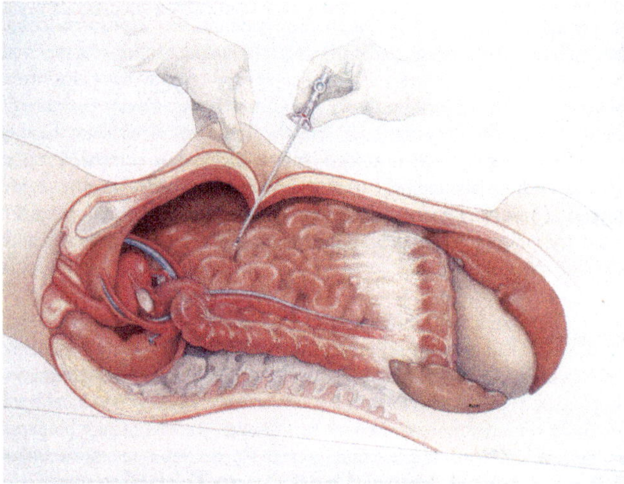

Fig. 3.1 Closed introduction of the Veres needle (Reproduced with permission from Wolters Kluwer, Surgical Laparoscopy, 2nd edition, Karl A. Zucker)

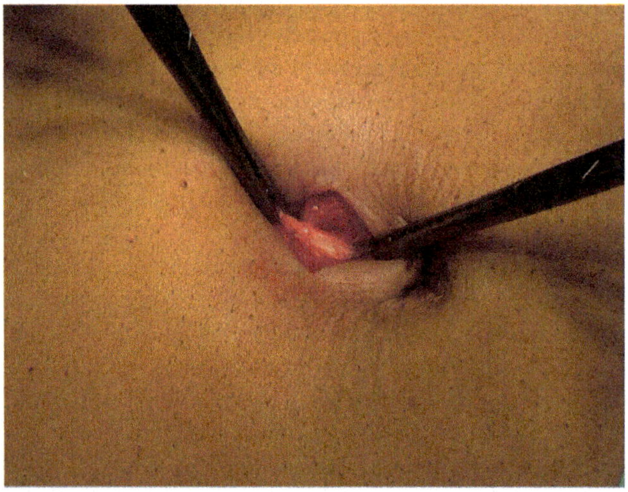

Fig. 3.2 The vertical raphe of the fascia is elevated with two Kocher clamps

the surgical team with an image of the layers of the abdominal wall during passage. Some surgeons first insufflate the abdomen through a Veres needle while others introduce the first trocar without a pneumoperitoneum.

The open method is performed under direct vision. The fascia is exposed through a 1–2 cm incision. The size of the incision depends on the habitus of the patient. The fascia is grasped with two Kocher clamps placed on the vertical raphe of the fascia. The fascia is incised transversely between these clamps and, thereafter, the peritoneum is picked up with forceps and opened under direct vision (Fig. 3.2). A Hasson's trocar with a cone, which can slide along the shaft to plug the opening in the fascia gastight, is inserted and secured with stay sutures to the fascia (Fig. 3.3). Alternately, disposable

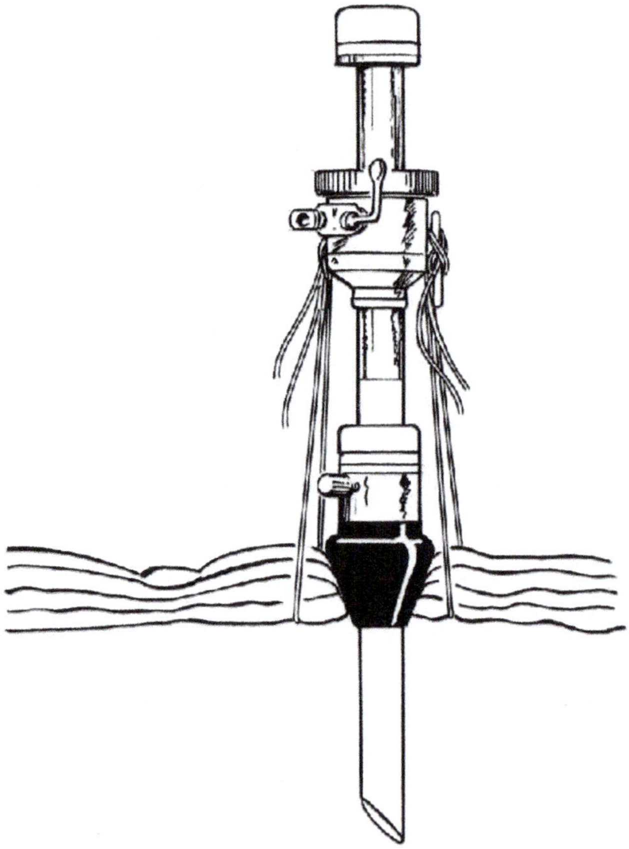

Fig. 3.3 Hasson's trocar secured to the fascia

Hasson's trocars with an inflatable balloon at the tip are available.

3.3 Selection of Technique

In children, there is consensus that the open method is preferable. However, in adult patients the debate persists with wide geographical variations [2]. The risk of the closed technique is blind insertion of the Veres needle and the first trocar (Fig. 3.4). Vascular and visceral injuries with in some cases fatal consequences have been reported below 0.1 %. Hence the incidence is very low but the impact is very high when an injury does occur. The hybrid technique does include use of the Veres needle in some centres and therefore is associated with its risks. Insertion of the first trocar under laparoscopic guidance appears to enhance safety but distinguishing the different layers of the abdominal wall can be difficult. The open technique is completely done under direct vision which eliminates the risk of vascular injury and is associated with very low risk of visceral injury. The disadvantage of the open technique is a larger incision, particularly in obese patients, than for the closed technique.

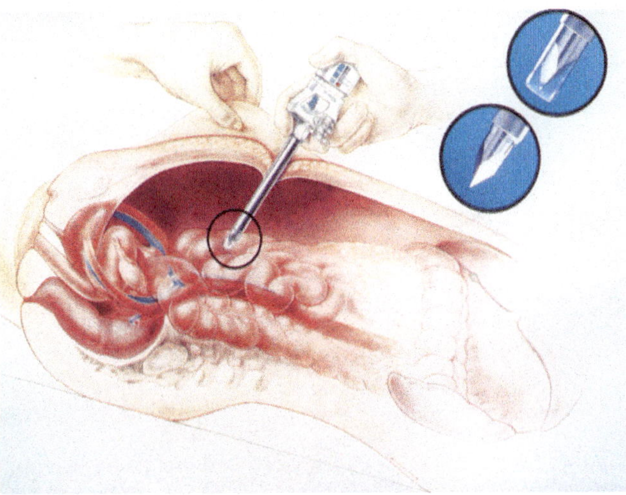

Fig. 3.4 Blind insertion of the first trocar (Reproduced with permission from Wolters Kluwer, Surgical Laparoscopy, 2nd edition, Karl A. Zucker)

3.4 Access to the Thoracic Cavity

This section is limited to access for thoracoscopic procedures of the lungs and disorders of the mediastinum [3]. To achieve adequate vision and working space, collapse of the ipsilateral lung is necessary, using a double lumen tube or a bronchial blocker. Some surgeons also use positive intrapleural pressure by insufflation of carbon dioxide combined with high frequency ventilation. Correct tube placement by a skilled anaesthesiologist and close communication between surgeon and anaesthesiologist throughout the whole procedure are of utmost importance. Controlled collapse of one lung has important physiological consequences for the patient. Significant hemodynamic and ventilatory changes may occur during the operation and these should be detected and managed promptly. Most pulmonary surgeries are done with the patient in a lateral decubitus position using a bean bag. Flexing the operating table at the level of the thoracolumbar junction puts the patients' hips out of the way and widens the intercostal spaces for easier access. The scope is usually positioned in the midaxillary line just above the diaphragm to allow for an optimal view of the ipsilateral pleural cavity. Additional trocars are placed in such a way that efficient dissection by triangulation of instruments is possible.

3.5 Safety

The most commonly used route to access the pleural cavity is via the intercostal spaces. Collapse of the lung will only occur after creating a pneumothorax by opening the pleura. The normally negative pleural pressure then becomes positive (atmospheric pressure) after which the lung will collapse through its elastic recoil if the lung is blocked and ventilation is limited to the contralateral lung. When creating a pneumothorax by opening the parietal pleura, iatrogenic injury to the lung parenchyma, diaphragm, intercostal vessels of nerves, or even heart and intraabdominal organs may occur. This risk is best avoided by dissecting in the intercostal space layer by layer under direct vision. This can be done through an incision of 1.5 cm over the superior border of one of the ribs, avoiding the intercostal vessels and nerves which run in the groove at the inferior border of the ribs. For thoracoscopy specially designed trocars are available which may be introduced through this incision allowing introduction of the scope. Under direct thoracoscopic vision more trocars may be inserted, depending on the procedure to be performed. Pleural adhesions may be encountered and these should be taken down if necessary. For lung resections a small auxiliary incision of 4–6 cm without rib spreading is used. This site allows extraction of the specimen. A wound protector is used at this site which makes introduction of instruments easy and avoids contamination of the wound edges.

3.6 Problems and Contraindications

Complete pleural fusion may occur after severe infectious pleuritis or surgical pleurodesis. In these circumstances a pneumothorax cannot be created. Even after converting to a thoracotomy using extrapleural dissection, surgery is difficult and has a higher risk of complications such as bleeding. In patients with severe lung emphysema the lung is much stiffer than normal and may not collapse sufficiently after creating a pneumothorax to allow for a safe surgical procedure. By gentle compression of the lung with a blunt instrument or a sponge stick, trapped air can be expressed in such a situation. Limited vision or access by the diaphragm, especially in obese patients, may be overcome by tilting the operating table and pressing the diaphragm downwards with a sponge stick. Patients with a severely limited lung capacity on spirometry also may not tolerate controlled collapse of one lung and surgery on a ventilated lung by thoracotomy may be necessary. The same applies of course for procedures in patients with only one lung after pneumonectomy.

References

1. Neudecker J, Sauerland S, Neugebauer E, Bergamaschi R, Bonjer HJ, Cuschieri A, et al. The EAES clinical practice guideline on the pneumoperitoneum for laparoscopic surgery. Surg Endosc. 2002;16(7):1121–43.
2. Bonjer HJ, Hazebroek EJ, Kazemier G, et al. Open versus closed establishment of pneumoperitoneum in laparoscopic surgery. Surg Endosc. 1997;11(5):491–4.
3. Satyapal KS, Singh B, Partab P, et al. Thoracoscopy: a new era for surgical anatomy. Clin Anat. 2003;16(6):538–41.

Part II

Abdominal Wall

4 Totally Extraperitoneal Endoscopic Inguinal Hernia Repair (TEP)

Marc J. Miserez

4.1 Introduction

There is no doubt that surgical techniques using mesh result in fewer recurrences than techniques that do not use mesh. The open Lichtenstein and endoscopic inguinal hernia techniques are the best studied. Endoscopic hernia repair can be performed by TAPP (TransAbdominal PrePeritoneal) or TEP (Totally ExtraPeritoneal) technique. Both minimally invasive techniques follow the principle of Stoppa, who promoted a giant prosthetic reinforcement of the abdominal wall in the preperitoneal plane in order to cover the whole myopectineal orifice on both sides. We prefer TEP since it preserves peritoneal integrity, although it is more difficult to learn because of the limited working space and a different appreciation of the usual anatomical landmarks.

Endoscopic hernia techniques allow an earlier return to normal activities or work, comparable recurrence rates in the long-term (>4 years postoperatively) and a lower chance of chronic pain/numbness than the Lichtenstein technique, at least in the first 3–4 years postoperatively. On the other hand, endoscopic techniques also result in a longer operation time than the Lichtenstein technique (8–13 min), a higher incidence of seroma and a higher rate of rare but serious complications. The latter are seen especially during the steep and long learning curve for endoscopic techniques. TAPP seems to be associated with higher rates of visceral injuries, port-site hernias and intestinal obstruction, while there appear to be more conversions with TEP. The learning curve for endoscopic inguinal hernia repair in general and TEP in particular ranges between 50 and 100 procedures, with the first 30–50 being the most critical.

It cannot be stressed enough that adequate training might minimize the risks for serious complications during the learning process. The most important variables in this learning curve are the presence of a structured training program, the laparoscopic experience of the trainee (can be junior resident but must be experienced in laparoscopic cholecystectomy), a suitable patient selection (no recurrent or scrotal hernia, no obese patients, no previous appendectomy for right-sided hernia), but especially the expertise and motivation of the trainer, who should be present during the procedure (i.e. intraoperative mentoring) and emphasize specific tips and tricks to perform the procedure smoothly and safely.

4.2 Indications

Both the open Lichtenstein and endoscopic techniques are recommended in the guidelines of the European Hernia Society (EHS) as the best-evidence based options for repair of a **primary** unilateral inguinal hernia providing the surgeon is sufficiently experienced in the specific procedure (Grade A recommendation) [1]. Although from the perspective of the hospital an open mesh procedure is the most cost-effective operation in primary unilateral hernia, hospital costs for an endoscopic procedure can be reduced by using reusable instruments as much as possible and mesh fixation only in selected cases. In our department, a large majority of hernia patients are treated on an outpatient basis.

From a socio-economic perspective, an endoscopic procedure is probably the most cost-effective approach for employed patients, especially for **bilateral** hernia. Moreover, for **recurrent** hernias after conventional open repair, endoscopic techniques result in less postoperative pain and faster reconvalescence than the Lichtenstein technique.

M.J. Miserez, MD, PhD
Department of Abdominal Surgery, University Hospital Gasthuisberg, Katholieke Universiteit Leuven, Leuven, Belgium
e-mail: marc.miserez@uz.kuleuven.ac.be

H.J. Bonjer (ed.), *Surgical Principles of Minimally Invasive Procedures*, DOI 10.1007/978-3-319-43196-3_4

For **women** we also use the TEP procedure as the first choice, since they have a higher risk for recurrence (inguinal or femoral) than men following an open inguinal hernia operation, because of a higher occurrence of femoral hernias.

For experienced surgeons, an endoscopic technique can also be used for **incarcerated** hernias in the absence of contamination in the surgical field. A diagnostic laparoscopy at the beginning of the procedure allows inspection and an attempt to reduce hernia content under visual control. Moreover, after a period of reperfusion (= at the end of the hernia repair), a reexploration for compromised bowel can be done, possibly limiting the need for intestinal resection.

Contraindications for us are a previous ipsilateral preperitoneal mesh placement in the groin, large scrotal (irreducible) inguinal hernias, major lower abdominal surgery, surgical prostatectomy and a patient who cannot undergo general anesthesia.

4.3 Pre-operative Work-Up

In case of an evident hernia, clinical examination is enough. Of course, the surgeon should be convinced that the hernia is the cause of the patient's complaints. With obscure pain or when no reducible swelling can be felt, additional studies can be helpful. If expertise is available, ultrasonography can be performed. MRI (with Valsalva) has a high sensitivity and specificity and is also useful for revealing other (musculotendineal) pathology. CT scan can be helpful in obese patients (e.g. detection of preperitoneal lipoma) or for diagnosis of other (intraabdominal) pathology. In case of doubt about the other side, a laparoscopic exploration before preperitoneal insufflation allows a thorough evaluation of the contralateral groin. Only a preperitoneal lipoma without a true peritoneal hernia sac can be missed, even with simultaneous compression on the groin from outside.

4.4 Operating Room Set Up

Recently, we proposed a standardised clinical training program in TEP emphasizing systematic dissection in ten consecutive steps, expert tips and tricks, and pitfalls to be avoided [2].

A video of the different steps is available at www.websurg.com. The complete procedure in a male patient with a right inguinal hernia is presented. Steps 1, 2, 4, 8 and 10 are more basic and steps 3, 5, 6, 7 and 9 more advanced.

The patient is placed in supine position after bladder emptying (Fig. 4.1). Make sure the hernia is reduced after induction of general anesthesia. The surgeon stands contralateral to the hernia side.

4.5 Surgical Technique

4.5.1 Step 1: Introduction of 1st Trocar

After disinfection and sterile draping, a small transverse incision for the first trocar is made just below the umbilicus on the contralateral side of the hernia; in this case, on the left (Fig. 4.2). With a bilateral hernia, we generally start with the largest hernia. After retraction of the skin and subcutis, the anterior rectus sheath is opened transversely just next to the midline in order to visualize clearly the medial edge of the rectus muscle, which is then retracted laterally until visualization of the posterior rectus sheath. Then a 10 mm trocar is bluntly inserted. The video shows a self-retaining blunt balloon trocar but this is not a dissection balloon. Another Hasson type trocar can also be used. Insufflation with CO_2 is started until 12 mmHg and the patient is placed in Trendelenburg position. A 0° or preferably 30° angled 10 mm endoscope is inserted and blunt dissection with the endoscope is continued in the retromuscular space up to the pubic symphysis.

4.5.2 Step 2: Introduction of 2nd Trocar

When the rectus muscle is nicely visualized, a second reusable 5 mm trocar is inserted under direct vision about three fingerwidths exactly under the first trocar. In the case of a bilateral hernia, this trocar is placed more towards the midline for more ergonomic working on both sides. During this step and the further dissection, care should be taken not to damage the epigastric vessels. If this happens, we apply a 5 mm clip proximally and distally to control the bleeding. The surgeon keeps the endoscope in one hand and starts dissection with the other hand.

4.5.3 Step 3: Dissection to Bogros' Space and Introduction of 3rd Trocar

A pair of scissors is introduced through the 5 mm trocar. In order to find the right plane, it may be necessary to cut some fibers of the arcuate line of Douglas. The correct preperitoneal dissection plane is easily found due to its angel hair appearance. The dissection is performed immediately laterally and as close as possible to the anterior abdominal wall between the hernia sac below and the epigastric vessels above. Also more laterally, it is very important to stay in this plane. Dissection is continued bluntly towards the lateral abdominal wall and the anterior superior iliac spine. This can be verified by lateral transillumination. Stay in this plane and do not dissect into the lateral abdominal wall itself. Dissect all attachments as close to the umbilicus as possible and move laterally. The purpose is to strip the peritoneum here sufficiently from the posterior rectus sheath in order to have enough space for the upper edge of the mesh to

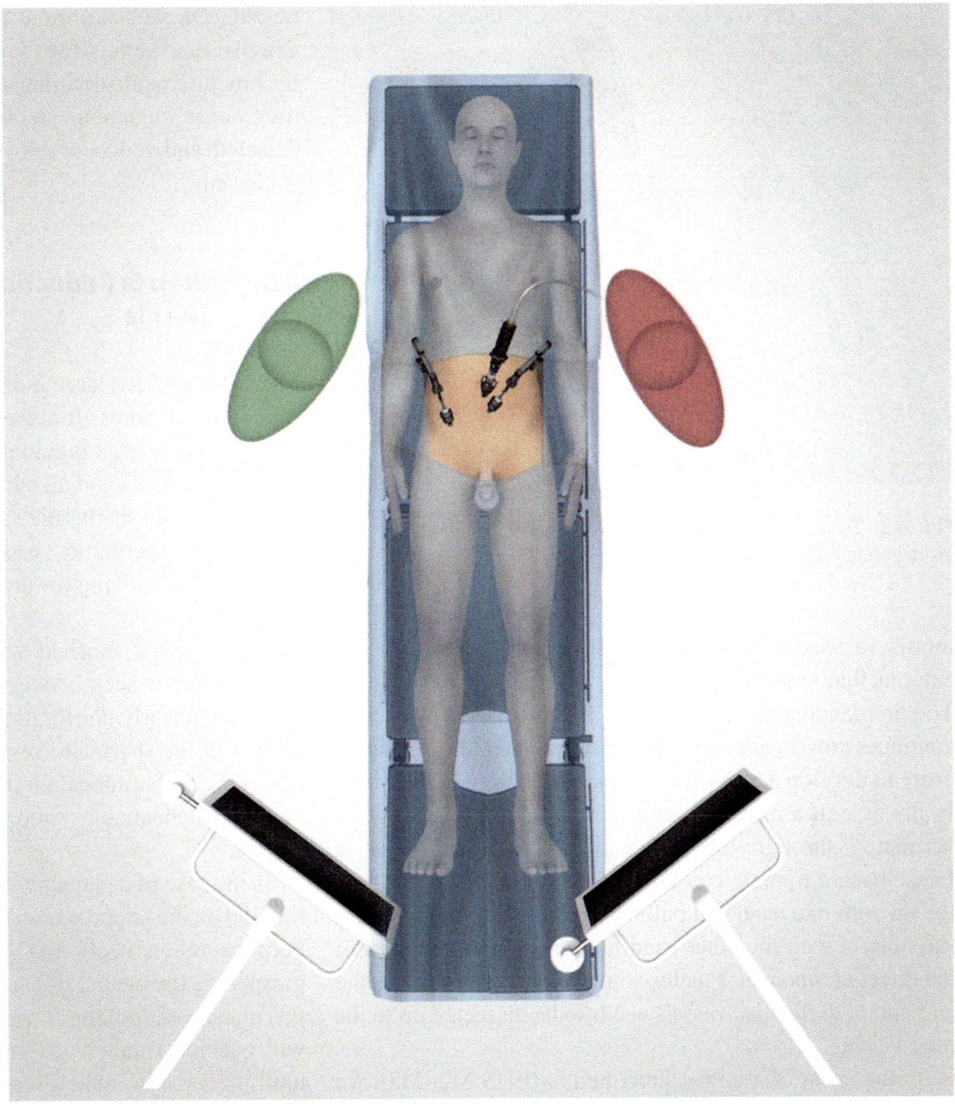

Fig. 4.1 Patient positioning for Totally ExtraPeritoneal (TEP) repair of right groin hernia

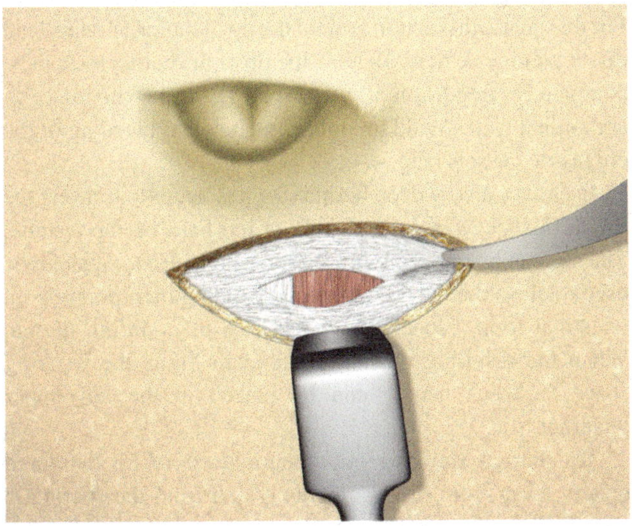

Fig. 4.2 Transverse incision of the anterior rectal sheath

be placed. Some sharp dissection may be necessary. The 3rd trocar, also 5 mm and reusable, needs to be introduced ideally at the level of the umbilicus cranially and medially to the anterior superior iliac spine (Fig. 4.3). This location can be verified by introducing an IM needle before putting in the trocar. Place the needle in the middle of the transilluminated spot and then the introduction of the 3rd trocar can be optimized while keeping the peritoneum away with the other hand. Do not put the trocar too obliquely through the anterior abdominal wall because this again will limit the expansion of the upper edge of the mesh.

4.5.4 Step 4: Reduction of a Direct Inguinal Hernia

Now the rest of the operation is performed with the assistant holding the endoscope. The Retzius space is dissected bluntly using two atraumatic graspers, avoiding the corona

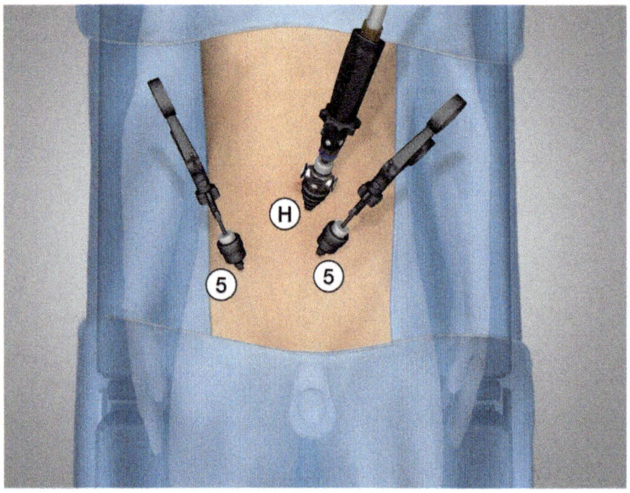

Fig. 4.3 Trocar placement for Totally ExtraPeritoneal (TEP) right groin hernia repair

mortis (a vascular connection between the obturator and external iliac systems close to the symphysis pubis) (Fig. 4.4). The first landmark is the Cooper's ligament. This dissection continues crossing the midline and deeper near the bladder in order to develop a nice place for the lower edge of the mesh. In the case of a direct inguinal hernia, the preperitoneal fat herniating through the defect of the inguinal floor at Hesselbach's triangle can be reduced by gently pulling on the fat with one hand and pulling on the weakened transversalis fascia with the other hand until complete reduction of the direct component. Finally, some preperitoneal fat cranial and lateral to the iliac vessels needs to be dissected up to the internal ring.

In the event of a larger direct hernia (EHS M2–M3), we prefer to fix the deepest point of the stretched transversalis fascia with one or two fixation devices on the upper part of Cooper's ligament to decrease the risk for seroma formation and for bulging of the prosthesis through the defect. The fixation instrument should be brought in via the medial trocar and a good stabilization of the instrument with two hands is very important to avoid slipping during firing. Fixation should be done not too laterally because of the external iliac vein and not too medially because of the pubic symphysis and the risk of pubic osteitis.

4.5.5 Step 5: Reduction of Femoral/Obturator Hernia

Always explore the femoral canal for the presence of a femoral hernia. In most cases, it will only be herniating preperitoneal fat, without a definite peritoneal sac, just medial to the external iliac vein. Please clearly differentiate in obese patients between herniating preperitoneal fat, which needs to be reduced, versus normal fat and lymph nodes around the external iliac vein. Always avoid direct traction on this fragile structure while dividing any fatty attachments. Just below the Cooper's ligament, an obturator hernia can sometimes be detected and reduced. Most of the time, this is clinically irrelevant.

4.5.6 Step 6: Reduction of Indirect Inguinal Hernia

The reduction of a large indirect inguinal hernia is one of the most difficult steps. It always starts with pulling the hernia sac near the internal inguinal ring medially and sweeping the spermatic vessels and all surrounding preperitoneal fat laterally away from the hernia sac. This will allow blunt dissection of the spermatic vessels from the hernia sac while progressively moving towards the internal ring and the tip of the hernia sac.

Dissection is finished when the small fascia with blue transparency is seen between the hernia sac posteriorly and the vas anteriorly. Perforating this fascia will allow full dissection of the spermatic vessels and the vas from the hernia sac. If the preperitoneal fat medial to the internal ring has not been freed adequately (step 4), this fascia will not be clearly visible.

In the case of a patient with a larger hernia sac, try to keep traction on the lateral part of the sac by constantly folding the peritoneum on itself and grasping it with an atraumatic grasper via the medial trocar. The angled scope can help with this maneuver, looking from lateral to medial. The hernia sac will become smaller and smaller. Continue this dissection until the vas is visible. Please note that the vas can be very adherent to the tip of the sac and in this case it needs to be gently dissected away from the sac. Never grasp the vas and avoid damaging its vascularization by skeletonizing the vas. For this gentle dissection around the tip of the sac, a Maryland dissector may be helpful. Now the tip of the hernia sac can be completely freed, bluntly or sharply, from the anterior abdominal wall. Avoid too much traction and bleeding of the epigastric vessels (Fig. 4.4).

In case of a very deep hernia sac, it is better to transect the sac at this stage instead of pulling too hard on the testicle. The sac can be opened with scissors and an Endoloop can be used to close the defect, of course avoiding incorporating an intestinal loop, especially in the case of a sliding hernia. When the resulting pneumoperitoneum limits the working space, a Veres needle can be placed in the left upper quadrant.

The hernia sac and peritoneum need to be dissected clearly away from the vas medially and from the spermatic vessels laterally, both of which are parietalized until these clearly diverge at the base of the so-called triangle of Doom.

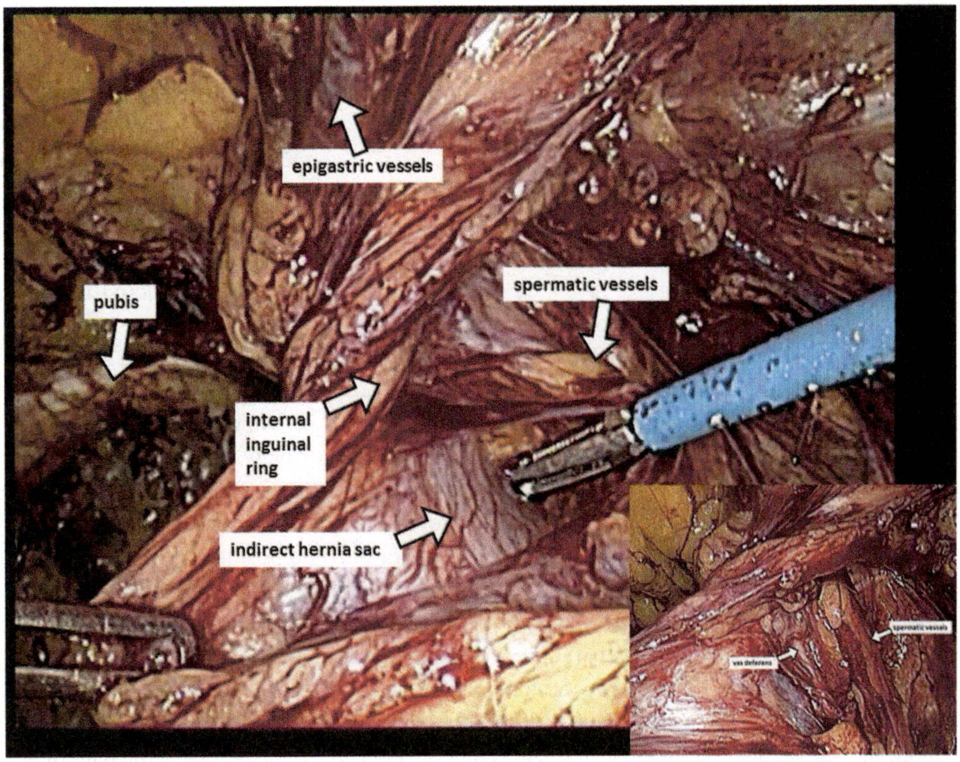

Fig. 4.4 Extraperitoneal anatomy of the right groin area (inset showing also vas deferens after further dissection)

Here also gentle manipulation of the peritoneum is important. Remember the peritoneum also needs to be reduced when there is no indirect component to allow proper placement of the mesh. In these cases, the peritoneum is extremely thin and fragile.

In the case of a female patient, we advocate transection and coagulation of the round ligament near the internal ring in most cases in order not to damage the peritoneum

4.5.7 Step 7: Lateral Dissection and Reduction of a Preperitoneal Lipoma

Lateral dissection is continued in the preperitoneal plane of angel hair. In order to have an adequate landmark, it is important to stay close to the edge of the peritoneum. The psoas muscle can be visualized and in some cases, the inguinal nerves running over it can be seen. The overlying fascia needs to be preserved. It is necessary to avoid tenting of the parietalized spermatic vessels. Systematic exploration for a preperitoneal lipoma originating laterally near the spermatic vessels is very important in all cases but especially in obese patients or in patients where no obvious hernia sac can be found. All this fat needs to be reduced adequately so that it can be placed deep to the prosthesis. In most cases, the lateral internal spermatic fascia between the peritoneum and the anterolateral abdominal wall needs to be transected by blunt and sharp dissection.

Ultimately, with adequate retraction of the peritoneal fold, a kind of groove or pocket is freed from the midline over the Cooper's ligament, the iliac vessels, the vas and the spermatic vessels towards the psoas muscle and the lateral abdominal wall for complete expansion of the lower edge of the mesh.

4.5.7.1 Contralateral Dissection

Because the unilateral dissection is now finalized, this is the moment to continue to the other side in the case of a bilateral hernia. No additional trocars are necessary and the surgeon changes sides. The different steps are identical to those described earlier without the need for an additional lateral trocar. Contralateral dissection is started in the same preperitoneal plane laterally with lifting of the epigastric vessels through the midline trocar and dissecting with the lateral one, again between the hernia sac below and the epigastric vessels above. During this step, it is very important to stay close to the muscles of the abdominal wall to avoid perforating the peritoneal sac.

4.5.8 Step 8: Preparation and Introduction of the Mesh

We use a polypropylene mesh 15 cm wide and 13 cm long with a small inferolateral cut for the psoas muscle. The mesh is rolled from below in a very tiny roll so that the free edge of the mesh is the upper part. Then the lateral part of the rolled mesh is grasped. The mesh is introduced blindly into the 10 mm trocar, which is stabilized until some resistance is encountered. Further introduction can be done while pushing the mesh down the trocar with the scope under direct vision.

4.5.9 Step 9: Placement of the Mesh and Fixation in Selected Cases

After introduction, the lateral part of the rolled mesh is grasped via the lateral trocar and the medial part via the medial trocar. The mesh is pulled laterally and is first positioned horizontally before it is unrolled. To unroll it, we take the free upper edge near the midline, which is pulled upwards, while unrolling it via the lateral trocar. The mesh is first positioned on the midline, overlapping the latter by some 2 cm, and then further laterally, ensuring that the lateral upper border of the mesh is adequately unfolded and that the lower edge of the mesh is adequately positioned in the preformed pocket over its entire length. In general, the mesh should ideally be positioned with the middle centred on the internal inguinal ring. This can be adjusted in large direct hernias (more medially), large indirect hernias (more laterally) or in large femoral hernias (deeper to the Cooper's ligament). Only in the case of large direct and femoral hernias we fix the prosthesis with one or two fixation devices on the upper part of Cooper's ligament, but never lateral to the spermatic vessels. Our strategy to fix the mesh is the same in unilateral and bilateral hernias. In the case of a peritoneal tear and potential adhesion of viscerae to the mesh, the peritoneal edges can be adapted with small clips just before desufflation. Closing the peritoneum earlier during the procedure might result in tearing of the clips during later manipulation.

4.5.10 Step 10: Desufflation

In order to avoid an early hernia recurrence, desufflation should be performed by pushing on the inferolateral border of the mesh with one hand and mainly by pulling upward on the deepest part of the hernia sac with the other. This position is kept until full desufflation and flat positioning of the patient. In the case of an accidental pneumoperitoneum, please make sure that the abdominal cavity is adequately desufflated to decrease the risk for postoperative pain. Then all trocars are removed and the anterior rectus sheath is approximated with an absorbable suture. The skin wounds are closed intradermally and approximated with Steristrips™ after local anaesthetic infiltration.

4.6 Postoperative Care

In order to decrease the risk for postoperative seroma formation and scrotal hematoma, we ask the patient to wear slim fit underwear for a week. The patient is free to resume activities "doing what he/she feels he/she can do". Probably only a limitation on heavy weight lifting for 2–3 weeks is enough. Early return to work (2–4 weeks postoperatively depending on physical activities) should be encouraged. This will require a change in attitude by surgeons, general practitioners and patients and may result in significant savings in health expenditures.

In case of a nonreducible groin swelling early postoperatively, an incarcerated recurrent hernia will most likely be excluded by history taking and physical examination; an ultrasound examination can be useful to distinguish this from a postoperative seroma/hematoma. In the case of a reducible groin swelling, the distinction is less clear, since also a seroma can be "reducible"; in those cases we prefer a conservative attitude in the first weeks.

Conclusion

In order to provide a surgery tailored to the patient, we believe all surgeons qualifying in general surgery should not only have profound knowledge of the anterior and posterior (preperitoneal) anatomy, but also be familiar with the technical aspects of an anterior approach (i.e. Lichtenstein) and a posterior approach. In our department, TEP inguinal hernia repair is the method of choice for unilateral or bilateral inguinal hernia repair. The application of endoscopic hernia techniques also in primary hernias allows, in addition to the advantages mentioned above, a large patient exposure for surgical trainees, provided training conditions are optimal. Only then, will surgeons be adequately trained to also perform laparoscopy in recurrent and bilateral hernias.

References

1. Simons MP, Aufenacker T, Bay-Nielsen M, Bouillot JL, Campanelli G, Conze J, de Lange D, Fortelny R, Heikkinen T, Kingsnorth A, Kukleta J, Morales-Conde S, Nordin P, Schumpelick V, Smedberg S, Smietanski M, Weber G, Miserez M. European Hernia Society guidelines on the treatment of inguinal hernia in adult patients. Hernia. 2009;13:343–403.
2. Miserez M, Arregui M, Bisgaard T, Hughe M, Van Bruwaene S, Peeters E, Penninckx F. A standardized resident training program in endoscopic surgery in general and in laparoscopic totally extraperitoneal (TEP) inguinal hernia repair in particular. Surg Laparosc Endosc Percutan Tech. 2009;19:125–9.

5 Inguinal and Femoral Hernia Trans-Abdominal Pre-peritoneal Patch Plasty (TAPP)

Jan F. Kukleta

5.1 Introduction

The event of laparoscopic cholecystectomy has facilitated the search for a laparoscopic solution of groin hernia repair. The adoption of a synthetic non absorbable mesh as an indispensable part of the procedure was the first precondition of the operative strategy. René Stoppa has recognized early the importance of the mesh size in relation to recurrence and the advantage of the posterior approach over the trans-inguinal one concerning the perfect placement of a large mesh in the pre-peritoneal space. Stoppa's Giant Prosthetic Reinforcement of Visceral Sac (GPRVS) became the fundament of the later developed Trans-Abdominal Pre-peritoneal Patch plasty (TAPP) as described by Arregui in March 1992 [1].

The rational of endoscopic hernia repair (TAPP and TEP) is the combination of physical and surgical advantages. The trans-abdominal route in TAPP offers an excellent exposure of the entire posterior wall of the groin. The posterior approach allows placement of a large prosthetic mesh with a technique of minimal tissue trauma. The mesh in pre-peritoneal space lies in the line of first defense, supported by the intra-abdominal pressure which distributes uniformly over the overall surface unlike in a mesh placed in pre-muscular position (Pascal's hydrostatic law). The tissue ingrowth into a large mesh immobilizes it more efficiently than in a smaller one so that permanent fixation of mesh is seldom necessary, resulting in smaller risk of recurrence and of less fixation-related pain. Covering and overlapping the whole myopectineal orifice with mesh reinforces the posterior wall of the inguinal canal without the defect closure. It is a true tension free repair with all its positive consequences: less acute and much less chronic pain, earlier resumption of daily activities and better patient's satisfaction.

J.F. Kukleta, MD, FMCH
Klinik Im Park, Hirslanden, Zurich, Switzerland
e-mail: jfkukleta@bluewin.ch

5.2 Indication

TAPP is a complex surgical technique with a demanding learning curve. It has a large indication range in hands of an experienced laparoscopic surgeon with very few relative or absolute contraindications. It can be performed in all types of groin hernias (inguinal and femoral, unilateral and bilateral, primary and recurrent, even in some incarcerated and strangulated ones).

The trans-abdominal approach requires general anesthesia (GA), although TAPP in regional anesthesia with sedation was reported as being feasible. Patients unfit for GA or with blood clotting disorders should get an open repair. In case of large inguino-scrotal hernias or after previous interventions in lower abdomen (adhesions), especially in pre-peritoneal space with or without prosthetic mesh already implanted (after cystectomy, prostatectomy,plug repair, Rives repair, PHS/UHS, TAPP/TEP, etc.) generally an open repair is advised. Such patients belong in experience hands. TAPP repair can be performed in those difficult scenarios too, if enough expertize is present. But one has to be very critical to his own abilities and respect the risk-benefit ratio keeping the patient in mind first.

5.3 Preoperative Work-Up

There is no specific work-up necessary for a TAPP repair. Although there is insufficient evidence for routine antibiotic prophylaxis and insufficient evidence for routine thromboembolic prophylaxis in laparoscopic hernia surgery (IEHS Guidelines 2011) [2]. I systematically use the single-dose of cephalosporin 30 min preoperatively and low molecular heparin subcutaneously according to the patient's weight in the evening prior to intervention.

Abdominal hair is clipped just before going to the operating room and the patient is asked to empty his bladder before surgery, as full urinary bladder can substantially increase the technical difficulty of TAPP repair. Perioperative catheterization of urinary bladder is very rarely necessary. If technical difficulties (e.g., after prostatic surgery, scrotal her-

H.J. Bonjer (ed.), *Surgical Principles of Minimally Invasive Procedures*, DOI 10.1007/978-3-319-43196-3_5

nia) or an extended operating time are expected consider using a urinary catheter during the intervention. Eventual retrograde instillation of methylene blue solution may help to rule out or to localize a bladder wall injury.

5.4 Operating Room

The patient lies in supine position with both arms tucked to his body, the arm rests have to be flat in order not to interfere with laparoscopic instruments. The patient is provided a simple peripheral IV line only, in most cases. As the operating surgeon I prefer to stand at patient's right shoulder for both left and right groin hernia with the primary monitor at patient's left leg (Fig. 5.1). The assistant stands opposite to surgeon with secondary monitor between surgeon and the scrub nurse on the right side. The skin disinfection and the drape allow free access to groin for the improbable case of conversion.

5.5 Instrumentation

I use a 10 and 5 mm 30° angled endoscope with the possibility of sterile exchange. The standard set consists of one 10 mm, one 5 mm and one 3 mm reusable conical trocar, 5 and 3 mm graspers, 3 mm scissors and 3 mm needle-holder. Small size gauze is ready for eventual cleaning of operating field.

5.6 Surgical Technique Step by Step

1. The first skin incision is a 10 mm infra-umbilical smiley. In case of very short lower abdomen consider discrete overstretching of the thoraco-lumbar spine or place the endoscope above umbilicus. Pneumoperitoneum is established with a reusable Veres needle insufflating 2.5–4.0 lt. of CO_2 up to intra-abdominal pressure of 12 mm of mercury. Prior the insufflation routine security tests are always performed (aspiration, drop test, etc.).

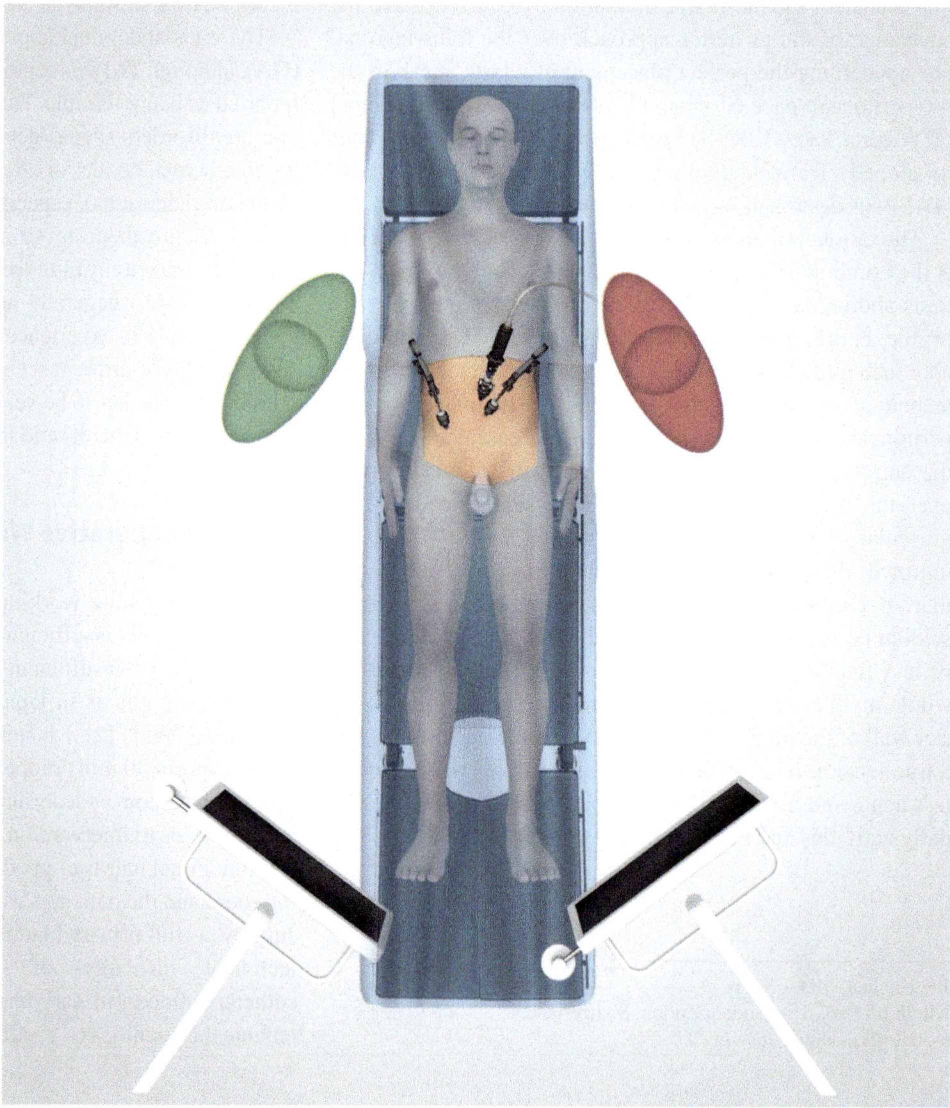

Fig. 5.1 Patient positioning for Trans-Abdominal Pre-peritoneal Patch plasty (TAPP) of groin hernia

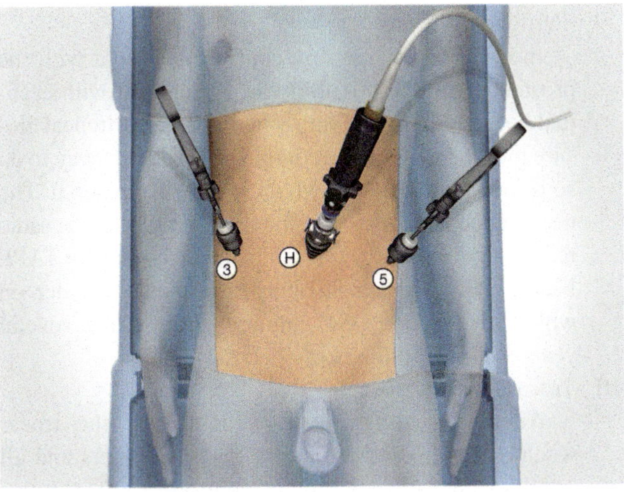

Fig. 5.2 Trocar positioning for Trans-Abdominal Pre-peritoneal Patch plasty (TAPP) of groin hernia

2. Insert the 10 mm endoscope (T1 = trocar nr. 1) and visualize the abdominal content in the theoretical reach of the Veres needle to rule out any injury. Explore the ipsilateral and the contralateral groin and inform the anesthetist of uni- or bilateral procedure. Complete the exploration of the entire abdominal cavity.

   The 5 mm trocar (T2) is placed lateral to semilunar line on the left side at the level of umbilicus and the 3 mm trocar (T3) on the right side at the same level further lateral of semilunar line for easier reach of the right groin. The trocars are always placed under direct visual control (Fig. 5.2). Mind the distance of the dominant hand-trocar to the bony structures (ribs and iliac crest) to prevent reduced mobility of your instruments.
3. Discrete Trendelenburg position(15°) increases the working space. Keep your endoscope lens clean to guarantee a perfect vision through the whole procedure. Don't compromise. Try to localize the well-known anatomical landmarks (medial umbilical ligament (MUL), anterior superior iliac spine (ASIS), inferior epigastric vessels, inner inguinal ring, spermatic vessels and vas deferens. Decide if you deal with direct, indirect or a pantalon hernia, don't forget the femoral, obturator and Spighelian hernias. It helps the primary orientation and the anticipation of dissectional difficulties. The other important structures(secondary orientation) become visible during the pre-peritoneal dissection: the ileopubic tract, the symphysis pubis, Cooper's ligament, and the femoral canal.
4. Horizontal or cranially convex peritoneal incision 3–4 cm above of all possible defects extending from ASIS to MUL is carried out from lateral to medial. Proceeding from lateral to medial facilitates the pneumodissection (tissue separation by gas penetration), which helps to identify and separate the visceral layer of the peritoneum from the parietal one. The parietal layer of peritoneum is not the transversalis fascia! In some individuals it can be very well developed as a kind of endo-abdominal fascia and it covers the entire floor, protects the epigastric vessels and continues as the spermatic fascia protecting spermatic vessels and the nerves in triangle of pain (lateral of spermatic vessels) and triangle of doom (over the extern iliac vessels). It is recommendable to preserve this layer to protect the nerves from contact with the prosthetic material. Crossing the "epigatrics" in this "spider-web"-like space lets you anticipate and prevent any damage to these vessels. The medial umbilical ligament doesn't need to be transected. If more space is needed, a cranial extension of the peritoneal incision parallel to MUL may be helpful. The extent of dissection reaches medially 1 cm beyond the symphysis pubis to the contralateral side, cranially 3–4 cm above the transversalis arch or any direct defect, laterally to ASIS, and caudally minimally 4–5 cm below the ileopubic tract at the level of psoas muscle and 2–3 cm below the Cooper's ligament at the level of superior arch of the pubic bone.
5. Indirect hernias

   The indirect hernia sac has to be retracted by separating the peritoneum from the spermatic fascia. Large and/or deep indirect sacs can be more difficult to dissect and may prolong the operating time, but complete retraction is possible in almost every case. Delicate dissection and good control of hemostasis do not increase the incidence of scrotal hematomas and seromas, but prevent the formation of chronic seroma/pseudo-hydrocele. Seldom there is a firm adherence of the sac to the spermatic structures at the level of the inner inguinal ring. In such condition it is much easier to separate the spermatic vessels from the overlying peritoneum far latero-caudally first, before starting the dissection along the vessels towards the inguinal canal and to the top of the indirect sac. In this manner, damage to the spermatic vessels can be safely prevented.

   The cord lipomas deserve a special attention. Quite often, substantial funicular masses of pre-or retroperitoneal fat prolapse into the enlarged hernia orifices. One has to look for them actively. Once retracted from the inguinal canal I prefer to resect them, because they may become symptomatic or mimics recurrent hernia.

   The search for or exclusion of such masses is an integral part of the endoscopic hernia repair.
6. Direct hernias

   The most direct hernia sacs are easily retracted with their preperitoneal fat and separated from the white appearing attenuated transversalis fascia. The incidence of postoperative seromas in direct hernias can be significantly reduced when the lax transversalis fasciais inverted and either ligated with endoloop or fixed to Cooper's ligament with a suture. The reduced "dead space" not only prevents seroma formation but eliminates an eventual prolapse of a light-weight mesh into the former hernia cavity creating a pseudohernia. Even in case of big direct hernias being successfully reduced, additional revision of the inner ring and an exclusion of a cord lipoma is mandatory.

7. Femoral hernias

   The standardized technique of dissection will never fail in recognition of a femoral hernia. The femoral canal is a kind of preexisting funnel surrounded by the pubic bone caudally, the femoral vein medially and a vascular arch cranially. Some of the symptomatic hernias don't even have a peritoneal prolapse – the hernia sac. The corresponding preperitoneal fat is often incarcerated (=non reducible). Gentle traction and respect to anatomy (cave corona mortis) help to reduce sometimes quite surprisingly big content.

8. Mesh choice, mesh size, mesh slit, mesh fixation

   The resulting pre-peritoneal space has to accommodate a mesh of adequate size (at least 10 × 15 cm or bigger). A macroporous polypropylene, polyester or PVDF mesh is unpacked after all the dissection is completed, additional surgeon's gloves may be put on and the mesh is trimmed with new instruments if necessary. The mesh is rolled-up along its longer axis and blindly introduced through the camera trocar (T1). The suture material for later peritoneal closure is handled the same way.

   The mesh must be meticulously conformed to the underlying tissues. Lateral or vertical slit in the mesh and encircling the spermatic structures was in the past believed to prevent the mesh dislocation. The experience has proven the opposite. So, no slit in the mesh, but extended parietalization (mobilization of peritoneum over the iliac fossa) is required in order to accommodate the mesh and not to lift it up when closing the peritoneum.

   Depending on the hernia type, hernia size, mesh choice and the surgeon's experience and skills, the need for mesh fixation can vary. Due to scar tissue in growth the mesh will be secured in place in the long term. Because the retention need is temporary, the nature of fixation choice can be temporary too. The least invasive and more secure (than the non-fixation) is the use of a sealantor of a glue. It can be fibrin-sealant or cyanoacrylate glue. In large hernias, especially the direct ones or after previous pre-peritoneal interventions the use of more rigid heavy-weight meshes (e.g. Prolene® or Optilene®) and absorbable fixation devices (Permasorb®, Absorbatack®, Sorbafix®, Securestrap®) or suture may be justified.

   My personal preference is Ultrapro® mesh, in general of 10 × 15 cm size. I use additional gloves and new instruments to handle the mesh and fix it with Glubran-2® or Histoacryl® (both being n-butyl-cyanoacrylates) since 2001. My infection rate since 1992 is 0.0 % and prolonged pain (not chronic) is extremely low.

9. Peritoneal closure

   In order to prevent any contact of viscera with the prosthetic and the possibility of entrapment with eventual bowel obstruction (inner hernia), the peritoneal closure must be perfectly accomplished. The best way to do so is the running suturewith an absorbable material. The neck of deeper hernia sacs should be closed for the same reason too (endoloop, suture). In the early years of TAPP I closed the peritoneum with EMS® stapler, later on with Vicryl®- or PDS® running suture. Since several years V-lock® suture is my favorite choice.

10. Trocar incision closure

   After evacuating the remaining CO_2 the trocar wounds bigger than 5 mm are closed in layers and all incisions are infiltrated with a long lasting local anesthetic (Naropine®).

Postoperative Care Ninety eight percent of all my patients leave the hospital the next day (Switzerland). The pain control measures are minimal. There are no weight-lifting restrictions. In contrary the patient is encouraged to be as active as the body feeling allows. The earlier "the normal way of life" is challenged, the shorter is the convalescence.

The patients have to be informed prior to- and after the surgery of several unimportant symptoms, which may appear in the early postoperative course:

1. "post-laparoscopy pain" in upper chest or shoulders,
2. swelling at the previous hernia site or
3. superficial hematoma of penis or scrotum

The first resolves mostly within hours.

1. Some patients develop a seroma or hemato-seroma in the site of the previous hernia. These mostly short lasting swellings ("pseudohernias") will resolve in days or 1–2 weeks and don't have to be aspirated. In some instances an aspiration reinforces the patient's confidence and gives a local relief.
2. In very few patients (temporary converts from per-oral anticoagulation, Aspirin users) a superficial hematoma of penis basis or scrotal neck can appear 2–3 days after surgery. Being sometimes quite impressive they resolve in much shorter time than a true hematoma would. Once again: adequate information before the operation is the key.

Around 10 days after the intervention the absorbable intra-cutaneous sutures are cut or removed and at 6 weeks postoperatively the patient gives his final feedback (by phone, seldom by e-mail) to confirm his/her well-being or a need for a clinical control.

5.7 Summary

The TAPP technique for the repair of nearly all forms of inguino-femoral hernias is a powerful tool in the repertoire of a modern surgeon.

The potential patient's benefits justify the longer learning curve. Even after reaching the expertize TAPP remains a more demanding procedure than the open repair. Correct indication, strict adherence to the principles of a well standardized surgical procedure, attention to details, delicate dissection and the readiness to turn any "everyday repair" to "the best ever repair" may offer your hernia patient his/her best Solution.

References

1. Arregui ME, Davis CJ, Yucel O, Nagan RF. Laparosocpic mesh repair of inguinal hernia using a preperitoneal approach, a preliminary report. Surg Laparosc Endosc. 1992;2(1):64–8.
2. Bittner R, Arregui ME, Bisgaar T, et al. Guidelines for laparoscopic (TAPP) and endoscopic (TEP) treatment of inguinal hernia (International Endo Hernia Society, IEHS). Surg Endosc. 2011;25(9):2773–843.

6 Laparoscopic Ventral Hernia Repair

Salvador Morales-Conde, María Socas, and Isaias Alarcón

6.1 Introduction

Laparoscopic surgery continues to advance in achieving further benefits over the conventional approach for certain pathologies. In 1992 LeBlanc, et al. carried out the first laparoscopic repairs of ventral hernias (LVHR) [1]. Although not originally considered to be a pathology that could benefit from this approach, laparoscopic repair of ventral hernias has attained wide acceptance in recent years because of the significant advantages afforded by improvements in prosthetic materials and in fixation devices, as well as in the surgical technique used. Even that the latest meta-analysis show similar recurrence rate between the two approaches, this technique offers as a great advantage compared to the open repair since a significant reduction of local morbidity has been observed, making it a procedure that solves a long-standing challenge for the surgeon.

Nevertheless, there are still certain points of controversy that should be clarified, starting with the simple fact of establishing more precise indications and contraindications for the use of this approach. In addition, a multitude of more specific technical details should be discussed, including if the defect should be closed or not, how to manage the seroma, how to choose the type of mesh and its size and how to fix the mesh. One of the most interesting points currently being debated is whether or not it is necessary to use sutures or tacks alone, following the "*Double Crown*" technique, or other additional methods of fixation, such us, glues or the new method of fixations available, such us absorbable tackers.

S. Morales-Conde • M. Socas • I. Alarcón (✉)
Unit of Innovation in Minimally Invasive Surgery, University Hospital "Virgen del Rocío", Sevilla, Spain
e-mail: smoralesc@gmail.com

6.2 Indications and Contraindications

Basically all ventral hernias can be repaired by laparoscopy as the standard procedure. Emergency operations performed in cases of strangulated hernias must be analyzed on an individual basis to assess whether or not laparoscopy should be used. However, various factors place limits on the indications for laparoscopic repair such as the size of the defect, the presence of skin problems, the physical characteristics and the clinical history of the patients and the site where the hernia is localized. Subxyphoid, suprapubic, lumbar and parastomal hernias are good indication for laparoscopy, although these techniques require special technical considerations to be analyzed.

At the lower limit of the size of the defect, hernias that can be repaired with local anesthesia, those under 3–4 cm, are usually excluded. However, in patients requiring laparoscopic surgery for other concomitant conditions, obese patients and multi-recurrent hernias, laparoscopic repair would be indicated despite the small size of the hernia. Regarding the upper limit of the hernia size, different authors has performed many successful repairs of massive abdominal wall defects, although those hernias that need to associate a dermolipectomy or those with loss of domain should be excluded of being repair by this approach. We, therefore, conclude that until the limits are clearly established, the degree of difficulty in managing the instruments within the abdominal cavity and the size of the meshes available are the only actual limit to the technique, as far as large hernias are concerned.

On the other hand, this technique is often criticized by surgeons who perform open ventral hernia repair because the posterior rectus sheath cannot be reapproximated laparoscopically. There is no data to determine whether patients with an important rectus diastasis associated to a ventral hernia or an incisional hernia with an important distance between the rectus sheath, should be repaired by laparoscopy or an anatomical repair by re- approximation of the anterior

H.J. Bonjer (ed.), *Surgical Principles of Minimally Invasive Procedures*, DOI 10.1007/978-3-319-43196-3_6

rectus sheath should be performed, to improve the physiopathological function of the abdominal wall. New techniques are being described proposing an approximation of the rectus muscle with a running sutures performed by laparoscopy or a combined approach using an endoscopic component separation dissection before to place the mesh.

Contraindications to laparoscopic ventral hernia repair would include pregnant patients, children and patients with intra-abdominal sepsis, while patients with portal hypertension, previous abdominal radiotherapy or previous abdominal tuberculosis should be considered relative contraindications for this approach. These last two cases should be considered as difficult situations together with incarcerated hernias or those patients with multi-recurrent hernias previously repair with polypropylene, since more adhesions are usually found.

On the other hand, the characteristics of the sac of the hernia are important to determine the contraindications of this technique, since the evolution and complication of the seroma and the cosmetic results would be different depending on the type of sac. Definitive contraindications for this approach include patients with skin problems and fistulas.

6.3 Laparoscopic Surgical Procedure

6.3.1 Preoperative Work-Up

It is controversial whether pre-operative imaging techniques are needed for any ventral repair to select patients for LVHR. There have been suggestions that imaging studies might be helpful in patients with recurrent hernias in unusual anatomic locations and to evaluate the sac content. Having these data preoperatively can aid with decision making, such as the best way to access the reoperative abdomen, or to determine the localization of the bladder, iliac crest, or other important structures relative to a hernia defect.

6.3.2 Instrumentation

- ***Optic***: a 30° angle view scope is essential to perform the laparoscopic approach of ventral hernias since offers an excellent view of the entire anterior abdominal wall, and of the defect that need to be covered.
- ***Trocars***: a 10–12 mm trocar is used for the 30° scope and to introduce the mesh, and two 5-mm trocars are used for introducing the the mechanical fixation devices and the standard laparoscopic instruments.
- ***Graspers, scissors, and other laparoscopic instrumentation***: atraumatic bowel graspers are needed to manage the bowel and to perform traction gently to reduce the content of the hernia sac. Sharp scissors are required for proper dissection and prevention of bowel injury. A needle holder should be also available in case of an enterotomy to suture the bowel and continue the procedure by laparoscopy.
- ***Energy source***: monopolar cautery is acceptable as long as it is used far away from the viscera. Adhesiolysis must be performed with extremely care since missed bowel perforation could be life-threatening for the patient. For that reason, electrocautery should be used in a bleeding area after the adhesions are freed since if the proper plane is maintained blood loss is not expected.
- ***Fixation devices***: meshes could be fixed with tacks alone, which guarantee a proper fixation of the mesh to the anterior abdominal wall if the Double Crown technique is followed, or with transfascial sutures alone or with a combination of both. The new absorbable tackers should be evaluated in the future in order to determine if they could substitute the conventional metal tacks.

6.3.3 Operating Room Set-Up

The description of the technique is based on a primary or incisional ventral hernia at the midline and about 5 cm far from the bone margins, the patient is placed in supine decubitus, with the surgeon and the assistant to the patient's left and the monitor in front of them to the patient's right. A Foley catheter is only used in patients with suprapubic hernias or hernias located at the middle third below the midline and if operation is likely to be prolonged.

6.3.4 Surgical Technique

Creation of Pneumoperitoneum and Placement of Trocars Due to the presence of adhesions in the abdominal cavity, surgeons recognize that there is a risk of intra-abdominal lesion when creating the pneumoperitoneum or introducing the initial "blind' trocar. This has led some authors to recommend open laparoscopy using a Hasson trocar in patients with previous surgeries who will undergo laparoscopy. Many authors, however, are not of this opinion, using systematically Veres needle. In these cases, pneumoperitoneum is created by placing the Veres needle in the left hypochondrium, since this is the area of the abdomen where we are likely to find fewer adhesions because of the lower frequency of inflammatory processes at this level introducing the first trocar in the left side of the patient. Once the pneumoperitoneum has been created, the initial trocar is placed in the patient's side (normally, the left abdomen) away from the proximal border of the hernia in this area, being recommended to use a bladeless or a optic trocar, since bowel injuries are often associated with blind insertion of the initial trocar rather than with the Veres needle itself.

In addition, a high percentage of patients presenting ventral hernias are obese, this factor being associated with the presence of incisional hernias and with their recurrence. In these patients, performing an incision on the side of the abdomen (where trocars for laparoscopic repair of this type of hernia are normally inserted) in order to place a Hasson trocar often involves performing a minilaparotomy, since the fat tissue is generally thicker at the sides than at the midline. This large incision can result in pneumoperitoneum leaks and other complications such as infections, incisional hernias, etc. On the other hand, placing the first trocar with the abdomen insufflated let to place this first trocar far from the hernia defect, allowing secure the mesh in an easier and safer way at this proximal side, avoiding an insufficient fixation and, therefore, recurrences.

Once the pneumoperitoneum is created, the cavity is generally approached from the patient's left side, placing three trocars drawing a line, introducing the 10–12 mm trocar first and then placing the other 5 mm trocars under direct vision (Fig. 6.1). An important thing to remember when placing the trocars is to stay as far as possible away from the defect margin closest to the surgeon. This will provide proper visualization of the margin, making it easier to achieve wide overlap with the mesh and perform any maneuvers needed to secure the prosthesis. When it is not possible maintain a suitable distance from this margin, it is recommended to introduce an additional 5 and 10-mm trocar in the patient's opposite flank in order to adequately fix the mesh on the margin closest to the initial trocar.

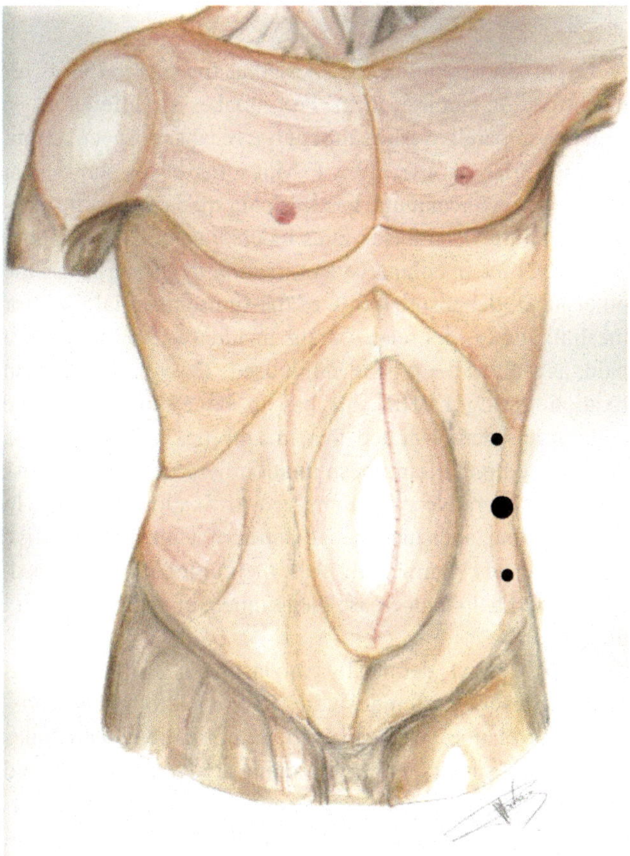

Fig. 6.1 Placement of trocars for ventral hernia repair

Adhesiolysis once the trocars are introduced, the adhesions are evaluated. Adhesiolysis is considered to be a key point of this procedure, since incorrect performance of the adhesiolysis process can have extremely serious consequences for the patient. Nevertheless, if we have any doubts regarding the possibility of bowel perforation the procedure should be converted to open, or at least one of the trocar must be enlarged to check the bowel. Missed perforation of the abdominal wall is associated with high morbidity and mortality. Hemostasis of the area of adhesiolysis should be checked in order to avoid complications.

Identification of the Defect and Selection of the Mesh Once the adhesiolysis process is completed, the actual defect of the hernia must be delimited by drawing them on the skin. A needle could be inserted through the skin, visualizing its tip inside the cavity under laparoscopic vision to detect and trace the hernia defect on the patient's skin. Then the abdomen is deflated and the exact measurements of the defect are determined, in order to select a mesh designed to be placed intra-abdominally, which should overlap at least 5 cm beyond the hernia orifice in all directions. Once the proper mesh is selected, several marks are traced on the patient's abdomen and on the mesh surface that will be placed in contact with the viscera, in order to facilitate orientation of the prosthesis within the cavity. Sutures could be placed at this point at the cardinal points to facilitate also orientation, being removed or let in place later. Afterwards, the mesh is rolled along its long axis, leaving the mesh side that will be in contact with the bowel rolled toward the inside, what will facilitate the maneuvers needed to extend the mesh. Meshes should be introduced through one of the trocars to prevent potential contamination that can occur when it is inserted through the skin. If a large prosthesis is needed, it is recommended to remove the trocar and insert the mesh wrapped in sterile plastic through the trocar hole, and then remove the plastic from inside the cavity.

Fixation of the Mesh Once the mesh is inside the cavity, the area where the cranial tack should be placed is localized either by the previous drawn on the mesh or by a suture at that place. A needle or the suture passer will set the place where the first tack should be placed. When this tack or suture is placed, we stretch the mesh in the caudal direction and perform the same maneuver, placing the second tack or suture at the lower cardinal point. Subsequently, the lateral tacks are placed following the same system, avoiding the tendency of the mesh to move in the opposite direction from the point where the scope is introduced. Once the mesh is fixed at the four cardinal points, we proceed to extend it adequately, adding an outer crown of tacks that are placed right on the margin of the mesh. These tacks are separated from each other by a distance of one-two centimeter, an adequate distance to ensure that the bowel do not slip between the tacks and cause acute incarceration. Once the outer crown is finished, the inner crown of tacks is added at the margin of the hernia sac, in order to ensure better attachment of the mesh, to perform the Double Crown technique (Fig. 6.2), adding extra-suture in case this technique is not followed. In case the technique proposed combined tackers and glue, the distance among the tackers could be increased to 3–4 cm [2].

While the crown of tacks is being placed, the surgeon must exert strong pressure against the tacker from the outside to ensure that the mesh is fixed to the fascia. Once all the tacks are placed, it is recommended to proceed to identify any of them that are left hanging from the wall or that are improperly placed, and insert them through the entire thickness of the mesh. Poorly positioned tacks will lead to adhesions, as it has been shown in differente experimental studies, and could cause major complications in the future, such as fistulas or occlusions.

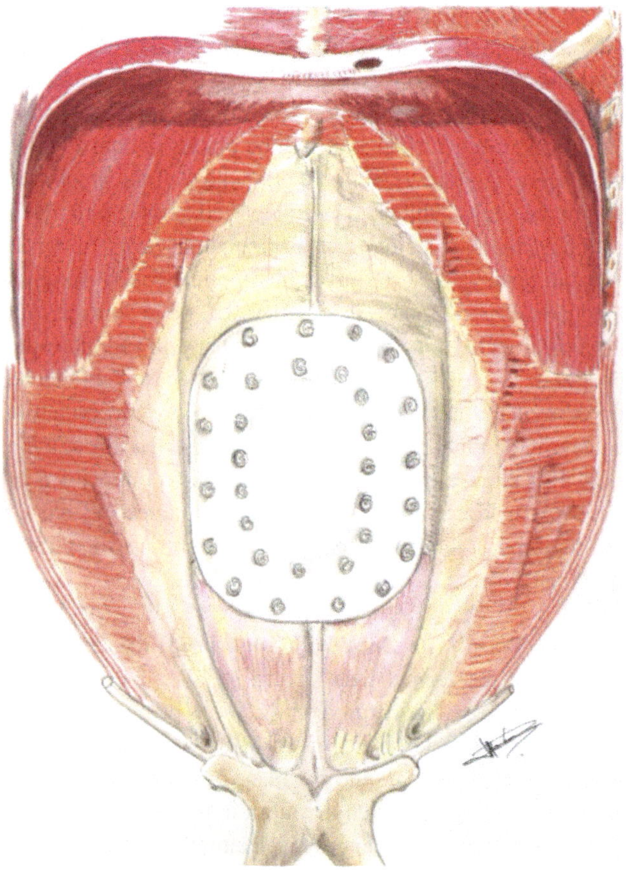

Fig. 6.2 Double crown technique

Finishing the Procedure Once the procedure is completed, the abdomen is deflated and the 12-mm trocars must be closed. A compression bandage is placed at the level of the hernia sac to reduce the space between the mesh and the sac and to prevent seroma, avoiding the use of drains. This bandage is kept on for 1 week and is withdrawn at the 7-day follow-up visit to remove the skin sutures.

6.3.5 Postoperative Management

Once the procedure is completed, we start the patient on fluid intake about 6–8 h after surgery, continuing to solid foods as tolerated. The patient is normally discharged within 24–48 h of the surgery. In terms of physical activity, we do not establish any limitation for the patient and only recommend gradual resumption of regular daily activities based on the patient's progress during postoperative recovery. Patient follow-up is carried out at 1 month, 3 months, 6 months and 1 year, with yearly visits thereafter.

6.4 Complications After Laparoscopic Hernia Repair

6.4.1 Postoperative Pain

Different studies published show that the method used for mesh fixation (sutures, tacks, both) makes no differences on acute postoperative pain, although a recent prospective randomized trial published by F Muysoms et al. shows that Double Crown technique has less pain than the use of transfascial sutures, and this sutures incurs a significantly longer operation time in comparison to fixation by tacks [3]. On the other hand, the absorbability of the suture material used for mesh fixation is not related to the incidence of postoperative pain, as well as the type of mesh used. The role of glues on fixation during LVHR still has to be established, some authors has demonstrated that in umbilical hernias with a defect size up to 5 cm, mesh fixation by glue results in less acute postoperative pain compared to fixation by tacks. In the meantime, and since the incidence of acute postoperative pain correlates significantly with the number of tacks used, glues could help to decrease the numbers of tacks used to fix the mesh.

Chronic pain is defined by pain lasting at least 3/6 months postoperatively. Different studies have tried to find any possible correlation between different fixation techniques (transfascial sutures and tacks, sutures only, tacks only) and the incidence of chronic postoperative pain. The median percentage incidence of chronic pain in the suture and tack fixation group were 2.75 %, 3.75 %, 6,35 % respectively showing no statistical differences.

6.4.2 Mesh Shrinkage

Beldi et al. has publishes a study by conventional abdominal X-ray examination comparing tacker (single crown technique) versus suture fixation of a mesh with an overlap of at least 5 cm, at the 2nd postoperative day, after 6 weeks and 6 months postoperatively. A significant decrease of mesh size was detected in horizontal direction in the tacker group, whereas no significant differences were found in vertical direction and mesh surface area. On the other hand, Schoenmaeckers et al. studied mesh shrinkage after use double crown fixation technique of ePTFE-meshes by CT measurements. A shrinkage rate of 7.5 % was found at 17.9 months postoperatively. Different studies have observed a high proportion of reduction of the size of the mesh in animals observed, while clinical studies in humans have shown less shrinkage.

6.4.3 Tack Hernia

Several case reports have been published how fixation device have induced incisional hernias. The first report in 2003 published by LeBlanc concerned the development of an incisional hernia at the site of a penetrating tacker and described as a "tack hernia". On the other hand, further reports by Muysoms et al., Khandelwal et al. and Barzana et al. have also described incisional hernias after suture fixation.

6.4.4 Recurrences

Since no differences has been found on hernia recurrence based on the method of fixation (Double Crown vs. sutures) other factors has been related to these recurrences. A proper overlap, of at least 5 cm in all directions, and the proper fixation of the mesh at the side of the initial trocar are factors that influence also in the presence of recurrences.

New hernias below original hernias have been described as a factor of recurrence after open repair. This factor has been also described after laparoscopic approach what has led to recommend to cover the entire incision even in those cases in which a weak area is not detected, since this damaged tissue could be involved in the presence of a new hernia. At present, it appears evident that when undertaking laparoscopic repair of an incisional hernia, adhesiolysis must cover the entire area of the previous scar in order to identify possible wall defects at this level, other than those originally destined to be repaired. This is precisely one of the advantages of laparoscopy over traditional open repair. Defects that were not identified during the clinical examination and that were the cause of recurrence or appearance of a new defect after open repair can be detected and repaired in the same surgical procedure.

6.4.5 Seroma

Seroma, defined as serous fluid retention between the mesh and the anterior abdominal wall, is presence in most of the cases after LVHR, as different series that analyzed its presence by radiological exams shows. Its presence cannot be considered a complication since patients do not even detect them in most of the cases. For these reasons, it is important to defined that seroma must be considered an incident after this surgery that may lead to complications. A new clinical classification of seroma has been published by S. Morales-Conde in order to establish the real incidence of seroma and its clinical significance [4].

The potential complications related to seroma formation include pain, discomfort to the patient, cellulites, being the most important complication of them the possibility of getting infected. The infection of a seroma is considered one of the most challenging complications since it might lead to mesh removal and recurrence. Seroma could also be related to recurrence, since the weight of this serous fluid between the mesh and the anterior abdominal wall could increase the tensile strength on the fixation of the mesh and therefore desattach tackers from its original fixation to the anterior wall and be responsible of an improper anchoring of the mesh right after surgery, which may influence in the presence of recurrence in the future.

The real importance of seroma formation and the influence of them in the quality of life in the postoperative period of the patient are also still to be determined. But it can be concluded that seroma is not really a key factor in the postoperative period after this surgery and its simple presence cannot be considered a complication. But, it would be better to avoid it since, in some cases, could be responsible for some of the complications described.

6.4.6 Missed Bowel Perforation

Lysis of adhesions is considered to be the most dangerous and rate limiting aspect of laparoscopic ventral hernia repair. Adhesiolysis must be performed with extreme care since missed bowel perforation could be life-threatening for the patient. The incidence of enterotomy during laparoscopic ventral hernia repair has been reported to be 1–6 %. But adhesiolysis complications are not only associated with laparoscopic surgery. Cases of intestinal perforation have also been reported after open surgery, with consequences similar to those occurring after laparoscopic surgery. In fact, in studies comparing laparoscopic and open surgery for the treatment of ventral hernias, higher rates of intestinal perforation due to adhesiolysis were reported in the open surgery group than in the laparoscopy group.

Minimal use of energy sources during adhesiolysis has been advocated to avoid bowel injury. Monopolar cautery is acceptable as long as it is not used in close proximity to any viscera.

6.4.7 Adhesions, Fistulas and Bowel Occlusion

Different factors have been related to this complication: inappropriate mesh being placed intra-abdominally in contact with the bowel and poorly positioned tacks will lead to adhesion, as it has been shown in different experimental studies, and could cause these major complications in the future.

It has been published a current review of the literature regarding safety measures such as adhesions, fistulas, and infections after LVHR. The only real concern based in this analysis is about using pure PPM in the intraperitoneal position. The use of intra-peritoneal PPM to repair incisional hernia has been demonstrated in clinical and experimental studies that carries the risk of adhesions and damage to the intra-abdominal viscera. Polypropylene is a material widely used in surgery but, because of its association with formation of enterocutaneous fistulae and adhesions, direct contact between mesh and intestine should be avoided. This study clearly points a very few mesh-related complications after a proper mesh placed intraperitoneally, and shows that experimental studies and theoretical considerations may argue for using a covered mesh, i.e., a composite mesh, or e-PTFE for LVHR in humans, although it is stressed that there are no human data at the moment to support this. Clinical information based on reoperative findings available in the literature about adhesions to prosthetic materials shows different data, but this information related to implanted e-PTFE mesh at reoperation in patients who had previously undergone LVHR shows no or minimal formation of adhesions in 91 % of cases, and no severe cohesive adhesions were found.

References

1. LeBlanc KA, Booth WV. Laparoscopic repair of incisional abdominal hernias using expanded polytetrafluoroethylene: preliminary findings. Surg Laparosc Endosc. 1993;3(1):39–41.
2. Morales-Conde S, Cadet H, Cano A, Bustos M, Martín J, Morales-Mendez S. Laparoscopic ventral hernia repair without sutures--double crown technique: our experience after 140 cases with a mean follow-up of 40 months. Int Surg. 2005;90(3 Suppl):S56–62.
3. Muysoms F, Vander Mijnsbrugge G, Pletinckx P, Boldo E, Jacobs I, Michiels M, Ceulemans R. Randomized clinical trial of mesh fixation with "double crown" versus "sutures and tackers" in laparoscopic ventral hernia repair. Hernia. 2013;17(5):603–12.
4. Morales-Conde S. A new classification for seroma after laparoscopic ventral hernia repair. Hernia. 2012;16(3):261–7.

Part III

Oesophagus

7 Motility Disorders

Giovanni Zaninotto and Mario Costantini

7.1 Introduction

Though a relatively rare disease (with an estimated prevalence of 0.5–1 new cases per 100,000 population a year, and with no clear age predilection), achalasia is the most common motor disorder of the esophagus. Its pathophysiology consists of the loss of esophageal body peristalsis and an impaired lower esophageal sphincter (LES) relaxation, resulting in a residual pressure gradient between the esophagus and the stomach during swallowing, which gives rise to a functional obstruction at the gastro-esophageal junction.

It is widely accepted that the partial or total absence of swallow-induced LES relaxation (the main functional anomaly in achalasia) is caused by a loss of the inhibitory innervation in the myenteric plexus; the exact mechanism behind this loss of inhibitory neurons is far from clear and treatment is still limited to mechanical or surgical disruption of the LES.

7.2 Indications

Dysphagia, for both solids and liquids, is the main symptom of achalasia and the swallowing behavior of achalasia patients (especially those with a dilated esophagus) is unique: they often make food pass through the cardia by drinking large quantities while eating, thus increasing the pressure in the gullet enough to overcome the LES resting pressure. Undigested food regurgitation occurs, especially at night, with corollary symptoms that may include respiratory complications (nocturnal cough and aspiration), chest pain, and weight loss.

Although the above-mentioned symptoms may seem rather obvious and diagnostic evaluation has certainly improved, there is often still a considerable delay between the onset of symptoms and the diagnosis of achalasia, due not to an atypical clinical presentation of the disease, but to the physician's misinterpretation of its typical signs and symptoms. Patients are often treated for suspected reflux disease, they are sometimes given sedatives and may even be referred to a psychologist.

There is a lively debate regarding the most effective treatment for long-term symptom relief. The relative rarity of achalasia means that most patients are treated according to local preferences and expertise. First-line achalasia treatment has traditionally been pneumatic dilation, reserving surgery for patients requiring repeated dilations or when this treatment fails. Currently, minimally invasive surgery – with its more limited related morbidity – is progressively employed in patients with achalasia.

Non-decompensated achalasia (grades I to III according to the radiological classification), i.e., with a maximum esophageal diameter of about 6 cm and a gullet that is still "straight" is suitable for laparoscopic myotomy. In cases of mega-esophagus (>6 cm in diameter and/or a sigmoid shape), laparoscopic myotomy can still be performed, but the success rate is lower; it may still be an option, nonetheless, before scheduling a patient for esophagectomy.

7.3 Alternative Treatment

Pneumatic dilation is a good alternative to surgery. It aims to disrupt the LES by forcefully dilating it with an air-filled balloon. To date, the most commonly used is the Rigiflex balloon (Microvasive, Boston Scientific, Cedex, France), which is available in three sizes (30, 35, and 40 mm in diameter). Briefly, the balloon is inserted over an endoscopically maneuvered guide wire, positioned across the LES, and inflated under endoscopic visualization. The immediate success rate of this procedure is 55–70 % with a single dilation,

G. Zaninotto, MD, FACS (✉)
Department of Academic Surgery, St Mary's Hospital, Imperial College, London W2 1NY, UK
e-mail: g.zaninotto@imperial.ac.uk

M. Costantini, MD
Department of Surgery, Gastroenterology and Oncology, University of Padova, School of Medicine, Padova, Italy

H.J. Bonjer (ed.), *Surgical Principles of Minimally Invasive Procedures*, DOI 10.1007/978-3-319-43196-3_7

but this figure can be improved with multiple dilations. The best results can be obtained by using increasing balloon sizes in a stepwise fashion over several months. The long-term results may be less positive, however, with about 60 % of patients still symptom-free after a year, but more than 50 % experiencing recurrent symptoms after 5 years. One of the major risk factors for recurrence is young age (<40 years old), with a 5-year remission rate of only 16 % for patients under 40, as opposed to about 60 % for older patients. Other predictors of failure after pneumatic dilation are male gender, a single dilation with a 30 mm balloon, and a post-treatment LES pressure >10 mmHg.

Esophageal perforation is the most important and potentially life-threatening complication of pneumatic dilation, occurring in up to 6.6 % of the patients. Other potential complications following pneumatic dilation include prolonged pain, gastroesophageal reflux, aspiration pneumonia, gastrointestinal hemorrhage, esophageal mucosal tears without perforation, and intramural esophageal hematoma.

7.4 Preoperative Work-Up

The conventional diagnostic work-up is based on functional studies, such as esophageal manometry and barium swallow. The radiographic features are esophageal dilation and minimal LES opening with a bird's beak appearance, sometimes with an air-fluid level in the gullet and no intragastric air bubble. These radiographic features may be missed by a conventional test, especially in the early stage of the disease. A "timed" barium swallow test has been proposed and is widely used in evaluating patients before and after treatment. A fixed amount of barium (200 ml) is ingested in 2 min, and pictures are taken after fixed intervals (0, 1′, 2′, 5′) to measure the height of the barium column at various times. At manometry, the typical findings are aperistalsis of the esophageal body and incomplete LES relaxation, sometimes with a high intra-esophageal pressure due to the stasis of food and saliva. LES resting tone is often elevated. Swallowing may trigger simultaneous low-amplitude pressure waves with a similar morphology in all channels in the esophageal body, called "common-cavity" waves.

Endoscopy is usually the first test to be performed in a patient with dysphagia. Findings may seem normal in patients with achalasia, especially in the early stages, when the gullet is only mildly dilated. Esophagitis ("stasis" esophagitis) may be identified and should not be confused with reflux esophagitis. Esophageal candidiasis, resistant to the usual treatments, can also be found, and is usually related to the functional obstruction. Malignant tumors can produce an achalasia-like syndrome called "pseudoachalasia" by infiltrating the gastro-esophageal junction and mimicking the clinical and manometric presentation of achalasia; they account for about 5 % of cases of misdiagnosis. In general, patients with pseudoachalasia are older and have a shorter history of dysphagia and weight loss. Endoscopy, with a careful examination of the cardiac and fundic region, is therefore mandatory as part of the diagnosis work-up to avoid this potential pitfall, and if the clinical suspicion is strong, computerized tomography (CT) and endoscopic ultrasound should be considered. These latter tests should be considered, particularly in elderly patients with symptoms of recent onset.

Finally, all of the tests routinely performed before surgery under general anesthesia (blood tests, chest X-rays, EKG) are required. Additional tests may be requested by the anesthesiologist for particular patients, but are rarely necessary.

7.5 Operating Room

The operation is performed under general anesthesia and oro-tracheal intubation. The patient is placed supine on the operating table with legs abducted on flat padded leg boards to minimize the risk of lower extremity neurovascular injury. Alternatively, the patient can be positioned in simple supine position, i.e. with the legs together on the operating table.

The right arm is tucked against the patient's side and the left arm remains on an arm board (Fig. 7.1). The patient should be well secured, as a steep reverse Trendelenburg position is needed to displace the intra-abdominal organs from the subdiaphragmatic area and bring the surgical site closer to the surgeon, who stands between the abducted legs to gain easy access to the upper abdomen. This position demands all the measures usually adopted to prevent deep vein thrombosis (stockings, heparin prophylaxis). Due to the brevity of the operation, a Foley catheter is unnecessary, unless it is requested by the anesthesiologist in the case of frail patients.

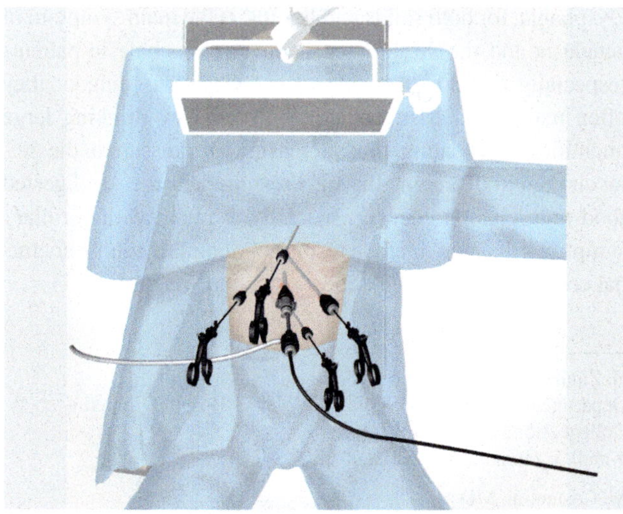

Fig. 7.1 Patient positioning for Heller's myotomy

The poor emptying of the achalasic esophagus makes the gullet retain saliva and ingested food, so there is a high risk of regurgitation and aspiration during the induction of anesthesia in these patients. Patients should be kept on a liquid diet for 48 h before the operation, and a dilated gullet should be mechanically washed and emptied via a naso-esophageal tube the night before the procedure.

The standard laparoscopic instrumentation is required: two 12 mm trocars and three 5 mm trocars are used; a 30° laparoscope offers the best view of the cardiac region; a device for lifting the left liver lobe, atraumatic forceps for pulling down the stomach, and a cautery hook and scissors are the instruments needed for the procedure, plus a couple of standard forceps for tissue handling and a needle holder for suturing. An ultrasonic scalpel or Ligasure are usually not necessary. Small bipolar cautering forceps may be useful to control bleeding from the edges of the myotomy.

During the performance of the myotomy the endoscope may be useful to facilitate the procedure and check for any mucosal lesions. We prefer to position a guidewire across the cardia through the scope before starting the operation: during the myotomy, a 3.0 cm Rigiflex balloon is placed across the cardia and gently inflated and deflated.

7.6 Surgical Technique

7.6.1 Trocar Positioning (Fig. 7.2)

We usually prefer the open technique when performing the pneumoperitoneum: the first 12 mm blunt trocar, used for the laparoscope, is inserted along the midline, halfway between the umbilicus and the xyphoid. A 5 mm trocar is inserted as laterally as possible on the patient's right side, immediately below the costal margin, to lift the left liver lobe. A 5 mm trocar inserted immediately below the xyphoid is used for the operator's left hand, while a 12 mm trocar inserted laterally below the left costal margin provides access for the surgeon's right hand. Finally, a 5 mm trocar, at the same level as the first trocar and on the midclavicular line, is used to pull down the gastric fundus.

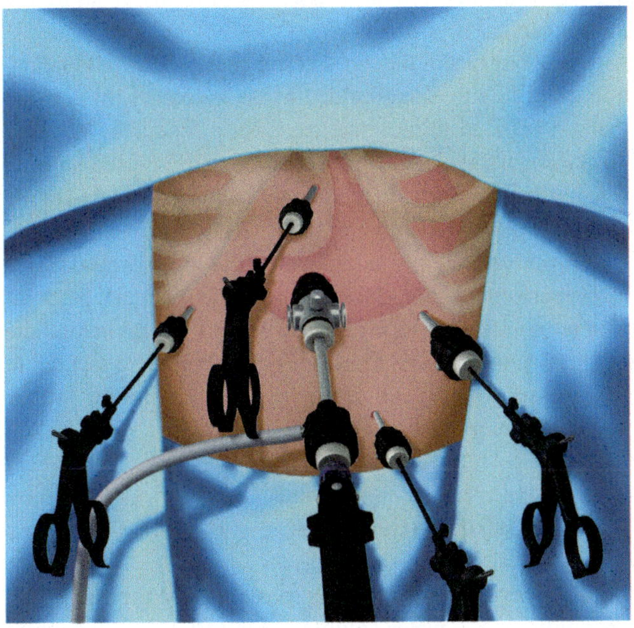

Fig. 7.2 Trocar positioning for Heller's myotomy

7.6.2 Exposure of the Anterior Wall of the Esophagus

An assistant on the surgeon's left-hand side lifts the left liver lobe using an atraumatic retractor, thus exposing the cardia region. It is not necessary to divide the left triangular ligament. An assistant on the surgeon's right-hand side grasps the gastric fundus with atraumatic forceps, maintaining a caudal traction on the esophagogastric junction. The operation begins with a minimal dissection of the anterior part of the esophagus. With the cautery hook, the peritoneum over the esophagogastric junction is divided to expose the anterior wall of the gullet. Any adipose tissue (usually found at this level) is removed, paying attention to the small vessels coming from the gastric wall, which should be coagulated with the bipolar forceps; they usually mark the inferior limit of the myotomy. The left vagus nerve, which becomes anterior at this level by crossing the anterior esophageal wall from left to right, is clearly evident and must not be damaged.

7.6.3 Myotomy

The myotomy is started with the cautery hook on the dilated part of the distal esophagus, above the lower esophageal sphincter that, in cases of long-standing achalasia, is often marked by a whitish, sclerotic area. The myotomy must in any case be started 2 cm above the esophagogastric junction to expose the esophageal submucosal layer with the least risk of perforation. The cautery power is reduced to 15 W to avoid transmitting its coagulating effect to the underlying mucosa. First the longitudinal muscle fibers are hooked, lifted, and coagulated, until the circular ones are exposed; then the latter are hooked, lifted, and divided using the same technique. Then the submucosal layer, which forms a slight bulge between the two margins of the myotomy, is exposed. At this point, using the forceps in the left hand, the margin of the myotomy is delicately lifted, and small scissors are used to bluntly dissect the muscle layer from the submucosal layer. The muscle tissue is then cut and minor bleeding from the edges of the myotomy can be controlled with a careful use of the cauterized scissors, or simply with the aid of mechanical compression using a small sponge. A myotomy 6–8 cm long is performed, extending it 1.5–2 cm on the gastric side below the oblique muscle fibers that represent the beginning of the gastric muscle, thus exposing the gastric submucosa, which is usually more vascularized than the esophageal mucosa (Fig. 7.3.). Scissors are used in the proximal part and a hook cautery is inserted downwards on the gastric side to lift and divide the circular muscle fibers. Care must be taken during the myotomy to avoid injuring the anterior vagus nerve and prevent any esophageal perforation or spiraling of the myotomy. A feature of our personal technique involves the intraoperative use of a 30 mm Rigiflex balloon. The balloon is placed inside the esophageal cavity at cardia level using an endoscopically-positioned guide wire. During the myotomy, the balloon is gently inflated and deflated with 40–60 cc of air using a syringe: this exposes the circular fibers, which can then be stretched and easily cut or torn apart (Fig. 7.3). The edges of the myotomy are separated and peeled away from the submucosal plane: any minimal bleeding from submucosal vessels is easily controlled by inflating the balloon, thus reducing the need to use the cautery. At completion of the myotomy, a flexible endoscope can be inserted to confirm sufficient dilatation and detect any perforation of the mucosa. Placing the patient in Trendelenburg position during endoscopic inspection and instilling the upper abdomen with saline allows recognition of a small perforation by the presence of air bubbles during endoscopic insufflation.

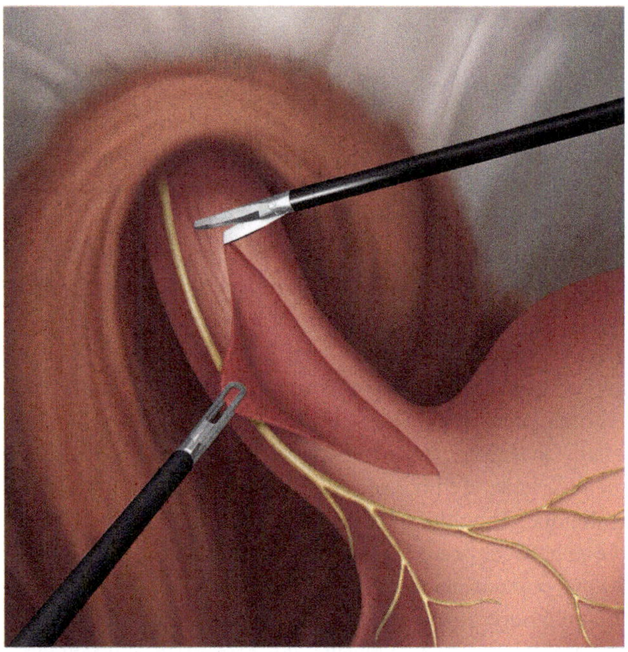

Fig. 7.3 The myotomy is being performed. The anterior vagus nerve must be identified and preserved from damage

7.6.4 Risks of the Myotomy

The main risk in performing esophageal myotomy is a mucosal lesion (perforation). This can be caused directly by an erroneous handling of the hook or scissors, or by the endoscope while checking the myotomy, or even by the Rigiflex balloon if it is inflated too vigorously. Indirect lesions can be caused by an excessive coagulation involving the mucosa, in which case the perforation occurs when the eschar falls out, 48–72 h after the operation. Direct lesions are usually detected during the operation and can be sutured directly with 4–0 interrupted reabsorbable stitches. This is usually done laparoscopically, but conversion to open surgery may be necessary. The suture line is then further protected with the anterior fundoplication. In the case of small indirect lesions, subsequently detected by Gastrografin swallow, a conservative treatment with gastric aspiration, NPO, TPN, and antibiotics usually suffices.

7.6.5 Antireflux Fundoplication

Although some authors perform only the myotomy as described above, a fundoplication is normally added to prevent postoperative gastroesophageal reflux disease, which may be a severe complication in patients with a poor esophageal clearing ability due to the absence of peristalsis. Given this lack of any propulsive peristaltic activity of the esophageal body, a partial fundoplication is usually performed, either anteriorly (Dor) or posteriorly (Toupet). The former has the advantage of protecting the exposed esophageal mucosa and can be performed without completely mobilizing the esophagus, thus preserving the natural antireflux mechanisms.

Using our technique, an anterior partial hemifundoplication according to Dor is added to the myotomy. In general, there is no need to mobilize the gastric fundus by dividing the short gastric vessels. Three stitches are inserted on each side, the proximal one to include the stomach, the edge of the myotomy and the diaphragm (Fig. 7.4).

If a posterior hemifundoplication (Toupet's procedure) is to be performed, the abdominal esophagus must be completely mobilized, and the gastric wrap is passed behind the esophagus: the right and left sides of the wrap are secured to the corresponding edges of the myotomy with three to four interrupted non-reabsorbable stitches.

7.6.6 Postoperative Care

A naso gastric tube is carefully positioned at the end of the operation. A water-soluble contrast esophagogram (Gastrografin) is obtained on the first postoperative day to

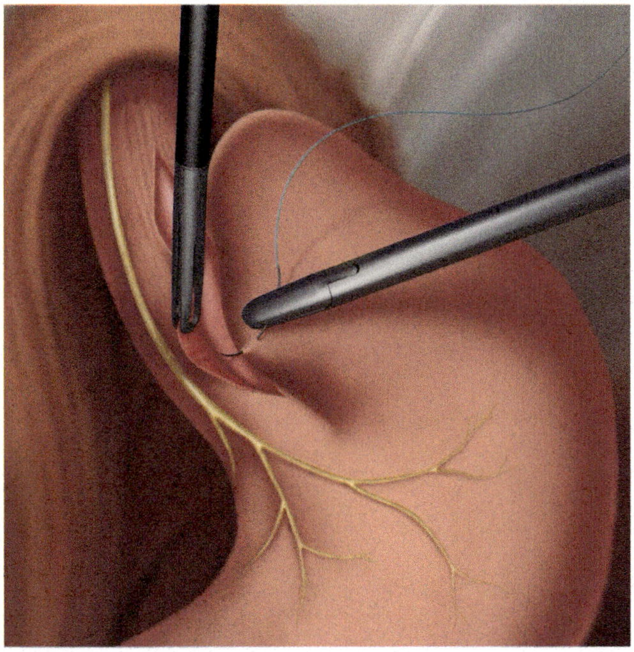

Fig. 7.4 A partial anterior fundoplication using the gastric fundus is added to the myotomy. Usually three stitches per side, securing the wrap to the myotomy edges, are needed, the most proximal ones also include the corresponding diaphragmatic pillar

rule out any mucosal perforation. In case of small perforation the NG tube is kept in position and the patients is maintained in parenteral nutrition for 6–8 days. If a large perforation is detected and the contrast freely diffuses in the abdomen or in the pleura, drainage and immediate suture are reccomended.

If no perforation are observed a liquid diet is started and the patient is discharged after another 24–48 h, once a soft diet has been started and depending on how far away from the hospital they live. A soft diet is recommended for 8–10 days, after which a normal diet is allowed.

Patients usually return to the outpatient clinic 1 month later for a barium swallow. Endoscopy and function tests are performed after 6 months to rule out any postoperative GERD. After that, endoscopy is recommended every 2 years to rule out any cancer growth.

Conclusions

Surgical myotomy is the most effective and durable treatment for achalasia, and since laparoscopy has reduced related morbidity, laparoscopic Heller myotomy has become the first-line treatment for this condition. A partial fundoplication should be performed in conjunction with the myotomy to minimize the risk of postoperative gastroesophageal reflux, a risk that must be avoided as far as possible in an esophagus with poor clearance capabilities. Although it is not clear which fundoplication is best in association with laparoscopic Heller myotomy (a prospective randomized trials is eagerly awaited), we have found the laparoscopic Heller-Dor combination a safe and effective treatment for achalasia.

References

1. Ancona E, Peracchia A, Zaninotto G, Rossi M, Bonavina L, Segalin A. Heller laparoscopic cardiomyotomy with antireflux anterior fundoplication (Dor) in the treatment of esophageal achalasia. Surg Endosc. 1993;7:459–61.
2. Spiess AE, Kahrilas PJ. Treating achalasia: from whalebone to laparoscope. J Am Med Assoc. 1998;280:638–42.
3. Torquati A, Richards WO, Holzman MD, Sharp KW. Laparoscopic myotomy for achalasia: predictors of successful outcome after 200 cases. Ann Surg. 2006;243:587–91; discussion 591–593.
4. Zaninotto G, Costantini M, Portale G, Battaglia G, Molena D, Carta A, et al. Etiology, diagnosis, and treatment of failures after laparoscopic Heller myotomy for achalasia. Ann Surg. 2002;235:186–92.
5. Zaninotto G, Costantini M, Rizzetto C, Zanatta L, Guirroli E, Portale G, et al. Four hundred laparoscopic myotomies for esophageal achalasia: a single centre experience. Ann Surg. 2008;248:986–93.

8 Gastroesophageal Reflux Disease (GERD) and Hiatal Hernia

Rudolph Pointner

8.1 Introduction

Gastroesophageal reflux disease (GERD) is primarily considered a motility disorder, because dysfunction of the antirefluxbarrier is a prerequisite for the development of the disease. The backward flow of gastric content into the esophagus, i.e., gastroesophageal reflux, is up to a certain extent a physiological phenomenon, in particular in the early postprandial phase. The primary pathophysiologic event occurs as a part of normal physiology, but results in GERD when symptoms or tissue damage occurs. Failure of the antireflux barrier is considered the most important factor in the pathogenesis of GERD. The antireflux barrier is composed of the lower esophageal sphincter (LES) and the crural diaphragm. The LES is a thickened ring of tonically contracted circular smooth muscle that generates a 2- to 4-cm high pressure zone at the gastroesophageal junction and serves as a mechanical barrier between the stomach and the esophagus. The crural diaphragm, the passageway of the esophagus through the diaphragm can contain a morphologic variation resulting in a hiatal hernia, which disrupts the physiology of the normal antireflux mechanism.

In the 1950s and 1960s a hiatal hernia was considered almost synonymous with GERD. Encouraged by studies by Cohen [1], attention shifted to the lower esophageal sphincter and investigators related sphincter function to the presence of GERD. It became evident that in patients with hiatal hernia, the altered geometry at the cardia could potentially affect lower esophageal sphincter function.

Recently, much work has been done to elucidate the effect of the hiatal hernia in the pathophysiology of reflux disease. We are now beginning to understand this complex relationship, showing that the crural diaphragm has its specific function in preventing gastroesophageal reflux and that the presence of a hiatal hernia interferes with this barrier function. The presence of a hiatal hernia is supposed to be associated with symptoms of gastroesophageal reflux and increased prevalence and severity of reflux esophagitis, although there are no data available regarding whether patients suffer more from symptoms corresponding to the insufficiency of lower esophageal sphincter pressure or hiatal hernia.

A hiatal hernia is defined as a proximal displacement of any abdominal organ other than the esophagus through a widening of the hiatus of the diaphragm. There are three different ways to describe a hiatal hernia:

- endoscopically, a hiatal hernia is present, when the Z-line can be identified above the crural ring with gastric folds between the crura and the Z-line.
- radiologically the hiatal hernia is described as four major types: the sliding hiatus hernia (Type I), the paraesophageal hernia (Type II), and the combination of Type I and Type II (Type III) with both the gastroesophageal junction and the fundus herniating through the hiatus. The fundus lies above the gastroesophageal junction. Type IV hiatal hernias are characterized by the presence of a structure other than stomach, such as the omentum, colon or small bowel within the hernia sac.
- intraoperatively the hiatal surface area (HSA) can be calculated by measuring the length of the hiatal crura and the diaphragm.

Unfortunately, none of these methods define the size of a hernia. Therefore, there is no exact definition of a preoperative hiatus hernia as the "normal" hiatus is well described in regard to its function but not its size regarding the anatomy.

Considering those pathophysiological connections, it becomes clear that the symptoms of patients with a hiatal hernia are the symptoms of patients with GERD.

Today GERD is a full-spectrum disease, i.e., a disease with many patient subgroups, ranging from those with asymptomatic disease without mucosal lesions to those with morpholic complications of erosive esophagitis. The concept

R. Pointner, PhD
Department of Surgery, A.ö. Krankenhaus Zell am See, Zell am See, Austria
e-mail: Rudolph.pointner@kh-zellamsee.at

H.J. Bonjer (ed.), *Surgical Principles of Minimally Invasive Procedures*, DOI 10.1007/978-3-319-43196-3_8

of the GERD clinical spectrum has changed tremendously during the last decade showing the GERD patient population to be a multifaceted one.

8.2 Symptoms

More than 40 % of adults of the western world experience symptoms of GERD at least once a month and approximately 10 % of adults experience daily symptoms. The most common symptoms of GERD are heartburn, regurgitation, and dysphagia. In addition to these typical symptoms, patients may complain of chest pain, globus sensation, respiratory symptoms (wheezing, aspiration, cough), ear, nose, and throat manifestations (sore throat, hoarseness), or even dental problems. All these symptoms are caused by injury of the esophagus, larynx, airways, pharynx, or mouth by a retrograde flow of gastric contents.

The therapeutic aim of antireflux surgery is the elimination of reflux-related symptoms and prevention of progression and complications of GERD. Traditional objective criteria to describe a successful surgical intervention are the normalisation of the lower esophageal sphincter pressure, normalisation of pH values, and the elimination of reflux symptoms including healing of esophagitis. Beside these factors, the patients' view of a successful intervention has become more important based on the fact that objective measurement of solely physiological outcome parameters does not correlate well with symptomatic outcome or patients' satisfaction with an intervention. Therefore, according to the definition of GERD by Dent et al. (GERD is likely present when heartburn occurs on 2 or more days a week), the efficacy of laparoscopic antireflux surgery should also be measured by quality of life data or patients' rating of satisfaction with surgery.

8.3 Indication for Antireflux Surgery

An improvement of a disease-related quality of life is the main indication for antireflux surgery. There is a general agreement in medical and surgical literature on the indications for antireflux surgery:

- patients with persistent or recurrent symptoms or complications who are resistant to proton pump inhibitor therapy (failure of medical management).
- young patients despite successful medical management (due to lifestyle modification, life-long medical therapy, escalating doses, costs of medication).
- patients who continue to suffer from regurgitation even if heartburn is effectively treated.
- well selected patients with atypical or extraesophageal symptoms, even if surgery is less successful than in patients with typical symptoms.
- patients with endoscopically or radiologically diagnosed hiatal hernias, and
- patients unwilling to accept long-term medication.

The best candidate for surgery is the patient who has complete resolution of symptoms when treated with modern antireflux medication such as proton pump inhibitors, which is related to patient compliance with prescribed medication. It must be pointed out that there is no general agreement among surgeons that the presence of a Barrett's esophagus is considered an indication for surgical intervention.

8.4 Pre-surgical Evaluation

The aim of an adequate and complete preoperative evaluation is to:

- diagnose GERD and exclude other disorders, such as lesions of esophagus or stomach,
  - measure severity of reflux (in quantity and quality)
  - define anatomy of esophagus and gastroesophageal junction.

In general, these objectives are accomplished by several tests, of which contrast studies (with barium swallows and endoscopy are most widely used:

- esophagogastroduodenoscopy including biopsy at the gastroesophageal junction and histological examination,
- esophageal manometry (for excluding primary motor disorders e.g. achalasia, and defining the exact position of the gastroesophageal junction)
- 24-h esophageal impedance pH monitoring to characterise the frequency, duration and extent of any kind of reflux including the possibility to correlate the patients symptoms to the reflux activities
- Contrast studies with barium swallow, an x-ray cinematography for a better documentation of sliding or paraesophageal hernias completes an exact evaluation of the disease.
- CT scanning can be helpful especially when obstructive of volvulized paraoesophageal hernia is suspected.

8.5 Principles of Surgery

Based on the pathophysiological findings underlying GERD and hiatal hernias, it is clear that the most effective way to permanently restore the competency of the gastroesophageal junction and the diaphragmatic crura is to close any kind of hernia and perform some kind of wrap over the esophagus just proximal to the gastroesophageal junction. The following aspects must be observed for a long-term effective antireflux procedure:

- The wrap must be constructed over the distal esophagus, just proximal to the gastroesophageal junction, and must be fixed to the esophagus to remain in that position permanently.
- The wrap must be constructed without tension using the fundus of the stomach.
- The total wrap (e.g. "floppy" Nissen fundoplication) should be approximately two centimeters in the length in its anterior aspect (longer in its back). The partial wrap (anterior or posterior, e.g. Toupet fundoplication) is usually between one and a half to twice the length of the total wrap.
- The wrap must lie below the diaphragm without tension.
- Hernia must be corrected if one is present. The diaphragmatic hiatus must be gently attached to the esophagus, above the wrap.

8.6 Surgical Technique

The two procedures most commonly used today are modifications of the fundoplication described by Nissen [2] and Toupet [3]. These modifications led to a shortening and a loosening of the wrap which led to a substantial improvement of potential side effects such as a dysphagia. The main differences between the Nissen and the Toupet fundoplications are that in the Toupet fundoplication, the edges of the stomach are attached to the anterior wall of the esophagus, rather to each other, leaving space in between, and the wrap is fixed to the right hiatal crus.

General agreement exists that the hiatus has to be restored in every case of GERD or hiatal hernia therapy. The surgical technique is almost exactly the same as it was described by Phillip Allison in 1951: "After a complete dissection of the left and right crus, both crura are approximated with two or more nonresorbable sutures". The simple sutured cruroplasty is performed as close as appropriate, with the esophagus lying loose between the crura with no narrowing. In case of an HSA of more than 6 cm^2, it can be considered to place a C-shaped mesh on the diaphragm and the approximated crura with its free side at the right crus. It is fixed circumferentionally with a hernia stapler. Fixation has to be performed with great care to avoid tack injury. Attention must be paid to the fact that the free edges of the mesh do not touch the esophagus.

8.7 Laparoscopic "Floopy" Nissen Fundoplication

The laparoscopic Nissen fundoplication is carried out under general anaesthesia. After optimal positioning of the patient (lithotomy position and head up) (Fig. 8.1), a pneumoperitoneum is established and 5–10 mm ports should be placed as shown in Fig. 8.2.

The best position for the surgeon is between the legs of the patient to allow comfortable access to the abdominal esophagus through the upper midline and left midsubcostal ports. The first step is to retract the left lobe of the liver using a liver retractor introduced through the right trocar. Then the gastrohepatic omentum is divided close to the liver and an incision is made into the peritoneum along the free edge of the right crus, the circumference of the diaphragmatic crura and to the left crus. Knowledge of the presence of an aberrant left hepatic artery, which may be found in about 12% of the patients, is very important for this step. Ligation of this vessel may result in hepatic necrosis. Circumferential mobiliza-

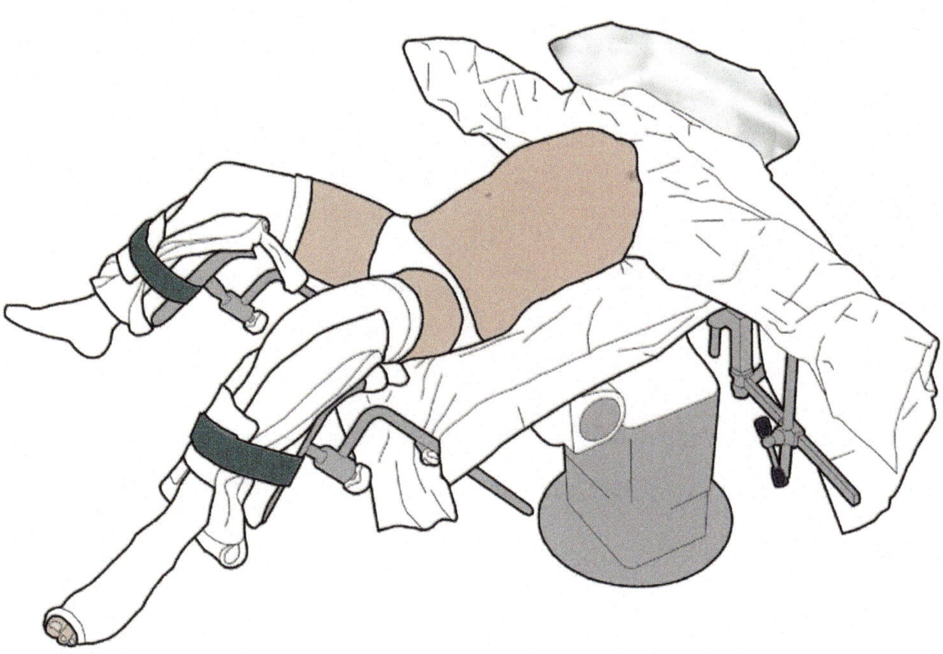

Fig. 8.1 Positioning of the patient: lithotomy and head up

tion of the esophagus is achieved by careful dissection of the anterior and posterior soft tissues within the hiatus. With traction of a Babcock clamp, which is positioned at the cardia, the mediastinal dissection of the esophagus is completed and the esophagus is freed from the pleura, the aorta, and the crural muscles. This procedure guarantees a wide dissection of the esophagus far up intrathoracically and results in a retroesphageal channel large enough to allow easy passage of the fundic wrap.

The anterior and posterior vagus nerves are identified without dissecting them. In the next step the HSA is calculated by measuring the length of the crura and the diameter from one to another edge.

According to the size of the HSA, the crura are approximated behind the esophagus with one or more non-absorbable sutures (Fig. 8.3).

In addition one or more sutures can be placed at the diaphragm above the esophagus especially in case of a weak pars flaccida. In case of an HSA ≥6 cm^2, a mesh

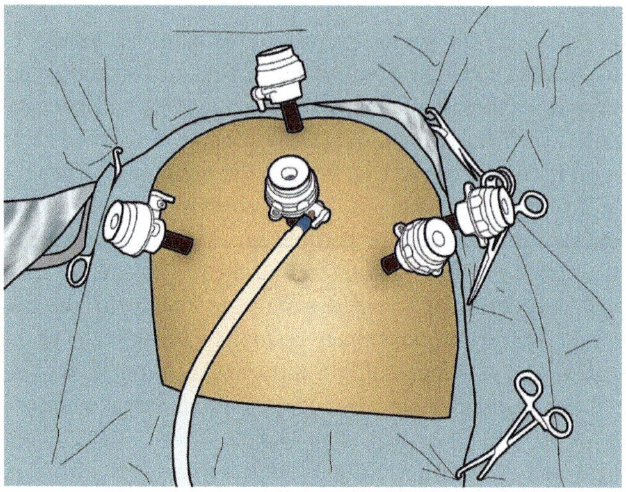

Fig. 8.2 Trocar placement for laparoscopic Nissen fundoplication

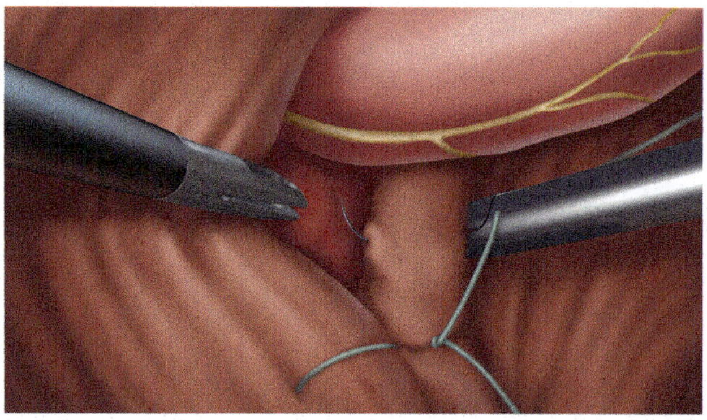

Fig. 8.3 Approximation of the crura with nonabsorbable sutures behind the esophagus

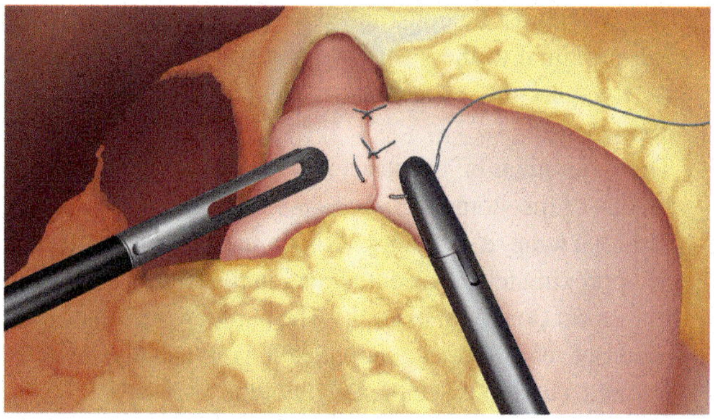

Fig. 8.4 Complete wrap (3 stitches)

prothesis can be used to reinforce the crura. The mesh is cut in a C-shape and positioned over the sutured crura with the arms of the C coming from the left side and lying over the sutures below and above the esophagus. Then the mesh is fixed by tacks. As the wrap should be made without tension to prevent postoperative dysphagia or disruption of the fundoplication, it is important to mobilize the fundus. The short gastric vessels are transected using a harmonic scalpel to mobilize the greater curvature of the stomach beginning approximately 10 cm distal to the angle of His. The rear cavity is opened and all the posterior attachements of the fundus are divided until the left crus is reached. The well mobilized fundus can be easily pulled by a Babcock clamp passed behind the esophagus from right to left. The left limb of the fundoplication should be carefully selected by using a part of the proximal fundus of the stomach close to the divided short gastric vessels to avoid rotational torsion of the cardia. To avoid a too tight or too loose wrap, the so-called "shoeshine-manoeuvre" is carried out, measuring the length of the fundus, which should result in the circumference of the wrap. With a length of the circumference of the wrap of 10–12 cm, the diameter of the wrap is at least 3 cm. A close 360° wrap around the abdominal esophagus is held in place using a U-stitch passed through the stomach and the esophagus. The next two stitches completing the wrap are positioned at maximum 1 cm above and 1 cm below this first U-stitch. They approximate the right pulled through part of the fundus with the left part of it, resulting in a floppy wrap with a length of about 2–3 cm (Fig. 8.4).

8.8 Laparoscopic Toupet Fundoplication

The beginning of the procedure is similar to the above described method of a Nissen fundoplication. After the complete dissection of the crura and the mobilization of the esophagus intrathoracically a tunnel between the crura, the stomach and the esophagus is created from the right to the left side. At that point the fundus is freed from the short gastric vessels beginning at the angle of His to the upper edge of the spleen. Thus the posterior part of the fundus can be freed from adhesions. This dissection is done through the tunnel under the esophagus coming from the right side. The evaluation of the HSA as well as the closure of the hiatus is performed in the same way as in a Nissen fundoplication. In the next step the well mobilized fundus is pulled through behind the esophagus from the left to the right side, and the posterior wall of the pulled through fundus is fixed to the right crus with three stitches. Thus the line of the former dissected short gastrics is positioned parallel to the esophagus at the right side. Close to this line the anterior wall of the fundus at the right side is fixed with two stitches to the right side of the esophagus. In the same way, the fundus laying at the left side of the esophagus is fixed with two stitches to the left side of the esophagus excluding the anterior vagal nerve.

Conclusion

Laparoscopic antireflux surgery and modified techniques have substantially improved the outcome of surgical treatment for gastroesophageal reflux disease. Therefore, laparoscopic fundoplication should be considered as a reasonable alternative to treat this very common disorder and not a method of last resort. An adequate preoperative evaluation of the disease helps to design an appropriate procedure. The laparoscopic approach improves exposure and enhances recovery. An improvement in control of symptoms and subsequent quality of life are achieved in the vast majority of the patients. Complications and surgical side effects are rare if the operation is performed by an experienced surgical team following the basic principals of sound operative technique.

References

1. Wolf BS, Heitmann P, Cohen BR. The inferior esophageal sphincter, the manometric high pressure zone and hiatal incompetence. Am J Roentgenol Radium Ther Nucl Med. 1968; 103(2): 251–76.
2. Nissen R. A simple operation for control of reflux esophagitis. Schweiz Med Wochenschr. 1956; 86(Suppl 20):590–2.
3. Toupet A. Technic of esophago-gastroplasty with phrenogastropexy used in radical treatment of hiatal hernias as a supplement to Heller's operation in cardiospasms. Mem Acad Chir (Paris). 1963; 89:384–9.

9 Minimally Invasive Esophageal Resection

Donald L. van der Peet and Miguel A. Cuesta

9.1 Introduction

In 1991, Dallemagne introduced the right thoracoscopic approach for oesophageal cancer with total lung block, thereby mimicking the conventional approach [1]· Initial reports showed a high conversion rate to thoracotomy and a high respiratory morbidity. Searching for reduction of the conversion rate and the respiratory infection rate, Cuschieri et al. designed the thoracoscopic approach in prone decubitus position so that a total collapse of the lung was no longer necessary for dissecting the oesophagus and thereby possibly reducing the rate of respiratory infections [2].

After a feasibility period, the Minimally Invasive Esophagectomy (MIE) approach in prone or lateral position is widely implemented and increasingly performed all over the world for patients with resectable esophageal cancer to reduce postoperative respiratory complications and enhance the quality of life by avoiding a right thoracotomy and laparotomy [3–5].

Another important development has been introduced in esophageal surgery in recent years: the systematic use of neoadjuvant treatment, such as chemoradiotherapy (CROSS scheme) or the use of chemotherapy (MAGIC trial scheme) [6, 7]. Neoadjuvant therapy for stages 2 and 3, significantly increases 5-year survival of patients with esophageal cancer in both squamous cell as well as adenocarcinomas.

9.2 Surgical Anatomy

Based on the information gathered by MIE a new surgical anatomy of the thoracic esophagus has been described. Distal of the carina, all structures (vessels, nerves and lymph vessels) to the esophagus are found to come from the side of the thoracic aorta. The envelop in which these structures are contained has been called meso-esophagus. From the thoracic outlet to the carina vessels and nerves are coming to the esophagus from both sides. Importantly is to consider that during esophageal resection by MIE this anatomical concept may help to standardize the MIE resection. Moreover still is discussion about which bronchial vessels has to be preserved during resection to prevail enough vascularisation to trachea and bronchi and at which level the vagal nerves should be cut in order to preserve pulmonary function [8, 9].

9.3 General Considerations. Choice of Approach. Mediastinal Lymph Nodes and Lymphadenectomy

Furthermore, question arises how to choose for transthoracic or transhiatal resection. According to the HIVEX trial performed in the Netherlands in 2002, which compared the transhiatal and transthoracic approach for esophageal cancer, it seems that transthoracic approach had a better survival on the long term with the only exception for the gastro-esophageal junction (GEJ) cancers [10]. At the same time we know that the possibility to metastasize to the mediastinum is high (40 %) even in middle and distal located cancers [11]. Both arguments point out that in principle all intrathoracic cancers will be approach through the thorax after neoadjuvant therapy, reserving the transhiatal approach for Siewert type 2 and in frail patients with distal located tumors [12].

Concerning the extent of lymphadenectomy it seems clear that if esophageal cancer at any location can metastasize at any level in the lymph nodes in the mediastinum, a complete mediastinal lymphadenectomy will be performed. Moreover, the introduction of neoadjuvant therapy, the preoperative imaging studies and the increased numbers of distal adenocarcinomas in the Western World have changed this concept at least in the West. Esophageal cancers in the West and East have different types and location, being the middle and proximal thoracic squamous cell cancer (SCC) more frequent in

D.L. van der Peet (✉) • M.A. Cuesta, MD
Department of Surgery, VU University Medical Center, Amsterdam, The Netherlands
e-mail: dl.vanderpeet@vumc.nl; ma.cuesta@vumc.nl

H.J. Bonjer (ed.), *Surgical Principles of Minimally Invasive Procedures*, DOI 10.1007/978-3-319-43196-3_9

the East and distal Adenocarcinomas (Adc), frequently in combination with obesity, in the West. The rate of SCC in the West is still around 15–20 %. According with this the lymphadenectomy we perform in the Western World may be quite different, especially after neoadjuvant therapy. Whereas 2 or 3 field lymphadenectomy is still standard in the East for middle and proximal SCC, in the West lymphadenectomy of the periesophageal and subcarinal lymph nodes is standard, being lymphadenectomy along the recurrent laryngeal nerves performed in SCC and if suspect lymph nodes are found preoperatively in those areas. In the rest of the cases the extent of lymphadenectomy is still in discussion.

9.4 Indications for Esophageal Resection and MIE

A minority of esophageal resections are performed for benign diseases mostly at terminal stages of the disease and frequently after different previous surgical interventions, making them not ideal patients for MIE. Majority of the indication are the considered resectable patients with all types of esophageal cancer, after preoperative work up to confirm that local resection is possible and exclude metastases. Endoscopy, endoscopic ultrasound, CT scan of thorax and abdomen, neck ultrasonography and the increasingly used PET CT scan will discriminate which patients are considered resectable.

Important is to know, not only the type of cancer and its stage, but also precisely the location and length of the tumor. According to this, neoadjuvant therapy can be decided in a multidisciplinary meeting. Currently in Europe the two modalities, chemotherapy and chemoradiotherapy are used in different countries [6, 7]. Moreover if the tumor is located in the GE junction many oncologists will choose for neoadjuvant chemotherapy. According to location we distinguish thoracic esophagus (upper, middle and distal) and gastroesophageal junction (GEJ) cancer. This GEJ may be classified according to Siewert, type 1 at the side of the esophagus, type 2 between the distal esophagus and the stomach and type 3 at the cardias [12]. Whereas for type 1 and 3 is clear what to do: for type 3 a total gastrectomy and for type 1 a transthoracic esophageal resection; for type 2 the choice of the approach remains difficult; possibilities are to perform an extended total gastrectomy with esophagojejunostomy at higher level or an Ivor Lewis operation.

9.5 Minimally Invasive Esophagectomy (MIE)

All type of resections performed in the past by open approach have been implemented by MIE: the 2 and 3 stage esophageal resection (Ivor Lewis and MacKeown), both in lateral and prone position. But also, the transhiatal (Orringer), and the robot assisted thoracoscopic resection [3–5].

Between lateral and in prone position differences are slight. In lateral position it is considered obligatory to block the lung by means of selective intubation whereas in prone position for the 3 stage operation no specific selective intubation is necessary. Using a thoracic CO2 insufflation of between 6 and 8 mmHg the right lung is compressed enough to permit an optimal visibility of the mediastinum whereas the lung is still partially ventilated.

Patients operated on previously by right thoracotomy are excluded for this approach. Frail patients with distal or GEJ tumors should be approached by transhiatal route.

Many people ask if it is difficult to perform MIE after neoadjuvant therapy. Esophagectomy is considered feasible and probably without added technical difficulties. Operating between 6 and 8 weeks after chemoradiotherapy permits a good resection through the proper planes.

Surgeons who want to introduce MIE have to make a plan in which the Surgical Department and the Hospital will support their wish. Moreover the Department will have enough volume of patients per year, at least 20 patients/year, the possibility of two surgeons working (and operating together) and enough experience in minimally invasive surgery. The choice of a mentor will facilitate this plan.

Learning curve is not yet determined. People think that at least 30 interventions are necessary to be confident with this approach.

Concerning evidence for MIE, there are published already four meta-analyses and one CRT, the TIME trial [14–18]. All of them indicate that a postoperative decrease of pulmonary infections can be accomplished if you operate by MIE whereas an increase will be found in Quality of Life (QoL) questionnaires in favor of MIE. Reduction of intraoperative blood loss, postoperative pain, and reduction in hospital stay have been also observed. Completeness of resection and number of LN retrieved are not different between the two approaches [13–15].

Moreover, at 1 year postoperatively, the most differences between the two approaches have disappeared with exception of QoL questionnaires, indicating the persistence of pain due to the post-thoracotomy syndrome. Survival after 1 year is not different between the two approaches [18].

In conclusion, all patients with esophageal squamous cell carcinoma or adenocarcinoma (stage 2 and 3) may be considered candidates after neoadjuvant therapy for MIE.

9.6 Surgical Procedure [17–20]

Three types of operations are widely employed and are described.

1. **Transhiatal resection with cervical anastomosis**

   Laparoscopy, cervical dissection of the esophagus, retrieval of specimen, formation gastric tube, and cervical anastomosis

For distal esophageal carcinoma and cardia carcinoma a transhiatal resection can be used. The conventional technique has been described by Orringer and consists of a laparotomy with celiac trunk lymphadenectomy, gastric tube formation with cervical anastomosis. For the minimally invasive approach the midline incision is replaced by 4–5 ports. To retract the left liver lobe several devices can be used. After resectability has been confirmed, the lesser omentum is opened along the liver. If an aberrant left hepatic artery is present it should be divided. To make sure that a curative resection is possible the crura should be dissected free. Now that this is done the omentum along the greater curvature is opened taking care that the right gastro-epiploic artery is left intact. This artery can usually be seen but can be difficult to identify especially in obese patients. To avoid injury a safe margin is used. Whilst dividing the omentum the assistant should provide traction with respect for the spleen. Dissection in the splenic hilum can be difficult when traction is not adequate. Lifting the stomach and approaching the splenic hilum from 'below' can facilitate dissection. Everting the fundus may aid in the final dissection of the stomach to left and anteriorly of the crus. The next step involves truncal dissection with lymphadenectomy and division of the left gastric artery and vein. This can be done by lifting the stomach and approaching through the gastrocolic ligament. In some cases dissection through the lesser omentum can be more easily. The truncal dissection is usually started by over the pancreas opening the peritoneum. The cautery hook can be very useful. The base of the left gastric artery and vein should be dissected free before ligation. Several energy devices can be used for dissection, also clips can be applied. After transection of the artery and vein the dissection continues up to the crura. To dissect along the cardias plane the anterior crus should be opened according to Pinotti. Now it is possible to dissect the esophagus up to the left pulmonary vein. Peri-esophageal dissection can now be completed; the pleura can be opened in this phase of the procedure. Now the neck of the patient is opened and the esophagus identified. This can be done on the left or right side as preferred by the surgical team. To facilitate dissection of the neck, the head of the patient should be turned away. Using a stitch the distal part of the cervical esophagus is put under traction. A loop is positioned proximal. Now the esophagus is opened and the stripper introduced. With advancement of the stripper during direct laparoscopic visualization the stomach is opened and the stripper grasped. A small incision is made along the umbilicus. The wound is protected using a port and the hand of the surgeon inserted. After complete transection of the esophagus the stripper is pulled towards the abdomen taking the esophagus along. This part of the operation can have hemodynamic consequences and the anesthesiologist should be notified in advance. A loop is tight to the stripper to facilitate gastric conduit positioning pre vertebral. The esophagus/stomach is retrieved extra-corporally and the gastric conduit created. Several staplers are used to create a gastric conduit. The optimal size is approximately two fingers. The tip is connected to the loop and by pushing the conduit up using minimal traction on the loop, it is positioned pre-vertebral and the esophagogastrostomy is fashioned according to local protocol. The use of drains and feeding jejunostomy is also according to local protocol. Fast track protocols can be applied with success in esophageal surgery.

2. **Transthoracic resection with cervical or intrathoracic anastomosis**
   Minimally invasive McKeown three stage esophageal resection
   Thoracoscopy
   Laparoscopy
   Cervical incision and anastomosis
   Minimally invasive Ivor Lewis 2 stage esophageal resection
   Laparoscopy
   Thoracoscopy
   Intrathoracic Anastomosis

When a more extensive dissection is warranted the transthoracic approach is utilized. Depending on the type of anastomosis the operation is started either by thoracoscopy or laparoscopy. The transthoracic resection with cervical anastomosis has been described by McKeown. The intra-thoracic anastomosis is associated with the technique described by Ivor Lewis. The extent of lymphadenectomy is subject to debate and needs to be elucidated in the era of neoadjuvant chemoradiotherapy. When an intra-thoracic anastomosis is fashioned the lymphadenectomy is limited to the subcarinal area whereas the McKeown approach facilitates an extended lymphadenectomy up to the upper mediastinum (Fig. 9.1).

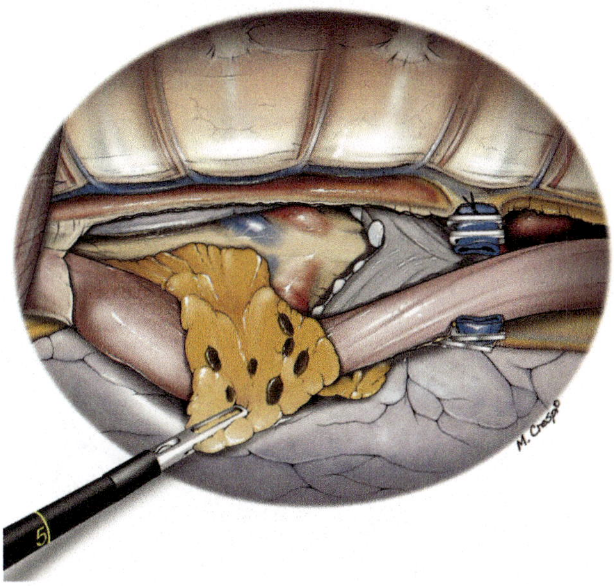

Fig. 9.1 Esophageal resection and mediastinal lymphadenectomy. (Reproduced with permission of Prof. Guy-Bernard Cadière, illustrator: Massimiliano Crespi)

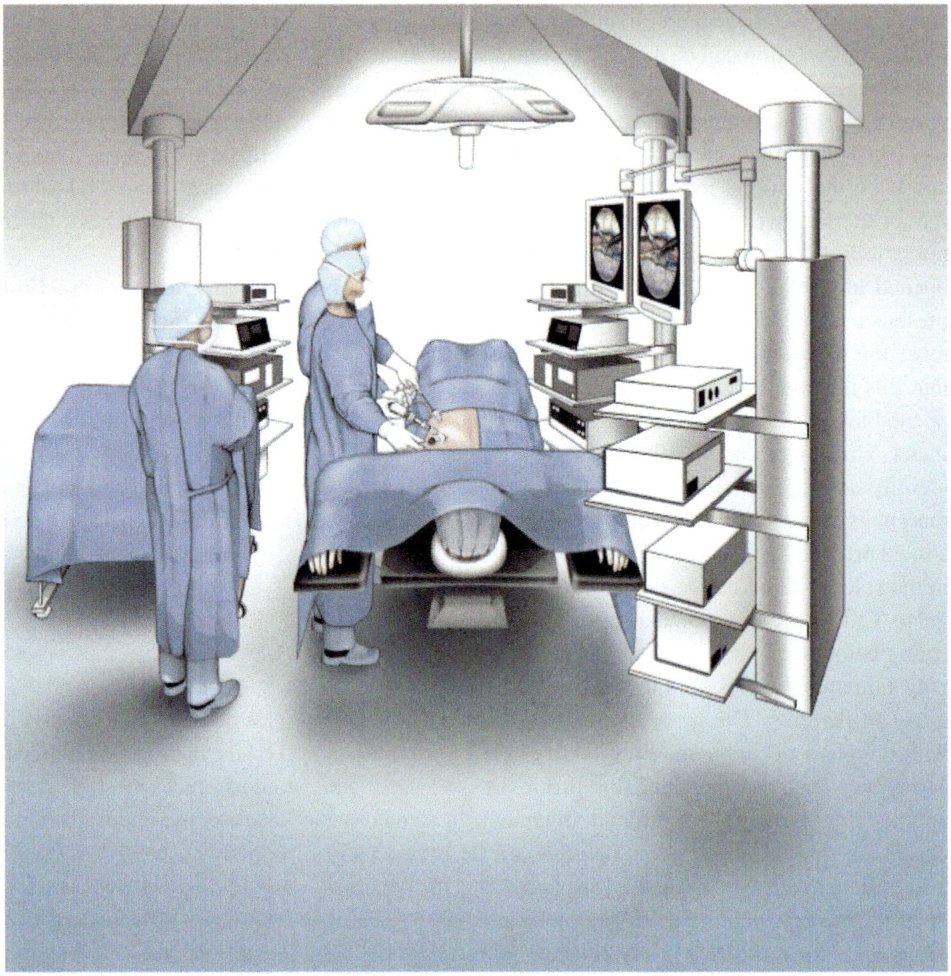

Fig. 9.2 Operating room setting for right thoracoscopy in prone position. (Reproduced with permission of Prof. Guy-Bernard Cadière, illustrator: Massimiliano Crespi)

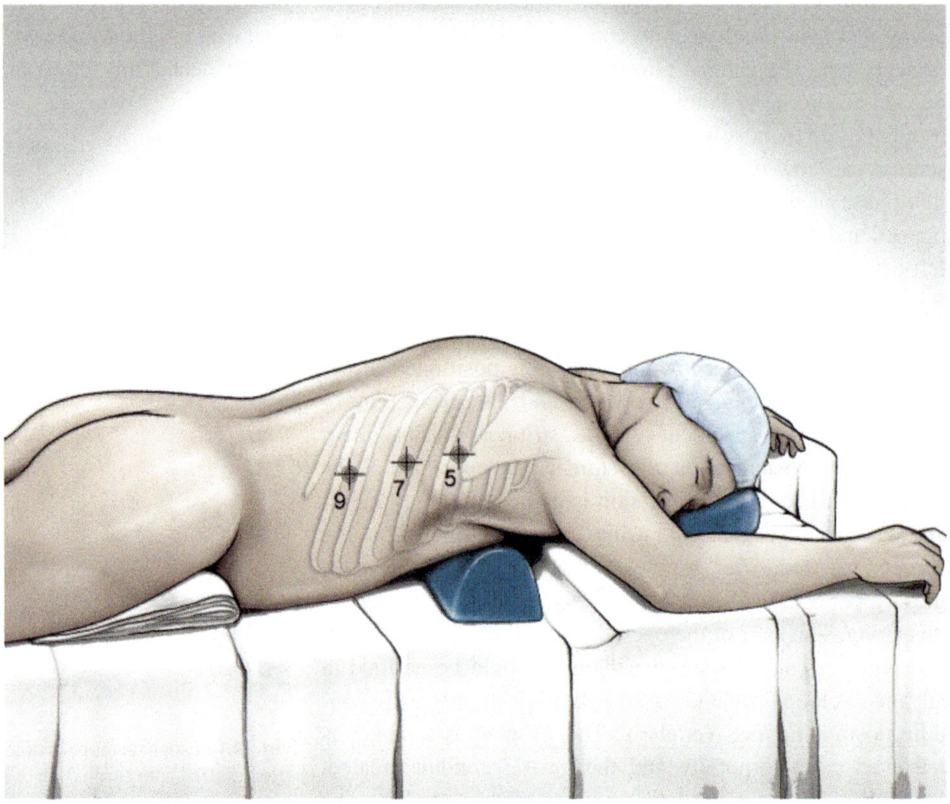

Fig. 9.3 Position of trocars. (Reproduced with permission of Prof. Guy-Bernard Cadière, illustrator: Massimiliano Crespi)

The abdominal phase in these techniques differs from the transhiatal in the intra-abdominal creation of the gastric conduit. In the case of an intra-thoracic anastomosis the resected specimen can be removed via a limited thoracotomy whereas in the so-called McKeown procedure a limited abdominal incision is often used. The thoracic phase can be done in left lateral, semi-prone or prone position. All approaches can be done using minimally invasive techniques. Most frequent used technique in the Netherlands is the prone position. Advantages are the use of single lumen intubation and the good visibility due to depression of the lungs with potential loss of blood not interfering with the operation-field.

After the abdominal phase the patient is placed in prone position using pads on the operation table (Fig. 9.2). Usually 3–4 ports are used, the position depended upon technique used (Fig. 9.3). After introduction of the ports the thoracic cavity is explored and dissection is started by incising the inferior pulmonary ligament (Fig. 9.4). The pleura is incised along the esophagus taking into account that the pulmonary vein is at risk of damage. The next landmark is the right bronchus, opening the pleura give access to the subcarinal station. Dissection of this station can be difficult as these lymph nodes are vulnerable and course anteriorly of the bifurcation of the trachea. The left bronchus is ideally approached after mobilization of the esophagus at the dorsal side. When dissecting this plane the so-called meso-esophagus can be appreciated. With the intra-thoracic anastomosis the level of transection is just proximal from the carina. The usefulness of resection of the azygos vein is questionable as is transection when an intra-thoracic anastomosis is made (Fig. 9.5). In case of the so-called McKeown procedure an extended dissection of lymph nodes along the esophagus and the recurrent laryngeal nerves are feasible. Identification of the recurrent nerves is mandatory in order to avoid injury. The procedure is completed by turning the patient in supine position and commencing with the abdominal part and cervical anastomosis. In case of the Ivor Lewis procedure the gastric conduit has already been formed and is pulled into the thoracic cage. The level of resection is determined by positioning the conduit in line with the proximal esophagus. As the tumor is now resected the specimen is removed through a small incision by enlarging one distal port. The use of a wound protector is recommended. Regarding anastomotic techniques the use of circular and linear staplers has been described [19]. In a review the feasibility of both the transthoracic as the oral staplers was shown. With increasing numbers of Ivor Lewis procedures performed, prevention of leakage plays a very important role. The anastomosis should be without tension nor torsion and are be taken to avoid a siphon-like situation by using a stitch placed at the level of the first staple line of the gastric conduit. This stitch is used as a marker to identify the position of the antrum. A thoracic drain can be left in situ when indicated.

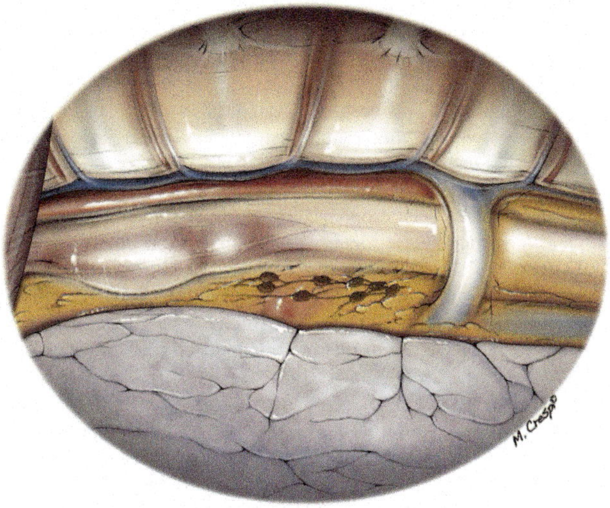

Fig. 9.4 Aspect of the posterior mediastinum in prone position, visualizing the esophagus (and tumor), the spine, azygos vein and right lung. (Reproduced with permission of Prof. Guy-Bernard Cadière, illustrator: Massimiliano Crespi)

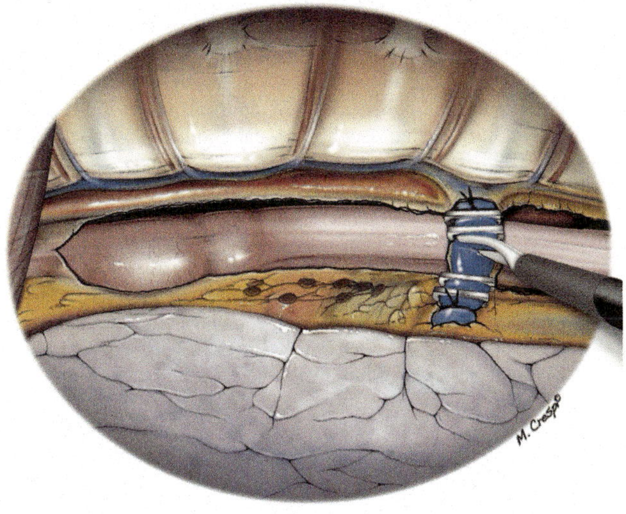

Fig. 9.5 Division of the azygos vein. (Reproduced with permission of Prof. Guy-Bernard Cadière, illustrator: Massimiliano Crespi)

9.7 Conversion

Extensive adhesions in the thoracic cavity, precluding an adequate partial collapse of the right lung will indicate conversion to right conventional thoracotomy.

Conversion has to be considered for oncological reasons such as possible ingrowth of the tumor in other organs in order to assure this and contemplate the possibility of no resection. Moreover important bleeding can be an indication to convert to thoracotomy. Question arises in which position conversion has to be accomplished. Most of surgeons will choose for a lateral thoracotomy. When conversion is anticipated the use of the semi-prone position has the advantages of easier access by means of a right thoracotomy.

9.8 Postoperative Care

Postoperative care in esophageal surgery is subject to discussion. As the frequency and complications of complications is high, strict protocol adherence is mandatory for successful management if complications occur. The use of drains and tubes has been shown to be associated with decreased quality of life and extended postoperative recovery. By using fast-track principles the mean length of stay after MIE can be decreased without compromising safety. Early enteral feeding has been shown to be safe and effective [21]

9.9 Complications

Many complications have been described after esophageal cancer. In general MIE will reduce the rate of pulmonary infections increasing quality of life because of the avoidance of thoracotomy. Technical complications such as leakage of anastomosis, chylothorax and recurrent laryngeal nerve palsy will not be different between open and MIE because the extent of resection is the same [22].

9.10 Quality of Life

As resection of the esophagus carries a high risk of severe complications, it may have a negative effect on health related quality of life. This quality can be expressed by means of Patient Reported Outcome Measures and are of increasing importance in decision making in esophageal cancer treatment [23]. Regarding cervical versus intra-thoracic anastomosis recent research did not find a difference in quality of life [14]. A randomized trial concerning this subject is underway.

References

1. Dallemagne B, Weerts JM, Jehaes C. Thoracoscopic esophageal resection. In: Cuesta MA, Nagy AG, editors. Minimally invasive surgery in gastrointestinal cancer. Edingburgh: Churchill Livingstone; 1993. p. 59–68.
2. Cuschieri A. thoracoscopic subtotal esophagectomy. Endosc Surg Allied Technol. 1994;2:21–5.
3. Luketich JD, Alvelo-Rivera M, Buenaventura PO, et al. Minimally invasive esophagectomy: outcomes in 222 patients. Ann Surg. 2003;238:486–94.
4. Palanivelu C, Prakash A, Senthilkumar R, et al. Minimally invasive esophagectomy: thoracoscopic mobilization of the esophagus and mediastinal lymphadenectomy in prone position-experience of 130 patients. J Am Coll Surg. 2013;2006:7–16.
5. Scheepers JJ, Veenhof XA, van der Peet DL, et al. Laparoscopic transhiatal resection for malignancies of the distal esophagus: outcome of the first 50 resected patients. Surgery. 2008;143:278–85.
6. Van Hagen P, Huslhof MC, van Lanschot JJ, et al. Preoperative chemoradiotherapy for esophageal or junctional cancer. N Engl J Med. 2012;366:2074–84.
7. Cunningham D, Allum WH, Stenning SP, et al. Perioperative chemotherapy versus surgery alone for resectable gastroesophageal cancer. N Engl J Med. 2006;355:11–20.
8. Cuesta MA, Weijs TJ, Bleys RL, et al. A new concept of the anatomy of the thoracic esophagus: the meso-esophagus. Observational study during thoracoscopic esophagectomy. Surg Endosc. 2015;29:2576–82.
9. Weijs TJ, Ruurda JP, Luyer MDP, et al. Preserving the pulmonary vagus nerve branches during thoracoscopic esophagectomy. Surg Endosc. 2016.30(9):3816–22. (Epub ahead of print).
10. Hulscher JBF, van Sandick JW, de Boer AG, et al. Extended transthoracic resection compared with limited transhiatal resection for adenocarcinoma of the esophagus. N Engl J Med. 2002;347:1662–9.
11. Akiyama H, Tsurumaru M, Ono Y, et al. Background of lymph node dissection for squamous cell carcinoma of the esophagus. In: Sato T, Lizukan T, editors. In color atlas of surgical anatomy for esophageal cancer. Springer-Verlag; 1992, p. 9–24.
12. Siewert JR, Stein HJ. Carcinoma of the cardia: carcinoma of the Gastroesophageal junction. classification, pathology and extent of resection. Dis Esophagus. 1996;9:173–82.
13. Biere SS, Cuesta MA, Van der Peet DL. Minimally invasive versus open esophagectomy for cancer: a systematic review and meta-analysis. Minerva Chir. 2009;64:121–33.
14. Biere SS, Maas KW, Cuesta MA, van der Peet DL. Cervical or thoracic anastomosis after esophagectomy for cancer: a systematic review and meta-analysis. Dig Surg. 2011;28:29–35.
15. Biere SS, van Berge Henegouwen MI, Maas KW, et al. Minimally invasive versus open esophagectomy for patients with esophageal cancer: a multicentre, open –label, randomised controlled trial. Lancet. 2012;379:1887–92.
16. Maas KW, Cuesta MA, van Berge Henegouwen MI, et al. Quality of life and late complications after Minimally Invasive compared to open esophagectomy: results of a randomized trial. World J Surg. 2015;39:1986–93.
17. Cuesta MA, van der Peet DL, Biere SSAY, Scheepers JJG, Heijnen BHM. Laparoscopic transhiatal esophagectomy. In: Puntambeker S, Cuesta MA, editors. Atlas of minimally invasive surgery in esophageal carcinoma. Springer; 2010. p. 171–89.
18. Cuesta MA, Scheepers JJG, Oosterhuis W, Biere SSAY, Van der Peet DL, Heijnen BHM. Thoracoscopic esophageal resection for cancer in prone decubitus position: operative technique. In: Puntambeker S, Cuesta MA, editors. Atlas of minimally invasive surgery in esophageal carcinoma. Springer; 2010. p. 149–69.
19. Maas KW, Biere SS, Scheepers JJG, et al. Minimally invasive intrathoracic anastomosis after Ivor Lewis Esophagectomy for cancer. A review of transoral or transthoracic use of staplers. Surg Endosc. 2012;26:1795–802.
20. Puntambekar S, Patil AM, Rayate NV, Joshi S N. Thoracoscopic and laparoscopic esophagectomy with two field nodal clearance. In: Puntambeker S, Cuesta MA, editors. Atlas of minimally invasive surgery in esophageal carcinoma. Springer; 2010. p. 33–109.
21. Weijs TJ, Berkelmans GHK, Nieuwenhuijzen GAP, et al. Routes for early enteral nutrition following esophagectomy. A systematic review. Clin Nutr. 2015;34(1):1–6. doi:10.1016/j.clnu.2014.07.011. Epub 2014 Aug 1. Review.
22. Blom RLGM, van der Peet DL, van Berge Henegouwen MI. Chapter 8. Prevention and treatment of major complications after esophageal surgery. In: Cuesta MA, Bonjer HJ, editors. Treatment of postoperative complications after digestive surgery. Springer; 2014. p. 53–73.
23. Straatman J, Joosten PJ, Terwee CB, Cuesta MA, Jansma EP, van der Peet DL. Systematic review of patient-reported-outcomes-measures in the surgical treatment of patients with esophageal cancer. Dis Esophagus 2015. doi:10.1111/dote.12405. (Epub ahead of print)

Part IV

Stomach

Laparoscopic Gastrectomy

10

Wiley Chung and Teodor P. Grantcharov

10.1 Anatomy

The stomach is roughly J-shaped and its size and shape depends on whether it is full or empty, on the position of the body, and on the phase of respiration. The stomach is divided into four portions: cardia, fundus, corpus, and pylorus. The stomach has an anterior and posterior surface. It also has two curvatures, the greater and lesser. The junction of the body with the pyloric antrum is marked by a distinct notch on the lesser curvature known as the incisura angularis. The thickened pyloric sphincter is easily palpated and surrounds the lumen of the pyloric canal. The greater omentum is attached along the greater curvature of the stomach meanwhile the lesser omentum is attached along the lesser curvature. The omentum contains the vascular and lymphatic supply of the stomach.

The arterial supply of the stomach includes the left gastric artery – from the coeliac axis; the right gastric artery – from the hepatic artery; the right gastro-epiploic artery – from the gastroduodenal branch of the hepatic artery; the left gastro-epiploic artery – from the splenic artery; and the short gastric arteries – from the splenic artery. The corresponding veins drain into the portal system.

The lymphatic drainage of the stomach accompanies its blood supply and consists of an extensive network organized into three drainage zones. Area I, the superior two-thirds of the stomach, drains along the left and right gastric vessels to the aortic nodes. Area II, the right two-thirds of the inferior one-third of the stomach, drains along the right gastro-epiploic vessels to the subpyloric nodes and then to the aortic nodes. Area III, the left one-third of the greater curvature of the stomach, drains along the short gastgric and splenic vessels lying in the gastrosplenic and lienorenal ligaments, then, via the suprapancreatic nodes, to the aortic group. This extensive lymphatic drainage and the technical difficulty of its complete excision is one of the great challenges in dealing with stomach cancer.

The anterior and posterior vagi enter the abdomen through the esophageal hiatus. The vagus nerve constitutes the motor and secretory nerve supply for the stomach. The stomach is innervated by terminal branches from the anterior and posterior gastric nerves.

10.2 Indications for Gastric Resections

10.2.1 Gastrointestinal Stromal Tumours of the Stomach

Previously known as leiomyomas and leimyosarcomas, gastrointestinal stromal tumours (GISTs) comprise only 3 % of all gastric malignancies and arise from mesenchymal components of the gastric wall. There is a slight male predominance and the median age at diagnosis is 60 years. GISTs often exhibit prominent extraluminal growth and can attain large sizes before becoming symptomatic. The presentation of such tumours are extremely varied and can range from asymptomatic masses found incidentally on physical exam or radiographic studies to vague abdominal pain and discomfort secondary to mass effect. When overlying mucosa becomes necrotic, GI hemorrhage may occur but perforation is not a common presentation. GISTs are diagnosed using endoscopy and radiologic imaging. They are graded according to their tumour size and histologic frequency of mitoses. Treatment is surgical resection into grossly normal gastric wall to ensure negative histologic margins. En bloc resection of any structures involved by local invasion should be attempted, although lympadenectomy is not indicated because lymph node metastases are rare. Metastasis occurs by hematogenous route, and hepatic involvement is common, as is local recurrence after resection. Unfotunately, GISTs are not radiosensitive nor responsive to traditional chemotherapy. However, most GISTs express the c-kit receptor which is a tyrosine kinase that acts as a growth fac-

W. Chung, MD • T.P. Grantcharov, MD, PhD, FACS (✉)
Department of General Surgery, St. Michael's Hospital, Toronto, ON, Canada
e-mail: grantcharovt@smh.ca

H.J. Bonjer (ed.), *Surgical Principles of Minimally Invasive Procedures*, DOI 10.1007/978-3-319-43196-3_10

tor receptor. Imatinib mesylate (Gleevec^{TM}) is a small-molecule inhibitor of the c-kit receptor that has become first-line therapy for metastatic or recurrent GIST.

10.2.2 Benign Gastric Outlet Obstruction

Gastric outlet obstruction can occur as a chronic process due to fibrosis and scarring of the pylorus from chronic ulcer disease or as a consequence of acute inflammation superimposed on previous scarring of the gastric outlet. In general, gastric outlet obstruction secondary to peptic ulcer disease has become exceedingly rare with modern medical antisecretory therapy. Patients may present with recurrent vomiting of poorly digested food, dehydration, and hypochloremic hypokalemic metabolic alkalosis. Management consists of adequate volume resuscitation and correcting electrolyte abnormalities, nasogastric suction, and intravenous antisecretory agents. Esophagogastroduodenoscopy (EGD) is necessary for evaluating the nature of the obstruction and for ruling out malignant etiology. Endoscopic hydrostatic balloon dilation can also be performed at the same time as EGD. Indications for surgical therapy include persistent obstruction after 7 days of nonoperative management and recurrent obstruction. Distal gastrectomy including the ulcer is the preferred operation for most patients.

10.2.3 Adenocarcinoma

Gastric adenocarcinoma is the fourth-most common cancer worldwide and the tenth-most common malignancy in the United States. Adenocarcinomas arise from mucous-producing cells in the gastric mucosa and comprise of 95 % of gastric malignancies. The anatomic pattern of gastric cancer is changing, with proximal cancers comprising a greater proportion of gastric cancers. Approximately, one third of gastric cancers are metastatic at presentation. The overall 5-year relative survival rate is 17 % for gastric cardia cancers and 25.6 % for noncardia gastric cancers [1].

Case selection is very important and the indications are still evolving. Early gastric cancers limited to the mucosa are suitable for laparoscopic or endoluminal local resection. Early gastric cancer with extension into the submucosa requires gastrectomy with removal of the greater omentum and level 1 lymph nodes (D1 gastrectomy) which can be performed safely laparoscopically [5]. Advanced gastric cancer involving the muscularis propria but not the serosa (T2 tumour) requires a more extensive regional lymphadenectomy [12]. Although not widely established in practice, D2 gastrectomies can be performed safely laparoscopically or using the hand-assisted laparoscopic surgical (HALS) technique. The role of laparoscopy in locally advanced tumours is still a matter of debate. Similarly, the role of palliative resection is still not clearly established. Most authors currently agree that distal gastrectomy can be performed with palliative intent, while the value of palliative total gastrectomy is controversial [6, 7].

10.3 Preoperative Evaluation of Gastric Adenocarcinoma

10.3.1 Endoscopy

Although diagnosis can be made by double-contrast upper GI barium contrast studies or by EGD, the later is generally the diagnostic method of choice because it permits direct visualization and biopsy of suspicious lesions. Screening examination by endoscopy is not cost-effective for the general North American population, given the low incidence, but may be warranted in high-risk individuals. These individuals would include patients more than 20 years post-partial gastrectomy, immigrants from endemic areas, patients with pernicious anemia or atrophic gastritis, and patients with familial or hereditary gastric cancer. Interestingly, massive endoscopy screening in Japan, a country with a high incidence of gastric cancer, resulted in an increase in the detection of gastric cancer confined to the mucosa and led to improvements in 5-year survival rates [8].

10.3.2 Endoscopic Ultrasound

Once the diagnosis of cancer is established, computed tomography (CT) and endoscopic ultrasonography (EUS) are the primary modalities employed for staging. EUS adds to the preoperative evaluation of gastric cancer in several ways. It is superior to CT in delineating the depth of tumour invasion in the gastric wall and adjacent structures and is of great value when endoscopic mucosal resection (EMR) is considered. EUS is superior at identifying perigastric lymphadenopathy. In fact, EUS is the most accurate method available for T staging of gastric cancer, and accuracy for N staging approaches 70 %. Addition of fine needle aspiration (FNA) of suspicious nodes increases accuracy even further and brings specificity to near 100 %.

10.3.3 CT Scan of the Thorax, Abdomen and Pelvis

CT scan of the thorax, abdomen and pelvis is the best noninvasive modality for detecting metastatic disease in the form of malignant ascites or hematogenous spread to distant organs, most commonly the liver. The overall accuracy for tumour staging is 60–80 % depending on the protocol used, but accuracy for determining nodal involvement is more limited and variable. Positron emission tomography (PET)/CT combines the spatial resolution of CT with the contrast resolution of PET. It is most useful for its specificity in detecting nodal and distant metastatic disease not apparent on CT scan alone. Preliminary studies suggest that the use of PET/CT in staging patients with gastric cancer leads to upstaging in 6 % and downstaging in 9 % of patients.

10.3.4 Staging Laparoscopy and Laparoscopic Ultrasound (LUS)

Laparoscopy significantly enhances the accuracy of staging in patients with gastric cancer. Routine use of staging laparoscopy has been shown to detect small-volume peritoneal and liver metastases in 20–30 % of patients believed to have locoregional disease, thereby avoiding unnecessary laparotomy in these patients. Staging laparoscopy is not indicated in patients with T1 and T2 lesions given the low incidence of metastases with these tumours.

10.3.5 CT Gastrography and Multi-planar Reformating

CT has become a valuable imaging study in the preoperative planning for gastric tumour resections, especially as more surgeons have gained expertise in laparoscopic surgery and have recognized a role for limited gastric resection for some tumors. Computed tomography gastrography (CTG) is a non-invasive technique which produces endoluminal images which can show subtle mucosal abnormalities which is comparable in quality to conventional optical gastroscopy [9]. CTG and multi-planar reformating (MPR) can offer valuable information about gastric tumors including morphology, location, size including both intraluminal and extramural components, distance of proximal lesions from the esophagogastric junction, distance of distal lesions from the pylorus, and assessment of localized versus extensive resection [9–11].

Early experience with CTG and MPR have shown them to be useful adjuncts to the conventional abdominal CT scan in the preoperative planning of laparoscopic gastric resections [10]. Correlation has been excellent between preoperative imaging and intraoperative findings [9, 11]. The utility of CTG and MPR in vascular road mapping has yet to be determined.

10.4 Surgical Procedure

10.4.1 Patient Position and Setup

The patient is placed in a supine, split leg position (Fig. 10.1). It is important to secure the patient to the operating table as steep reverse Trendelenburg position is necessary during the procedure. Antibiotic and DVT prophylaxis with subcutaneous heparin and sequential compression devices is recommended.

An alternative setup is to have the patient in the supine head-up tilt position with the surgeon operating from the right side of the operating table and the main video monitor facing the surgeon.

10.4.2 Team

For optimal operating conditions and comfort, the operating room should be arranged in an ergonomic manner. The surgeon stands between the patient's legs while the first assistant stands on the patient's left. The second assistant stands on the patient's right while the scrub nurse stands on the surgeon's left. The anesthesia unit and monitors are positioned at the head of the table.

10.4.3 Trocar Placement

The first trocar is introduced 15 cm below the xyphoid and accommodates the laparoscope. Two additional 12 mm trocars are positioned in the right and left paramedian areas below the costal margins. Both these trocars will accommodate the linear stapling devices and used for intracorporeal suturing. A fourth trocar is positioned on the left anterior axillary line just below the costal margin and is used for

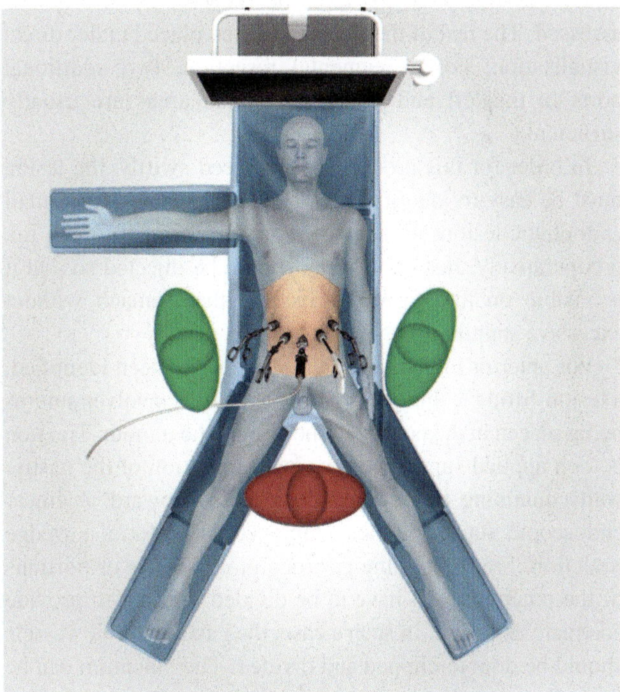

Fig. 10.1 Patient positioning for laparoscopic gastrectomy

retraction. In case of a total gastrectomy with Roux-en-Y reconstruction, a fifth trocar may be necessary in the left lower quadrant. It is used for the intracorporeal suturing of the jejuno-jejunostomy. Lastly, a sixth trocar is introduced below the xiphoid process which accommodates the liver retractor.

10.5 Segmental Wedge Resection for Benign Gastric Tumours and GIST

The surgical resection of benign gastric tumours allows establishment of a histological diagnosis, assess the risk of recurrence, indication of adjuvant treatment and need for continued surveilance. Segmental wedge resection without lymphadenectomy is indicated for small areas of high-grade dysplasia and subepithelial tumors, such as GISTs. Patients with dysplasia may be followed with serial endoscopy and biopsy to rule out histologic progression. In recent years Endoscopic mucosal/submucosal resections have been utilized with great success and minimal morbidity.

Segmental wedge resection is technically feasible for tumours located away from the GI junction, lesser curvature or the pylorus. For the rest, a formal resection with intestinal reconstruction may be necessary. Therefore, an accurate pre-operative localization is of crucial importance for planning of the procedure.

After pneumoperitoneum is established, the supra-umbilical port is inserted. The 30° scope is then passed into the port and an evaluation for potential intra-abdominal injury secondary to the Veres needle or port insertion is assessed. The rest of the trocars are then placed under direct visualisation. For a segmental resection, two additional ports in the left and right paramedian areas are usually sufficient.

In order for this procedure to proceed swiftly, the lesion must be easy to identify in the OR. It is advised that small endophytic lesions are identified and marked with India Ink preoperatively. Just enough ink should be injected so that it is visible on the serosal surface of the stomach without excessive staining.

For anterior tumours, once the lesion has been identified, a lesion-lifting technique is employed which involves sutures being placed in the normal tissue around the tumour. Traction is then applied superiorly, causing the portion of the gastric wall containing the tumour to be tented upward. A linear endoscopic stapler is then employed to perform a wedge resection. Frequently, the gastroepiploic vessels or portions of the omentum will have to be divided in order to provide adequate exposure. In such a case, the gastroepiploic vessels should be double-clipped and divided. The omentum can be divided using a laparoscopic energy device. Prior to the end of the procedure, endoscopy is employed to confirm hemostasis, ensure complete removal of the lesion, and establish that the gastric outlet is not significantly narrowed. For posterior tumours, the same approach as anterior tumours is employed with the exception of gaining exposure after mobilization of the greater curvature. In this variant of the procedure, the greater curvature is retracted anteriorly while the tumour is tented posteriorly.

Alternative technique involves excision of the tumour using an energy device and closure of the gastrotomy defect using a running absorbable suture.

The resected lesions should be sent to pathology for assessment of the margins. It is often difficult in laparoscopic removal to obtain generous margins. For this reason, the liberal use of pathologic frozen section evaluation to ensure negative margins is advised.

10.6 Distal and Subtotal Gastrectomy

Distal and subtotal gastrectomy is performed for benign lesions associated with gastric outlet obstruction and for treatment of gastric malignancies with curative or palliative intent.

10.6.1 Incision and Exposure

A 30° forward-oblique or 0° laparoscope is placed through a supra-umbilical trocar. The additional ports should be placed as described previously in Sect. 10.4.3.

A thorough exploration of the peritoneal cavity is undertaken to assess the extent of the cancer involvement and potential metastatic lesions. In cases of a locally advanced disease involving surrounding structures, the patient should be evaluated for neo-adjuvant regimen and in case of therapeutic response – a subsequent curative resection. Presence of distant metastases or peritoneal deposits confirm advanced disease but do not preclude palliative resection unless there is extensive involvement. The decision for palliative resection should be weighed against potential morbidity which may ultimately delay or prevent chemotherapy.

10.6.2 Separation of Omental Bursa and Mobilization of the Greater Curvature

Using atraumatic graspers, the omentum is retracted anteriorly while the colon is gently retracted inferiorly by the assistant. The omental bursa is then separated from the transverse mesocolon with a laparoscopic energy device. This area is mostly avascular. During the dissection, special care must be taken near the middle colic vessels which run posterior to the plane of dissection and are difficult to identify in case of adhesions between the omentum and the transverse colon mesentery. The correct plane may be easier to identify on the left and right aspects of the omental attachments to the colon.

After the gastrocolic omentum has been transacted and the lesser sac entered, the stomach is retracted anteriorly. This exposes the right gastroepiploic pedicle. The right gastroepiploic vein and artery are then dissected and ligated at their origin using hemoclips or vascular load of a linear stapler device. The greater curvature is mobilized up to the resection margin, preserving the short gastric vessels.

10.6.3 Mobilization and Division of the Duodenum

A vascular sling is passed along the posterior aspect of the stomach and then through an avascular window in the lesser omentum. This sling is then used to pull the stomach up and away from the lesser sac and pancreas to help improve exposure and dissection of the right gastric artery from behind the stomach. The right gastric artery should be ligated using hemoclips high up at the origin from the hepatic artery prior to division to ensure removal of the suprapyloric nodes. The division of the right gastric artery will free the duodenum just beyond the pylorus. The paraduodenal veins are then secured and the fibrous attachments between the first part of the duodenum and the head of the pancreas are divided.

10.6.4 Billroth II

The duodenum is divided with an endoscopic linear stapler beyond the pylorus. The staple line is inspected and reinforced with interrupted sutures if needed.

10.6.5 Billroth I

Duodenal continuity is maintained until the stomach is ready for resection

The dissection continues until it reaches the inferior border of the pancreas. The pancreatic capsule is then freed and elevated superiorly.

10.6.6 Ligation of the Left Gastric Vessels

Depending on the location of the tumor, the left gastric vessels may need to be ligated. The left gastric vessels' pedicle can be exposed by elevating the stomach anteriorly, away from the retroperitoneum. The artery and vein are then dissected down to their origin from the celiac trunk and secured using hemoclips or a vascular load of a linear stapler device.

10.6.7 Celiac Axis and Splenic Artery Lymph Node Dissection

The sling previously placed around the esophagus is used to retract the esophagogastric junction downward and to the left and a gentle downward force is applied on the superior margin of the pancreas. The nodal basins surrounding the hepatic artery and celiac axis are dissected. All major structures in the porta hepatis, including the hepatic artery and ducts, are carefully identified and the surrounding lymph nodes are removed. Dissection then proceeds along the hepatic artery in a distal-to-proximal manner toward the celiac axis including all the soft tissue surrounding the common hepatic, left gastric and splenic arteries.

10.6.8 Gastric Resection

The proximal transection site is selected and the appropriate areas on the greater and lesser curvatures are cleared from fat and remaining blood vessels.

10.6.9 Billroth II

A 3.5 mm endoscopic linear stapler is used to transect the stomach from the lesser to the greater curvature.

10.6.10 Billroth I

A 3.5 mm endoscopic linear stapler is used to make the first application vertical from the lesser curvature. The second and third applications are at an angle to the first application so that the transection line reaches the lesser curvature more proximally. The duodenum is transected using a linear stapler.

The specimen is placed away from the operative field and removed after the reconstruction has been completed.

10.6.11 Extraction of the Specimen

The specimen is removed through an upper midline minilaparotomy or a Pfannensteil incision with a wound edge protector in place. The resected specimen is opened and inspected on a back table and it must be confirmed that the lesion is removed with sufficient margins prior to reconstruction.

10.6.12 Reconstruction

10.6.12.1 Bilroth II Gastrojejunostomy

Billroth II includes a side-to-side anastamosis between a loop of proximal jejunum and the gastric remnant. It can be performed safely intracorporeally. Gastrotomy is performed using electrocautery. A loop of proximal jejunum, 30–40 cm from the ligament of Treitz is brought up in an antecolic fashion A small enterotomy is then made at the antimesenteric side of the jejunum. A 3.5 mm linear cutting stapler is inserted into the stomach and the jejunum and then fired to create the side-to-side anastomosis. The defect is then closed using a running 3–0 absorbable suture in a single layer.

10.6.13 Roux-en-Y Gastrojejunostomy and Jejunojejunostomy

Reconstruction after distal gastrectomy for cancer can also be performed with a Roux-en-Y gastrojejunostomy. The Roux-en-Y gastrojejunostomy is superior to the Billroth II gastrojejunostomy because of a lower incidence of bile reflux, reflux gastritis, esophagitis, and carcinogenesis of the gastric remnant [2, 3].

After the specimen has been resected as described in steps 6.1–6.6, the jejunum is divided transversely approximately 30 cm from the ligament of Treitz using a linear stapler loaded with 2.5-mm cartridge and a roux limb of approximately 40 cm is prepared. To prepare the jejunojejunostomy anastomosis, the roux limb is followed up to 40 cm from its initial transected end and a small enterotomy is made on the antimesenteric border of the jejunum. Another small enterotomy is made at the antimesenteric corner of the proximal, bilio-pancreatic end of the jejunum. The jaws of the 45 mm, 2.5-mm linear cutting stapler are then inserted into each of the enterotomies and fired to create the anastomosis. The resulting enterotomy is then closed using a 3–0 absorbable running suture.

The Roux limb is then brought up to the gastric remnant via the antecolic route.

To prepare the gastrojejunostomy anastamosis, a small gastrotomy is made on the posterior wall of the gastric remnant. Another small enterotomy is made at the antimesenteric corner of the roux limb. The jaw of the 30 mm, 3.5 cm linear stapler is inserted into each of the enterotomies and fired to create the side-to-side anastomosis. The anastomotic defect is then closed using 3–0 absorbable suture in a running fashion.

10.6.14 Testing the Anastomosis

All anastomoses are inspected for adequacy of the lumen and hemostasis of the suture and staple lines. The integrity of the anastomosis can be tested using gastroscopy or intragastric methylene blue injection.

10.7 Proximal Gastrectomy

Advances in screening and diagnostic techniques for the stomach have increased the detection rate of early-stage gastric carcinoma in the proximal one-third of the stomach [13]. In cases of gastric carcinoma with submucosal invasion or carcinoma of more than 2 cm, gastrectomy with lymph node dissection is recommended by guidelines established by the Japanese Gastric Cancer Association [14]. However, the extent of the resection and the method of reconstruction of proximal one-third gastric carcinomas are controversial. In the past, total gastrectomy was recommended owing to its radicality and safety [15]. To this date, no significant difference has been reported in total gastrectomy and proximal gastrectomy in terms of survival [16]. Nevertheless, proximal gastrectomy has been recommended owing to its retention of the physiological function of the remnant stomach compared to that after a total gastrectomy [17, 18].

10.7.1 Patient Positioning and Set-Up

The patient placement, operative team set up and trocar sites are as described in Sects. 10.4.1, 10.4.2 and 10.4.3.

10.7.2 Mobilisation of the Proximal Stomach

The dissection starts along pars faccida of the lesser omentum toward the right crus of the diaphragm. The peritoneum overlying the crus and the gastro-esophageal junction is transected circumferentially and the disal esophagus is mobilised. The distal resection line is identified and the stomach is trasected using 3.5 mm linear stapling device towards the greater curvature. Once the stomach is divided, the proximal part is elevated anteriorly and the left gastric vessels pedicle is identified. The left gastric vessels are dissected towards their origin from the celiac trunk, then divided using endoclips or a linear stapling device. The left side of the greater omentum including the short gastric vessels is transacted using an endoscopic energy device. Once this is completed it is important to confirm adequate length of the distal esophagus in order to ensure a tension-free anastomosis. The right gastric artery and right gastroepiploic artery are both preserved.

10.7.3 Transection of Esophagus

A penrose drain is placed around the Distal esophagus and used to retract it in caudal direction. The esophagus is transected using a 3.5 mm. endoscopic linear stapler.

10.7.4 Creation of Esophagogastric Anastomosis

The anvil of a circular stapler is attached to an oro-gastric tube and introduced in the distal esophagus.

A 25 mm. circular stapler is introduced through a small anterior wall gastrotomy and the spike of the stapling device placed anterior to the proximal stapler line. An end-to-end anastomosis is performed. The gastrotomy defect is closed using a single firing of a 3.5 mm linear stapler or sutured using a 3–0 running absorbable suture in a single layer.

10.7.5 Extraction of the Specimen

The specimen is removed through an upper midline mini-laparotomy or a Pfannensteil incision with a wound edge protector in place

10.8 Total Gastrectomy

Laparoscopic total gastrectomy is usually performed with curative intent for cancers in the middle and upper third of the stomach.

Sections 10.8.1, 10.8.2, 10.8.3, and 10.8.4 (see Sects. 10.6.1, 10.6.2, 10.6.3, and 10.6.4 above)

10.8.1 Hiatal Dissection with Mobilization of the Esophagus

The hiatal dissection begins on the left with division of the gastrophrenic peritoneal reflection. Next, the esophagogastric junction is bluntly seperated from the right crus and the hiatal canal is entered. The plane between the posterior wall of the esophagus and the preaortic fascia is further developed and the posterior aspect of the esophagus is bluntly dissected until the left crus is exposed. This step mobilizes the esophagus. A penrose drain is passed around the esophagus and it is retracted away from the mediastinum. The posterior separation of the esophagogastric junction is then completed.

10.8.2 Celiac Axis and Splenic Artery Lymph Node Dissection

See Sect. 10.6.5 above

10.8.3 Proximal Transection of the Esophagus

The esophagus is divided proximal to the gastroesophageal junction using a 3.5 cm linear stapler.

10.8.4 Jejuno-Jejunostomy

The jejunum is divided transversely approximately 30 cm from the ligament of Treitz using a 2.5 mm linear cutting stapler and a roux limb of approximately 40 cm is prepared. In preparation of the jejunojejunostomy anastomosis, the roux limb is followed up to the 40 cm from its initial transected end and a small enterotomy is made on the antimesenteric border of the jejunum. Another small enterotomy is made at the antimesenteric corner of the proximal biliopancreatic limb of the jejunum. The jaws of the 2.5 mm linear stapler are placed into each of the enterotomies and fired to create the anastomosis. The resulting enterotomy is then closed using running 3–0 absorbable suture.

The jejunal limb is then brought up to the distal esophagus via antecolic route.

10.8.5 Esophagojejunostomy

The esophago-jejunostomy can be done laparoscopically or hand-assisted using a hand-port.

10.8.6 Side-to Side Esophagojejunostomy Using a Linear Stapler

A small esophagotomy is made on the stapled edge of the esophagus. Next, a small enterotomy is made at the antimesenteric corner of the jejunal roux limb. The jaw of the 30 mm, 3.5-mm linear cutting stapler is inserted into the esophagotomy and enterotomy and fired to create the side-to-side anastomosis. The anastomotic defect is then closed using running 3–0 absorbable suture in a single layer.

10.8.7 End-to-Side Esophagojejunostomy Using a Circular Stapler

The anvil of a circular stapler is attached to an oro-gastric tube and introduced in the distal esophagus.

An incision in the jejunum is made adjacent to the staple line and a 25 mm. circular stapler is introduced through it in the limen. A point approximately 5 cm from the free margin is selected and the post of the circular stapling device is extended through the jejunal wall. The anvil is then placed into the post of the circular stapler and the tissue is approximated before firing the circular stapler to complete the anastomosis. The redundant section of jejunum is excised using a 2.5 mm linear stapling device.

10.9 Postoperative Care

Recent evidence confirmed that implementation of the principles of enhanced recovery program in upper GI surgery is associated with a reduced morbidity and shorter hospital stay [4].

10.9.1 Postoperative Feeding

It has been a common practice to restrict postoperative oral intake until passage of flatus because of fear for gastric distension and stress on the anastomosis threatening its integrity. Recently, there has been emerging evidence that early feeding after colorectal surgery reduces catabolism and morbidity. A recent large multi-institutional randomized controlled trial compared nil-by-mouth versus normal food on day 1 after major open upper gastrointestinal procedures confirmed the feasibility and safety of the early per-oral feeding and indicated that this regimen may be associated with enhanced recovery and reduction of hospital costs.

10.9.2 Drains and Nasogastric Tubes

Nasogastric tubes have traditionally been used for decompression after gastric surgery and still remain a routine part of the postoperative care in many centers. It has been a common belief that this could prevent aspiration and reduce postoperative ileus and anastomotic breakdown. A meta-analysis of randomized trials comparing nasogastric/nasojejunal decompression versus no decompression has demonstrated shorter time to flatus, no difference in anastomotic leak rate, pulmonary complications, hospital stay, morbidity and mortality rates in the no-tube group. Multiple studies have demonstrated that drains are unnecessary after gastrointestinal surgery and that prolonged use of urinary bladder catheters should not be recommended [19]. A systematic review assessed the value of prophylactic drainage in gastrointestinal surgery indicated that drains did not reduce complication or may even be harmful after hepatic, colorectal surgery and after appendectomy [20]. Similar observations have been made in pancreatic surgery [21]. However, the authors identified no randomized controlled or prospective trials assessing the value of prophylactic drainage in upper gastrointestinal surgery. One of the advantages of the minimally invasive approach is the low morbidity of early diagnostic laparoscopy in case of clinical suspicion of anastomotic leak. Therefore, the potential benefits of prophylactic drainage after laparoscopic resections may be limited.

10.9.3 Postoperative Pain Control

Effective analgesia is one of the key components in the postoperative care. Epidural analgesia has been demonstrated to be the most effective method after open abdominal procedures. In our experience non-steroidal anti inflammatory drugs and acetaminophen with supplementation of intravenous morphine if needed can provide adequate pain control after laparoscopic resection.

References

1. Altekruse SF, Kosary CL, Krapcho M, Neyman N, Aminou R, Waldron W, Ruhl J, Howlader N, Tatalovich Z, Cho H, Mariotto A, Eisner MP, Lewis DR, Cronin K, Chen HS, Feuer EJ, Stinchcomb DG, Edwards BK, editors. SEER Cancer Statistics Review, 1975–2007. Bethesda: National Cancer Institute; 2010. http://seer.cancer.gov/csr/1975_2007/, based on November 2009 SEER data submission, posted to the SEER web site.
2. Collins BJ, Miyashita T, Schweitzer M, Magnuson T, Harmon J. Gastric bypass: why Roux-en-Y? a review of experimental data. Arch Surg. 2007;142(10):1000–3.
3. Csendes A, Braghetto I, Burdiles P, Korn O. Roux en Y limb diversion as the first option for patients who have Barrett's esophagus. Chest Surg Clin N Am. 2002;12(1):157–84.
4. Grantcharov TP, Kehlet H. Laparoscopic gastric surgery in an enhanced recovery programme. Br J Surg. Article first published online: 21 Jul 2010. doi:10.1002/bjs.7184.
5. Cuschieri A. Gastric resections. In: Cuschieri A, editor. The SAGES manual – fundamentals of laparoscopy, thoracoscopy, and GI endoscopy. New York: Springer Science & Business Media; 2006.
6. Saidi RF, Remine SG, Dudrick PS, Hanna NN. Is there a role for palliative gastrectomy in patients with stage IV gastric cancer. World J Surg. 2006;30(1):21–7.
7. Pugliese R, Maggioni D, Sansonna F, Scandroglio I, Ferrari GC, Di Lernia S, Costanzi A, Pauna J, de Martini P. Total and subtotal laparoscopic gastrectomy for adenocarcinoma. Surg Endosc. 2007;21(1):21–7.
8. Mori Y, Arita T, Shimoda K, Yasuda K, Yoshida T, Kitano S. Effect of periodic endoscopy for gastric cancer on early detection and improvement of survival. Gastric Cancer. 2001;4(3):132–6.
9. Kim JH, Park SH, Hong HS, et al. CT Gastrography. Abdom Imaging. 2005;30:509–17.
10. Kim AY, Kim HJ, Ha K. Gastric cancer by multidetector row CT: preoperative staging. Abdom Imaging. 2005;30:465–72.
11. Kim JH, Eun HW, Hong SS, et al. Early gastric cancer: virtual gastroscopy. Abdom Imaging. 2006;31:507–13.
12. Dulucq JL, Wintringer P, Perissat J, Mahajna A. Completely laparoscopic total and partial gastrectomy for benign and malignant diseases: a single institute's prospective analysis. J Am Coll Surg. 2005;200(2):191–7.
13. Salvon-Harman JC, Cady B, Nikulasson S, Khettry U, Stone MD, Lavin P. Shifting proportions of gastric adenocarcinomas. Arch Surg. 1994;129:381–9.
14. Nakajima T. Gastric cancer treatment guideline in Japan. Gastric Cancer. 2002;5(1):1–5.

15. Papachristou DN, Fortner JG. Adenocarcinoma of the gastric cardia: the choice of gastrectomy. Ann Surg. 1996;192:58–64.
16. Harrison LE, Karpeh MS, Brennan MF. Total gastrectomy is not necessary for proximal gastric cancer. Surgery. 1998;123:127–30.
17. Adachi Y, Inoue T, Hagino Y, Shiraishi N, Shimoda K, Kitano S. Surgical results of proximal gastrectomy for early-stage gastric cancer: jejunal interposition and gastric tube reconstruction. Gastric Cancer. 1999;2:40–50.
18. Shiraishi N, Adachi Y, Kitano S, Kakisako K, Inomata M, Yasuda K. Clinical outcome of proximal versus total gastrectomy for proximal gastric cancer. World J Surg. 2002;26:1150–4.
19. Kehlet H, Wilmore DW. Evidence-based surgical care and the evolution of fast-track surgery. Ann Surg. 2008;248:189–98.
20. Petrowsky H, Demartines N, Valentin R, et al. Evidence-based value of prophylactic drainage in gastrointestinal surgery. A systematic review and meta-analyses. Ann Surg. 2004;240:1074–84.
21. Kawai M, Tani M, Terasawa H, et al. Early removal of prophylactic drains reduces the risk of intra-abdominal infections in patients with pancreatic head resection: prospective study for 104 consecutive patients. Ann Surg. 2006;244:1–7.

11 Laparoscopic Repair of Perforated Peptic Ulcer

Jonathan B. Yuval and Amir Szold

11.1 Introduction

Save for perforated appendicitis, perforated peptic ulcer (PPU) is the most common intra-abdominal hollow viscus perforation that requires surgical intervention [1]. The estimated annual incidence is approximately 5–10/100,000 [2, 3]. Perforation occurs in 2–10 % of patients with peptic ulcer disease and is the leading cause of death due to PUD [3].

Ulcer perforation is most commonly found in the anterior portion of the first part of the duodenum and usually is of a diameter smaller than 5 mm [3].

11.2 Clinical Presentation and Diagnosis

Patients with perforated peptic ulcers most commonly present with sudden severe epigastric pain that may radiate to the shoulder and is often associated with nausea and vomiting [3]. Presentation also typically entails acute abdomen, peritonitis and free air in abdominal plain films and/or in computerized tomography. Diagnosis is made both clinically and radiologically.

11.3 Pre-operative Management

Patients diagnosed with PPU should receive a well-monitored fluid resuscitation as well as intravenous antibiotics [4]. A naso-gastric tube is commonly recommended and narcotics may be administered for pain after the diagnosis is made. Following these initial stabilizing measures these patients should be promptly taken to the operating room.

11.4 Patient Selection

The Boey's shock score on admission (i.e. blood pressure below 90 mmHg, ASA class III or IV, and symptoms present for over 24 h) has been found reliable in selecting patients inappropriate for a laparoscopic intervention. If the patient has a Boey's score of 3, is over 70 years old or if symptoms have been present for over 24 h regardless of Boey's score, intervention by laparotomy should be considered [5].

11.5 Patient Positioning and Room Preparation

Positioning for PPU repair is similar to that used in laparoscopic cholecystectomy. A comfortable supine position with slight reverse Trendelenburg draws the operative field from under the costal margin and avoids leakage of gastric contents into the subphrenic space. Some authors advocate the use of a Lloyd-Davis position allowing for the surgeon to stand between the patient's legs [4] (Fig. 11.1).

11.6 Trocar Position and Laparoscope Angle

A 10 mm Trocar should be placed in the umbilicus for the video laparoscope. Additional working ports should be placed in the right and left midclavicular lines at the level of the transpyloric plain [4, 6] (Fig. 11.2). If needed an additional subxiphoid or right lateral subcostal trocar can be inserted for liver retraction. Alternatively a totally internal liver retractor such as the Endolift can be used [7]. An angled laparoscope (30° or 45°) is more commonly preferred for optimal visualization [4].

J.B. Yuval, MD
Department of Surgery, Hadassah-Hebrew University Medical Center, Jerusalem, Israel

A. Szold, MD (✉)
Assia Medical Group, Assuta Medical Center, Tel Aviv, Israel
e-mail: amikisz@gmail.com

H.J. Bonjer (ed.), *Surgical Principles of Minimally Invasive Procedures*, DOI 10.1007/978-3-319-43196-3_11

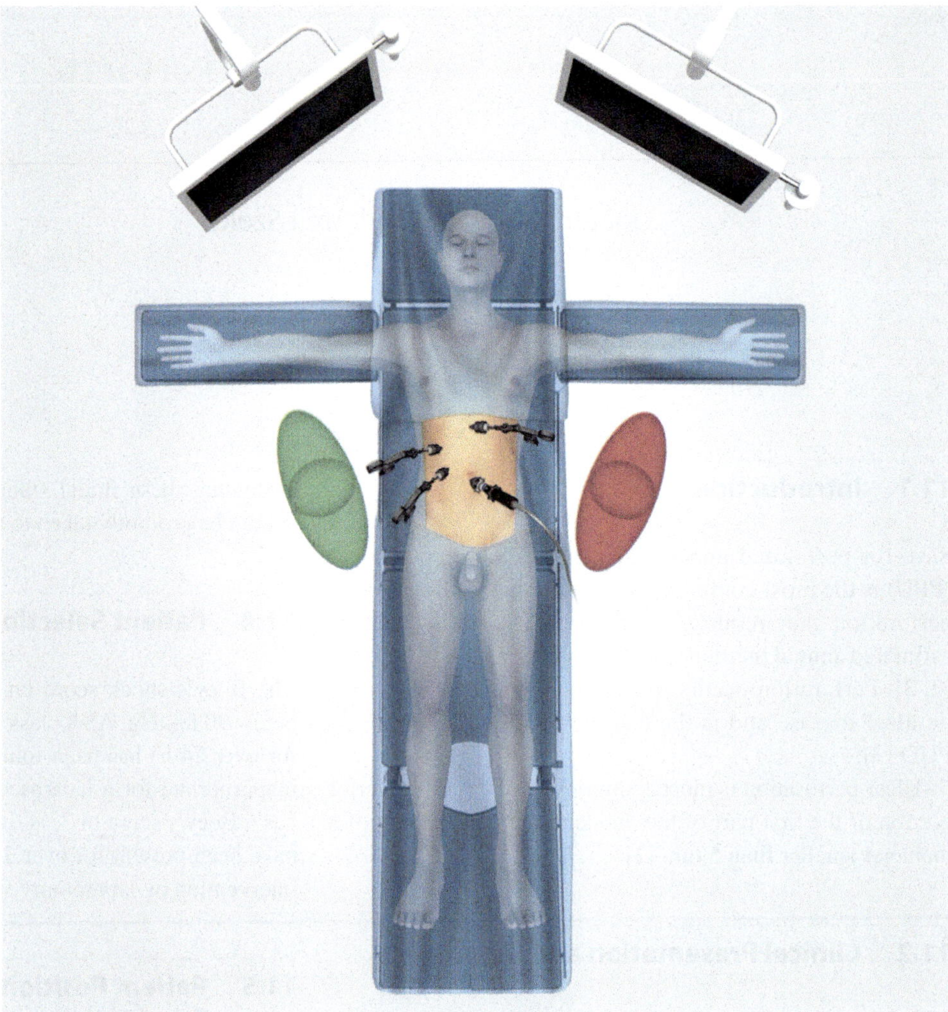

Fig. 11.1 Patient positioning for laparoscopic repair of perforated duodenal ulcer

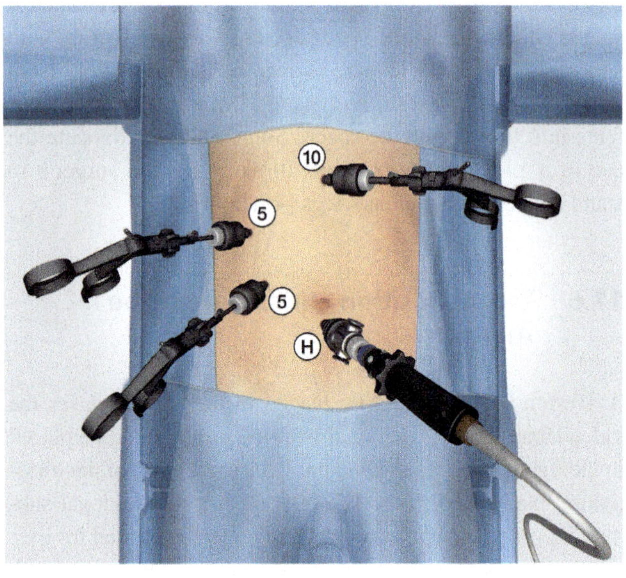

Fig. 11.2 Trocar positioning for laparoscopic closure of perforated duodenal ulcer

11.7 Details of the Procedure

The entire abdominal cavity should be thoroughly explored and the abdominal fluid sampled for microbiological culture. A warm isotonic solution should be used in large quantities to carefully lavage the abdominal cavity and suction out all exudate and food particles. Special care should be taken to expose and lavage the pelvis and subphrenic spaces, and open and drain possible inter-loop pockets of debris. If the omentum or liver have sealed off the perforation, it is advisable not to move them until lavage of the entire abdominal cavity has been performed in order to avoid any unnecessary soiling. The area of perforation should be thoroughly irrigated to wash off any fibrin or debris.

Gentle dissection should be used to expose the pyloroduodenal area to identify the perforation and any attached omentum or liver gently pulled off. Gentle compression of the antrum with an atraumatic instrument may aid in finding the location of the perforation by causing air bubbles to escape through it.

Identifying a perforation may not be straightforward. For example, a perforation of the dorsal stomach body may only become apparent after entering the lesser sac through the gastro-colic ligament. In many cases it is advisable to insert a liver retractor, which may entail insertion of an additional trocar as previously explained.

After the site of perforation has been verified, the size and probable etiology of the perforation is assessed. Due to the likelihood of a malignant perforation in gastric ulcers, a small biopsy from the margin of the ulcer should be taken before repair. If an obvious tumor is visualized and the patient's condition permits, a definitive procedure should be considered.

Two techniques are commonly used to close the perforation. In perforations smaller than 5 mm, a primary closure may be used with additional placement of omentum on top of the repair. In larger perforations it is commonly impossible to close the perforation by sutures because of edema and tissue fragility, and an omentopexy is required. A pedicled omental flap is placed on top of the perforation and secured with 3 or 4 horizontal sutures 10 mm from the edge of the ulcer. The sutures should be placed parallel to the pyloric plain in order to avoid stenosis or stricture. A pedicled flap from the falciform ligament may be used if the omentum is insufficient [8]. After completion of the omentopexy, air should be insufflated via naso-gastric tube to assess patency of the closure. In most cases it is advisable to leave a soft drain near the repair. If the perforation is bigger than 10 mm, is extra-pyloric or if technical difficulties are encountered consider conversion to laparotomy.

11.8 Post-operative Management

The patient is placed in Fowler's position. Naso-gastric suctioning and intravenous antibiotics are continued for several days until there is reasonable assurance that the pylorus is not obstructed by edema. Intravenous proton pump inhibitors are given as well. Fluid volume is maintained by intravenous fluids. After 72 h some perform upper gastro-intestinal radiography, if normal the patient can resume oral nutrition.

Abdominal abscesses can often complicate the post-operative period and should be treated accordingly. 6–8 weeks after surgery an esophago-gastro-duodenoscopy should be performed to assess ulcer healing and presence of Helicobacter Pylori (H. Pylori). Consider biopsy if healing is not adequate to rule out malignancy and eradicate H. Pylori if found.

If multiple ulcers were found in surgery, or if hypercalcemia is noted on laboratory results, consider eventual gastrin measurement. For accurate gastrin level testing the patient should not be taking any proton pump inhibitors.

11.9 Complications

30 day post-operative mortality is estimated at around 10% for hospitalized patients with PPU [9], but can be as high as 50% for patients with a Boey's score of 3 [9]. Morbidity is estimated at around 30%, the most common complications being respiratory deterioration, abdominal abscess and wound infection [9]. Additional common complications include ileus and post-operative ventral hernia. Suboptimal surgical technique can cause gastric outlet obstruction. Conversion rate to laparotomy is around 10% [1, 6]. Common reasons for conversion are inability to find or clearly visualize the ulcer defect and a large perforation diameter [6].

References

1. Sanabria A, Villegas MI, Morales Uribe CH, Laparoscopic repair for perforated peptic ulcer disease. Cochrane Database Syst Rev. 2013;2:CD004778.
2. Thorsen K, et al. Trends in diagnosis and surgical management of patients with perforated peptic ulcer. J Gastrointest Surg. 2011;15(8):1329–35.
3. Bertleff MJ, Lange JF. Perforated peptic ulcer disease: a review of history and treatment. Dig Surg. 2010;27(3):161–9.
4. Siu WT, et al. Laparoscopic repair for perforated peptic ulcer: a randomized controlled trial. Ann Surg. 2002;235(3):313–9.
5. Agresta F, et al. Laparoscopic approach to acute abdomen from the Consensus Development Conference of the Societa Italiana di Chirurgia Endoscopica e nuove tecnologie (SICE), Associazione Chirurghi Ospedalieri Italiani (ACOI), Societa Italiana di Chirurgia (SIC), Societa Italiana di Chirurgia d'Urgenza e del Trauma (SICUT), Societa Italiana di Chirurgia nell'Ospedalita Privata (SICOP), and the European Association for Endoscopic Surgery (EAES). Surg Endosc. 2012;26(8):2134–64.
6. Bertleff MJ, et al. Randomized clinical trial of laparoscopic versus open repair of the perforated peptic ulcer: the LAMA Trial. World J Surg. 2009;33(7):1368–73.
7. Elazary R, et al. A novel totally internal laparoscopic liver retractor. Surg Laparosc Endosc Percutan Tech. 2013;23(6):e222–4.
8. Munro WS, Bajwa F, Menzies D. Laparoscopic repair of perforated duodenal ulcers with a falciform ligament patch. Ann R Coll Surg Engl. 1996;78(4):390–1.
9. Lohsiriwat V, Prapasrivorakul S, Lohsiriwat D. Perforated peptic ulcer: clinical presentation, surgical outcomes, and the accuracy of the Boey scoring system in predicting postoperative morbidity and mortality. World J Surg. 2009;33(1):80–5.

Part V

Bariatric Surgery

Selection of Bariatric Procedures

12

G.-B. Cadière, Jacques Himpens, and Ramon Vilallonga

12.1 Introduction

The socioeconomic circumstances in the Western nations, as well as the profusion of food have drastically changed in the second half of the last century. As a result, the prevalence of morbid obesity has increased rapidly and in some countries obesity has reached an epidemic magnitude. Obesity is a multifactorial entity with aggregation of excessive body fat leading to harm to general health. Basically, morbid obesity is based on an imbalance between calorie uptake and calorie consumption. The causes for this imbalance may differ from patient to patient. For an exact definition/classification and gradation of obesity, the body mass index (BMI) was introduced. BMI is calculated as weight in kilograms divided by the square of height in meters (kg/m^2.). Based on BMI, obesity is divided into three severity grades: A BMI of 30–35 is considered as grade I obesity, 35–40 as grade II and a BMI >40 as grade III.

The basic treatment of obesity is psychological therapy, diet measures and increasing physical activities.

For patients with a BMI > than 40, the only efficient treatment for weight loss at long term is surgery. The endpoint in evaluating all bariatric surgery is: does the procedure allow the patient to resume physical activities and to maintain a healthy attitude towards food.

Laparoscopic bariatric surgery has been shown to be a safe and effective treatment option causing long-term weight loss in the morbidly obese patient

G.-B. Cadière, MD, PhD
European School of Laparosocpic Surgery, Centre Hospitalier Universitaire Saint-Pierre, Brussels, Belgium

J. Himpens, MD, PhD (✉)
Obesity Department, AZ Sint Blasius, Dendermonde, Belgium
e-mail: Jacques_himpens@hotmail.com

R. Vilallonga, MD, PhD
Endocrine-Metabolic and Bariatric Surgery Unit, Robotic Surgery, EAC-BS Center of Excellence, Vall d'Hebron Hospital, Universitat Autònoma de Barcelona, Barcelona, Spain
e-mail: vilallongapuy@hotmail.com

12.2 Surgical Indications

The selection criteria for bariatric surgery are clearly defined by EAES guidelines.

General indication: Obesity surgery should be considered in adult patients with a documented BMI greater than or equal to 35 kg/m^2 and related comorbidity, or a BMI of at least 40 kg/m^2. All patients must fully understand the proposed procedure and agree with postoperative care. Adults with a BMI between 30 and 35 accompanied by substantial obesity-related comorbidity or after prolonged medical treatment should undergo obesity surgery only in the context of controlled clinical trials.

Based on this precondition the following directives are further formulated by the obesity societies:

1. Age of the patients is between 18 and 65 years.
2. The patients must have received intensive medical/conservative treatment for weight loss in an obesity treatment center.
3. The patients should have undergone conservative therapy for weight reduction under medical supervision with all suitable non-surgical therapies for a minimum period of 12 months.
4. Patients with an underlying endocrinological disorder should be excluded.
5. Patients should be suitable candidates for general anaesthesia.
6. Patients should be aware of the long-term (if necessary lifelong) need for medical follow-up.
7. Patients should be willing to change existing eating habits and life style.

National and international professional societies have defined the following as absolute contraindications for a bariatric procedure:

1. Abuse of alcohol or drugs
2. Concomitant psychiatric comorbidities such as schizophrenia, psychotic condition

H.J. Bonjer (ed.), *Surgical Principles of Minimally Invasive Procedures*, DOI 10.1007/978-3-319-43196-3_12

3. Noncompliance with regard to the necessary lifestyle modifications as well as the prescribed medical aftercare
4. Manifest malignancies
5. Manifest esophagogastric diseases (e.g. gastric ulcer)
6. Limited tolerance to anaesthesia
7. Pregnancy

12.3 Choice of Bariatric Procedure

Available procedures in our department are: adjustable band gastroplasty (AGB), sleeve gastrectomy (SG), Roux-en-Y gastric bypass (RYGB) and biliopancreatic diversion with duodenal switch (DS).

There is no consensus on the criteria of choice for one bariatric procedure over another.

The first laparoscopic bariatric procedure was realized in October 1992, and consisted of an AGB. The different procedures experienced successive waves of popularity in Europe: the AGB reached a peak in terms of number of procedures performed in 2004, only to decline rapidly to the benefit of the RYGB that reached a peak in 2007. In turn, the RYGB witnessed a decline from 2010 to the benefit of SG. Conversely, for the DS, the specific indication of the procedure has limited the numbers throughout the years.

There are four criteria to evaluate a bariatric procedure :

1. long term efficacy in terms of weight loss : the procedure should in addition allow a healthy attitude towards food
2. operative mortality and morbidity (MM): should be less than the MM of the obesity disease.
3. late complications including (but not restricted to) GERD, pouch dilation, band erosion, marginal ulcer, stenosis and internal hernia
4. quality of life evaluated by subjective and objective parameters including the number and severity of reinterventions

Based on these criteria one can identify the procedures as follows:

1. efficacy in terms of weight loss : weight loss varies with the performed procedure, with in decreasing order of efficacy the DS, the RYGB, the SG and the AGB; moreover the latter two procedures may facilitate poor alimentary behavior
2. operative MM : procedures involving stapling and/or an anastomosis are likely to carry more morbidity and mortality than AGB. MM figures are, in declining order, linked with DS, RYGB, SG and AGB
3. late complications are not amenable to be classified as such because of the inherent complications characteristic for each procedure:
   For the AGB: band erosion and pouch dilation with GERD
   For the SG: GERD
   For the RYGB: anastomotic ulcer and stenosis; dumping, no longer considered a desired side effect, nutritional deficiencies
   For the DS: protein malnutrition and nutritional deficiencies.
4. quality of life : the procedures may be ranked in decreasing order : RYGB, SG, AGB. There are to our knowledge no data available yet for the DS.

The above mentioned criteria will orient the surgeon in his/her choice of procedure for the individual bariatric patient depending on the patient's characteristics.

Hence, in presence of severe eating disorders such as binge eating (BED), a merely restrictive procedure (AGB, SG) should not be chosen and a malabsorptive operation (DS) preferred.

In case of GERD, SG and AGB should not be chosen because they may worsen the condition, wheres the RYGB is known to improve GERD.

In case of type 2 diabetes (T2DM) (likely the most weight sensitive comorbidity), the most effective procedure should be favoured, i.e. DS and RYGB

In case of super-obesity (BMI >50 kg/m^2) the more effective procedure (DS, RYGB) will be chosen.

Decision of final patient procedure selection will additionally depend on the surgeon's experience, and on the patient's choice (Fig. 12.1).

12.4 Preoperative Assessement

Assessment and preparation of the bariatric patient requires a multidisciplinary team approach.

Psychological assessment will allow to rule out binge eating disorder (BED) and to detect anxiety and depression.

Dietary counseling will document past and current eating behavior (grazing, volume eating, sweets eating) and provide the history of weight loss.

Medical history must include previous surgeries and systemic diseases (such as arterial hypertension (AHT), T2DM, sleep apnea), life style and physical activity and present medication that might interfere with the surgery as well as with the weight loss process. Medication that might provide an issue is: anticoagulant drugs, orexogenic drugs such as antidepressants and drugs that cause weight gain such as Metformin and other antidiabetic drugs. Nicotine and alcohol abuse must be ruled out.

Physical examination shall include recording of weight, height (and BMI), neck circumference, blood pressure, examination of existing scars on the abdomen, and heart and lung auscultation

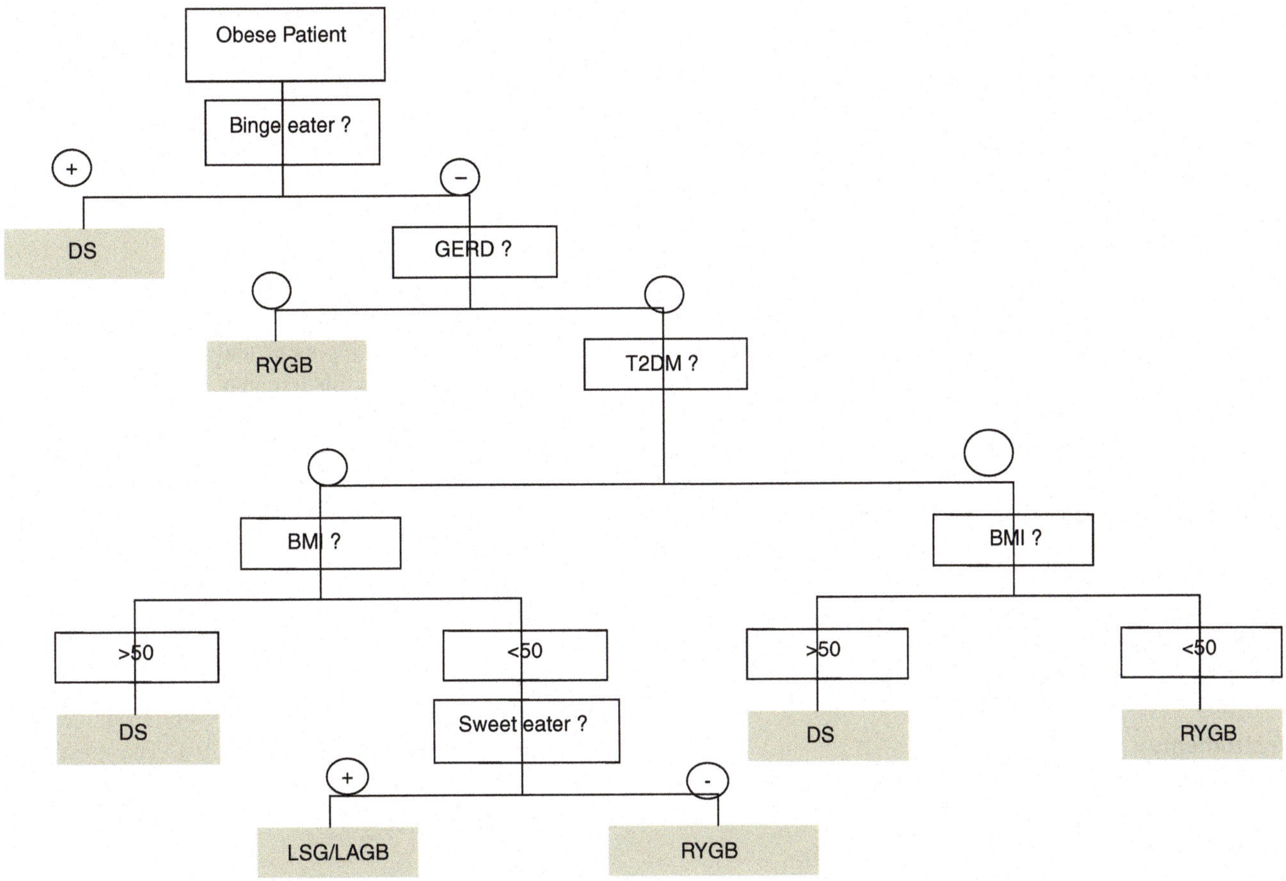

Fig. 12.1 Algorithm

Complete blood work should include: hemoglobin and hematocrit, thyroid hormones, serum cortisol, serum cholesterol and serum triglycerides, iron, Calcium, vitamin D and parathyroid hormone (PTH), liver function tests, Zinc, Magnesium, Selenium, vitamin A, K, E, B1, B6 and B12, fasting plasma Glucose, glycated hemoglobin A1c (HbA1c), Insulin and C peptide (to differentiate T2DM from T1DM).

Cardiovascular and pulmonary assessment is mandatory. This may include in selected patients a cardiac stress test, which should help exclude any contraindication to anesthesia, an echocardiogram to assess left ventricle ejection fraction, pulmonary function tests and arterial blood gas analysis.

An ultrasound examination of the abdomen should be done routinely merely to evaluate liver steatosis and to rule out gall bladder stones. If there are unclear findings, a CT scan or MRI should be performed. All patients should be screened for sleep apnea and treated consequently if needed.

Upper gastrointestinal evaluation should include an esophagogastroduodenoscopy with biopsies of the gastroesophageal junction and stomach to detect esophageal mucosal abnormalities (e.g. reflux esophagitis, Barrett's mucosa, esophageal/gastric malignancies, the presence of Helicobacter Pylori (HP)) and a barium swallow to detect hiatal hernia.

12.5 Patient Preparation

A good patient preparation is of the utmost importance to reduce the surgical aggression. Drugs interfering with the surgical procedure (anticoagulants) and substances of abuse (nicotine and alcohol) must be discontinued. Comorbidities should be addressed as needed. T2DM, arterial hypertension should be stabilized by adequate medication; sleep apnea should be treated preoperatively by a continuous positive pressure device (CPAP).

Patients routinely are put on a protein diet for at least 7 days prior to surgery to reduce steatosis

12.5.1 Different Types of Procedures

12.5.1.1 Adjustable Band

Principle of the Procedure

The satiety center is stimulated by gastric distension and suppresses the feeling of hunger. However, when one eats too fast, the satiety center does not obtain appropriate activation at an optimal time. The feeling of hunger then persists and encourages to continuing eating. With time the stomach adapts and becomes progressively distended which allows the individual to ingest increasingly larger quantities of food without feeling full. The principle of AGB is to reduce the stomach's volume by dividing it into two parts, similar to an hour glass. With AGB the first compartment has a volume of 25 cc, the equivalent of two tablespoons. The second compartment comprises the rest of the stomach. As soon as one ingests two spoonfuls, the first compartment is filled and one experiences a feeling of fullness. Since it takes a long time for the first compartment to empty because of the narrow outlet, more food can only be ingested after substantial time has elapsed. One must therefore eat at a much slower pace. Because of the slower emptying pace, the satiety center has the time to be stimulated. As the hunger sensation is no longer present, overall food intake is reduced. The outlet size of the first compartment can be adjusted as needed and the pace at which the stomach empties depends on the outlet size, as determined by the status of inflation of the band cuff, depending on the amount of fluid injected into a subcutaneous port which is connected to the cuff.

Instruments

- 5 trocars: 3 trocars of 5 mm, 1 trocar of 10 mm, 1 trocar of 15 mm
- 30° optical system
- Veres needle
- band
- 4 atraumatic grasping forceps
- coagulating hook
- suction device
- scissors
- needle-holder
- two stitches of Silk or Prolene 2/0
- two stitches of Ethibond 2/0

Technique

Patient, Team and Trocars Position

The patient is positioned supine with the legs apart and is carefully strapped to the operation table. The arms are placed in abduction. Shoulder supports are placed as well and extreme care is taken to pad the pressure points and articulations with foam cushions. The sequential calf compression devices are placed around the legs and activated. The surgeon (5) stands between the patient's legs, the cameraman to the patients right (C), the assistant to the patient's left (A). Abdominal insufflation up to 16 mmHg is obtained with the insertion of a Veres needle at the left upper quadrant, or, alternatively, at the umbilicus. Trocars are placed as follows: a 10 mm trocar (Ti) for the optical system (30° angled scope) just to the left of the midline, 10 cm distal to the xyphoid process; a 15 mm trocar (T2) on the left anterior axillary line 2 cm below the costal margin; a 5 mm trocar (T3) in the left upper quadrant on the mid clavicular line and between the 1″ and 2′d trocar; a 5 mm trocar (T4) in the right upper quadrant on the right mid clavicular line; a 5 mm trocar (T5), used for liver retraction, just distal and to the left of the xyphoid process.

Dissection of the Phrenogastric Ligament and of the Retrogastric Area

The grasper (T2) pulls the gastric fundus caudally in order to put the phrenogastric ligament under tension. A small window is now created in this ligament using the coagulating hook (T3). Location of this window is usually half way between the upper pole of the spleen and the esophagus just to the left side of the left crus (A). The gastrohepatic ligament is opened widely. The base of the right crus covered by the peritoneal sheet (posterior layer of the gastrohepatic ligament) is identified. The peritoneal sheet is incised (B).

Retrogastric Tunnel

A grasper (14) is advanced under direct vision from the right crus to the left staying close to the hiatus. The grasper is advanceed until its tip becomes visible in the dissection area of the phrenogastric ligament.

Introduction and Placement of the Band

An adjustable band with its tubing is introduced into the abdominal cavity through the 15 mm port (12). The band is grasped by the grasping forceps (14) and looped around the stomach at the level of the dissection. The tip of the tubing is introduced in the locking area of the band.

Calibration and Suture Stabilization of the Band

The anaesthesiologist introduces a balloon tiped orogastric tube inside the stomach, and 25 cc of air is insufflated in the balloon. The tube is pulled back until it fits snugly below the gastro-esophageal junction (A). The surgeon can now be ascertained of the correct positioning of the band, and the band is tightened around the stomach and locked. Four to five stitches (Silk or Prolene 2/0) are placed between the serosa of the stomach just above and below the band to avoid slipping (BC).

Placement and Injection of the Port

The 15 mm port is removed, and the non-kinking tube is cut to an appropriate length and connected to the injection port (A). The port is buried, convex side up, and stitched (Ethibond 2/0) to the parietal fascia overlying the costal margin to the left (B). The band is left deflated. Alternatively, a minimal amount of methylene blue can be infused into the band through the port, in order to facilitate subsequent fill-up sessions.

12.6 Postoperative Management

First postoperative day: a gastrograffin swallow is performed and provided good passage is demonstrated and the band is proven to be in a correct position, the patient can be discharged from the hospital.

The adjustment of the band is performed by the radiologist as it requires puncture under fluoroscopic guidance. Fill up sessions start 1 month postoperatively and are repeated as needed. The volume of injected fluid will depend on the pace of clearance of ingested contrast material. The band insufflation will be adjusted based on complications (reflux, food intolerance), on the obtained weight loss and on the radiographical findings

12.6.1 Gastric Sleeve

12.6.1.1 Principle of the Procedure

Sleeve gastrectomy is mainly a restrictive procedure of the stomach, aiming at making a gastric tube of 100–150 mL, with the preservation of the antrum. The mechanism of weight loss is to reduce the intake of food, by volume restriction and by reduction of appetite linked to a reduced ghrelin production. Other gastrointestinal hormones may intervene as well.

12.6.1.2 Instruments

- 5 trocars : 2 trocars of 5 mm, 1 trocar of 10 mm, and 2 trocars of 12 mm
- 30° optical system
- Veres needle
- 4 atraumatic grasping forceps (2 with 5–10 cm marks)
- coagulating hook
- suction device
- scissors
- needle-holder (5 and 10 mm)
- .1 Harmonic scalpel/Ligasure
- 60 mm (45 mm optional) linear stapler (5–6 blue/green/black cartridges)
- one or two stitches of PDS 1
- one stitch of Vicryl 2/0 and of Vicryl1

12.6.1.3 Technique

Patient, Team and Trocars Position

The patient is positioned supine with the legs apart. The patient is carefully strapped to the operation table and the arms are placed in abduction. Shoulder supports are placed and extreme care is taken to pad the pressure points and joints with foam cushions. The sequential calf compression devices are placed around the patient's legs and are activated. The patient is positioned in slight reversed Trendelenburg position with a 10° tilt. The surgeon (S) stands between the patient's legs, the cameraman to the patient's right (C) and the assistant to the patient's left (A). Abdominal insufflation up to 16 mmHg is obtained with the insertion of a Veres needle at the left upper quadrant, or at the umbilicus. Trocars are placed as follows: a 10 mm trocar (Ti) 20 cm distal to the xyphoid process for the 30° optical system; a 5 mm trocar (T2) on the left anterior axillary line, 5 cm distal to the costal margin; a 12 mm trocar (T3) in the left upper quadrant on the mid clavicular line just between the 1″ and the 2″d trocars; a 12 mm trocar (T4) in the right upper quadrant on the right mid clavicular line; a 5 mm trocar (T5), used for liver retraction, just distal and to the left of the xyphoid process.

First Technique

After identification of the pylrus, an area some 3–4 cm proximal to it is scored by cautery. The lesser sac is accessed through a window made in the greater omentum, across from the gastric angle, close to the greater curve of the stomach, within the epiploic arch. This window is extended in a caudal direction in order to devascularize the greater curve up to the marking (A). The dissection subsequently proceeds cranially in order to completely dissect the omentum off the greater curve. The dissection thus reaches the base of the left diaphragmatic pillar. The base of the right diaphragmatic pillar should be dissected as well to rule out all potential hiatal hernia. All retrogastric adhesions must be divided (B). A first firing of linear stapler (black or green load) (T4) divides the greater curve in the direction of the crow's foot. Other firings of linear stapler (black or green load) (13) transect the stomach parallel to the lesser curve, from the antrum up to the angle of His. Before the firing of the stapler, the anesthesiologist advances an orogastric tube of 34 Fr, in order to guide the gastric section (C). A running suture (PDS 1) reinforces the staple line (D). Alternatively, buttress material may be inserted on the staple loads The resected greater curve is extracted through the 12 mm left trocar site (T3).

Second Technique

After marking the stomach and opening the lesser sac as in the first technique, (A) a window is made in the greater omentum, close to the greater curve, across from the gastric angulus. The greater curvature is devascularized in a caudad direction until the score marks are reached. The stapler is inserted and using black or green load the stomach is transected, hereby guided by an orogastric tube of 34 French introduced by the anesthesiologist, but only up to the level of opening of the lesser sac. Further firings of the linear stapler (black or green load) are kept parallel to the lesser curve. All posterior gastric adhesions are divided. in the direction of the angle of His (C). Before the last firing of stapler (usually green load) (13) the angle of His is freed. In cases where no staple buttressing has been used, the staple line is reinforced by a running suture (PDS 1). The greater omentum is dissected from the now separated greater curve of the stomach, using the coagulating hook or the Harmonic scalpel or Ligasure (0). The resected stomach is then extracted through T3.

Leak-Test

The patient is placed in the Trendelenburg position. The operating field is immersed in saline solution. Compressed air is insufflated by the anaesthesiologist into the gastric sleeve. The absence of air bubbles is testimony to the integrity of the sleeve. Importantly, this manoeuvre allows to assess good symmetry of the sleeve as well. The procedure is concluded with the placement of a nasogastric tube and of a drain along the sleeve up to the upper pole of the spleen and the 12 mm left trocar site (T3) is closed with absorbable suture (Vicryl 1).

Postoperative Management

On the first postoperative day a methylen blue test is performed and provided there is no evidence of a leak, the nasogastric tube is removed and the patient allowed to drink water. On the third postoperative day the drain is taken out and the patient is discharged.

The patient is restricted to a semi-liquid diet for 1 week, followed by a pureed diet for another 4 weeks. An office visit is scheduled for around that time. When assessment is positive, the patient is advanced to a regular diet. Exercising is encouraged from the fifth postoperative week onwards. Patients are instructed to take either an H2 blocker or proton pump inhibitor, usually for up to 6 months.

12.6.2 Gastric Bypass

12.6.2.1 Principle of the Procedure

Biliopancreatic diversion with duodenal switch is primarily a malabsorptive procedure. The biliopancreatic diversion, pioneered in Genoa (Italy), is widely used in Europe and relatively sparingly in the United States. The duodenal switch is an adaptation of the biliopancreatic diversion developed in Canada and America. It consists of a combination of a sleeve gastrectomy and a biliopancreatic diversion. A Roux-en-Y limb is anastomosed to the first part of the duodenum at one end, and to the transeeted bowel some 75–100 cm proximal to the ileocaecal valve at its other end. With the duodenal switch the mechanism of weight loss is double:

1. sleeve gastrectomy ensures restriction in the amount of calories taken by mouth
2. the functional shortening capacity of the bowel reduces the absorption capacity of the latter since the exchange surface is smaller. Moreover fat can only be digested once the biliary and pancreatic juices are mixed with the food which obviously occurs only quite distally.

12.6.2.2 Instruments

- 5 trocars: 2 trocars of 5 mm, 1 trocar of 10 mm, and 2 trocars of 12 mm
- 30° optical system
- Veres needle
- 4 atraumatic grasping forceps (2 with 5–10 cm marks)
- coagulating hook
- suction device
- scissors
- needle-holder (5 and 10 mm)
- .1 Harmonic scalpel/Ligasure
- 60 mm (45 mm optional) linear stapler (5–6 blue/green/black cartridges)
- four stitches of PDS 2/0
- one stitch of Silk 2/0
- 2 stitches of Prolene 1

Patient Position and Disposition of Trocars

The patient is positioned supine with the legs apart and is carefully strapped to the OR table. The sequential calf compression devices are placed around the patient's legs and are activated. The surgeon stands between the patient's legs. The screen is placed above the patient's head. The patient is placed in steep reversed Trendelenburg. Abdominal insufflation up to 16 mmHg is obtained by the insertion of a Veres needle at the patient's left upper quadrant or at the umbilicus.

Trocars are placed as follows: a 10 mm trocar for the optical system, (a 30 ° angled scope) immediately to the left of the midline (trocar 1), 10 cm distal to the xyphoid, a 12 mm trocar in the right upper quadrant on the mid clavicular line (trocar 4), a 12 mm trocar in the left upper quadrant on the mid clavicular line at the same level as the optical trocar; a 5 mm trocar used for liver retraction just distal and to the left of the xyphoid (trocar 5) and finally a 5 mm trocar on the left anterior axillary line 5 mm distal to the costal margin (trocar 3).

Dissection of the His Angle

The liver is retracted with a 5 mm rod retractor inserted through the subxyphoid port. The root of the left diaphragmatic crus is exposed by caudad traction on the stomach fundus by the assistant to the patient's left, and the phrenogastric ligament is incised at the level of the angle of His with a coagulating hook (3) until visualization of the left diaphragmatic crus is obtained.

Dissection of the Lesser Curvature

Dissection is then initiated at the lesser curvature 5–6 cm under the esogastric junction. The third vessel (counting from proximal) is identified at this lesser curvature and a plane developed between Latarjet's pedicle and the serosa of the stomach. By continuing the dissection posteriorly the lesser sac is entered.

Gastric Pouch Manufacturing

The stomach is transected horizontally at that level by one firing of the linear stapler, blue load, introduced through the right upper quadrant 12 mm trocar. The posterior phrenogastric ligament is dissected until the previous dissection is reached.

The linear stapler (blue load) is introduced in the left upper quadrant 12 mm trocar and aimed from the left lateral horizontal section level towards the angle of His. Two or three vertical firings of the stapler are performed to reach the His angle. This allows for complete detachment of the gastric pouch from the remnant.

Latero Lateral Mechanical Linear Gastrojejunal Anstomosis

The transverse colon is lifted in upwards to visualize the Treitz Angle. The reversed Trendelenburg position facilitates the identification of the Treitz angle.

The intestinal loop is lifted in an ante-colic position over some 100 cm to reach the oesogastric junction. The patient is replaced in a neutral position. An opening is created in the loop with the coagulating hook which allows the introduction of a blue load linear stapler. The stapling is realized parallel and as close as possible to the vertical staple of the gastric pouch. The opening is closed with two running sutures (PDS 2.0). The superior running suture is initiated at the summit of the stapling line and comprises the gastric pouch and anastomosis stapling line.

70 cm of bowel are measured on the alimentary loop, from the gastrojejunal anastomosis. The alimentary loop at this point is secured to the biliopancreatic loop with a suture (silk 2.0). The suture is held by a grasper and is elevated to reach the upper part of the stomach.

Mechanical Side to Side Jejunojejusnostomy

A linear mechanical jejunojejunostomy is performed. The opening is closed by two converting running sutures (PDS 2.0). The jejunum in between the two anastomosis is sectioned with a linear stapler with white load.

Closure of the Mesenteric Defect and of the Petersen Space

The mesenteric defect, between the alimentary and the biliopancreatic limbs must be closed after conclusion of the jejunojejunostomy. A purse string stitch (prolene 2/0 or 1) is used for this purpose. A purse string is preferred over a running suture because it allows more mobility of the anastomosis, hence avoiding kinking which is the usual cause of blow out of the remnant stomach.

Postoperative Management

Provided there is no evidence of a leak, the patient is allowed to drink water. On the third postoperative day the patient is discharged.

The patient is restricted to a semi-liquid diet for 1 week, followed by a pureed diet for another 4 weeks. An office visit is scheduled for around that time. When assessment is positive, the patient is advanced to a regular diet. Exercising is encouraged from the fifth postoperative week onwards. Patients are instructed to take either an H2 blocker or proton pump inhibitor, usually for up to 6 months.

12.6.3 Duodenal Switch

12.6.3.1 Principle of the Procedure

Biliopancreatic diversion with duodenal switch is primarily a malabsorptive procedure. The biliopancreatic diversion (BPD), pioneered in Genoa (Italy), is performed mainly in Europe The duodenal switch is an adaptation of the BPD and was developed in Canada and America. It consists of a combination of a sleeve gastrectomy and a BPD. A Roux- limb is anastomosed to the first part of the duodenum at one end, and to the transected bowel some 75–100 cm proximal to the ileocaecal valve at its other end. With the duodenal switch the mechanism of weight loss is double :

1. sleeve gastrectomy ensures restriction in the amount of calories taken by mouth
2. the functional shortening capacity of the bowel reduces the absorption capacity of the latter since the exchange surface is smaller. Moreover fat can only be digested once the biliary and pancreatic juices are mixed with the food which obviously occurs only quite distally.

12.6.3.2 Instruments

- 6 trocars: 3 trocars of 5 mm, 1 trocar of 10 mm, and 2 loads linear stapler
- 30° degree optical system
- Veres needle
- 4 atraumatic grasping forceps (2 with 5–10 cm marks)
- coagulating hook
- suction device
- scissors
- needle-holder (5 and 10 mm)
- Harmonic scalpel/Ligasure
- 60 mm (45 mm optional) linear stapler (6–7 black/green cartridges and 3–4 white cartridges)
- two stitches of PDS 1
- two stitches of PDS 2/0
- two stitches of Prolene 1 or 2/0
- one stitch of white Vicryl 3/0
- one stitch of Silk 210

- one stitch of Vicryl 2/0 and 1
- one stitch of Ethibond 2

12.6.3.3 Technique

Patient, Team and Trocars Position

The patient is placed in the supine position with legs apart. The patient is carefully strapped to the operation table and the arms are placed in abduction. Sequential calf compression is used. Shoulder supports are placed as well and extreme care is taken to pad the pressure points and joints with foam cushions. The table is tilted head up at some 10°. The surgeon (5) stands between the patient's legs, the cameraman to the patient's right (C) and the assistant to the patient's [eft (A). Abdominal insufflation up to 16 mmHg is obtained with the insertion of a Veres needle at the patient's left upper quadrant, or at the umbilicus. Trocars are placed as follows: a 10 mm trocar (Ti) 20 cm distal to the xyphoid process for the 30° optical system; a 5 mm trocar (T2) on the [eft anterior axillary line; a 12 mm trocar (T3) in the left upper quadrant on the mid clavicular line just between the 1″ and the 2 trocars; a 12 mm trocar (T4) in the right upper quadrant on the right mid clavicular line; a 5 mm trocar (T5), used for liver retraction, distal and to the left of the xyphoid process; a 5 mm trocar (T6) just to the left of the linea alba, midway between the umbilicus and the pubis.

Sleeve Gastrectomy

This step constitutes the first part of the procedure and has been described in detail in chapter 5.

Duodenal Section and Cholecystectomy

A cholecystectomy is performed and the gallbladder is retrieved by T3. Two methods are available for transection of the duodenum.

- ANTERIOR APPROACH: After identification of the pylorus, the anterior peritoneal sheet at the lower border of the first duodenum, across from the common bile duct, is dissected with the coagulating hook (A). A passage between the duodenum and the pancreatic head is created under direct vision. This permits the introduction of the linear stapler (white load) (T3) (B) and the duodenum is transected (D). The gastroduodenal artery should become visible at this stage
- POSTERIOR APPROACH: The stomach is held up and all retrogastric adhesions at the distal end of the antrum are divided with the coagulating hook. With gentle dissection a passage is created just anterior to the pancreatic head and to the gastroduodenal artery. The anterior and posterior edge of duodenum are dissected (A) and a grasper is introduced between them and severs the peritoneal sheet from posterior to anterior. A tape (Ethibond 2) is looped around the duodenum at that level, and facilitates in holding the first part of the duodenum upwards. A firing of a linear stapler (white load) (T3) divides the duodenum (C).

Regardless of the approach, a stitch (white Vicryl 3/0) is placed at the inferior angle of the proximal sectioned duodenum.

Measurement of Common, Alimentary and Biliopancreatic Loops

The patient is positioned in a 10° Trendelenburg position with a 100 right tilt. Surgeon and assistants are now positioned to the patient's left (A-B). An appendectomy is performed and the appendix is retrieved by T4. The caecum is dissected off the parietal wall by the coagulating hook, in order to facilitate subsequent lifting of the alimentary loop. Starting at the ileo-caecal valve, the small bowel is measured for a distance of 75 or 100 cm. A PDS 2/0 stitch is placed on the bowel wall exactly at this level and fixed to the abdominal wall. The bowel distal to the stitch is marked gently with a coagulating hook (future common limb). From this point another 200 or 225 cm is measured, so that the sum of alimentary + common equals 300 cm. The bowel proximal to this point is marked with the coagulating hook (biliopancreatic limb) and a marking clip is placed just distal to this point (proximal end of the alimentary limb). A firing of stapler (white load) (T3) divides the bowel between the biliopancreatic and the alimentary limbs (C-D).

Jejunoileostomy: Semi-mechanical Side-to-Side

The bowel at the 75–100 cm marking (the marks will help to remain oriented) is sutured to the biliopancreatic limb, using the same stitch that was fixed into the parietal peritoneum. The common and biliopancreatic limbs are opened by the hook (A). A linear stapler (white load) (T3) joins the two limbs (B). The enterotomy opening is closed by a running suture (PDS or silk 2/0) with two separated suture lengths starting at each corner which are then tied together (CD).

Closure of the Mesenteric Defect

The mesenteric defect, located between the common and the biliopancreatic limbs, is closed after performance of their anastomosis. A purse string stitch (Prolene 2/0 or 1) is used to close this defect in order to prevent an internal hernia.

The patient is re-placed in the reversed Trendelenburg position. The surgeon returns between the patient's legs, the cameraman to the patient's right and the assistant to the patient's left (A-B).

Duodenoileostomy Totally Handsewn End- to-Side

The surgeon places himself again between the legs of the patients, the two assistants on either side. The alimentary limb is moved up in the direction of the duodenum. A running suture (PDS 1) is initiated on the superior corner of the transected duodenum and successive bites are taken alternatively on the duodenum and on the alimentary limb. This suture line constitutes the posterior layer of the anastomosis (A). A new running suture (PDS1) starting on the superior corner initiates the anterior layer of the anastornosis; the duodenum and the small bowel are opened with the coagulating hook (B). The posterior running suture is carried over the inferior corner of the anastomosis and is driven onto the anterior layer for a short distance (C). Finally the two running sutures are joined together halfway on the anterior layer and tied (D).

Closure of the Petersen's Space

The Petersen's space, a potential defect formed as a result of the procedure between the alimentary limb and the transverse rnesocolon, has to be closed in order to prevent an internal hernia. A purse string stitch (prolene 2/0 or 1) is used to this purpose.

Leak-Test of Both Anastomosis

A gastric tube is pushed down by the anaesthesiologist into the sleeve gastrectomy until it reaches the pylorus. The patient is placed in Trendelenburg position. The operating field is immersed in saline solution. Compressed air is insufflated into the gastric tube by the anaesthesiologist. The absence of air bubbles is testimony of the integrity of the sleeve gastrectomy and of the duo-denoileostomy. Subsequently the surgeon manipulates the entire alimentary limb until the air reaches the jejunoileostomy and compressed air is used again to test the integrity of the common, the alimentary and the biliopancreatic limbs. The procedure is concluded by the positioning of two drains, one near the sleeve and one near the duodenoileostomy and the 12 mm left trocar site is closed with absorbable suture (vicryl 1).

Postoperative Management

First postoperative day: methylen blue test is performed. If there is no evidence of a leak the patient may drink water.

Third postoperative day: gastrograffin swallow is performed only if there is suspicion of a leak. If not, the patient can start a liquid diet.

Fourth postoperative day: the drain is taken out and the patient is discharged if fit.

The patient is put on PPI IV for 24 h, followed by the same drug orally for 6 months. The patient is restricted to a semi-liquid diet for 1 week, followed by a pureed diet for another 4 weeks. An office visit is scheduled at around that time. If patient progress is good, the patient is allowed a regular diet. Sweets, alcohol and carbonated drinks are prohibited. Exercising is encouraged from the fifth postoperative week on. At 4 weeks, the patient receives follow up nutritional counseling for a protein-enriched diet and is given twice-daily multivitamins, oral calcium supplements, iron and fat-soluble vitamins (A, D, E, K). Laboratory evaluation for nutritional deficiencies is performed at each visit, including iron, ferritin, vitamin B12, folate, albumin, PTH, calcium, alkaline phosphatase, zinc, selenium, lipid profile, vitamin A and D levels, electrolytes, total proteins, and albumin. Liver enzymes and routine hematology are also included.

12.7 Follow Up

Obesity is a life long disease. "The fat cell never dies". Despite all surgical efforts, the patient will have a tendency to regain weight. The weight regain phenomenon usually occurs as of the third postoperative year. The weight regain issue as well as the potential complications linked with the surgery should be addressed by a multi disciplinary team that acts in synergy. To assure long term weight maintenance the team must encourage the persistence of the patient's life style changes initiated by the surgery, and, more specifically, help the patient to persevere in daily physical activity and good dietary choices. The following parameters should be monitored on the long term:

1. Nutritional management
2. Weight loss
3. Comorbidities that may have disappeared initially
4. Nutritional status to avoid malnutrition. Should be monitored especially: plasma protein, Potassium, Cholesterol
5. Vitamin and mineral deficiency. Should be monitored especially: Iron, Calcium, PTH, the water soluble vitamins A, D, E and K, the vitamins B1,B6 and B12, Zinc, Magnesium and Selenium
6. Medical symptoms after surgery: vomiting, dumping syndrome and hypoglycemia, neurological symptoms
7. Late surgical complications: gall stones, intestinal obstruction (internal hernia, trocar hernia), stoma complications (erosion, ulceration, dilation), candy cane formation, gastro-intestinal bleeding
8. Psychological issues (anxiety, depression)
9. Physical activity, if possible in cooperation with a trainer or physiotherapist

The patient should be seen by the surgeon at least once a year, by the medical nutritionist at least three times a year, and by the psychologist whenever needed.

Gastric Banding

13

Frank A. Granderath and Andreas Kirschniak

13.1 Introduction

The socioeconomic circumstances in the western nations, as well as the basic food situation have drastically changed in the second half of the last century. As a result of that, the prevalence rates of morbid obesity have increased rapidly. In some countries obesity has reached an epidemic magnitude meanwhile.

Obesity is a multifactorial entity with excessive aggregation of body fat leading to a general health damage. Basically, morbid obesity is defined as an imbalance between calory admission and the calory consumption. The causes for this imbalance usually differ from patient to patient. For an exact definition/classification and measurement of obesity, the body mass index (BMI) has been introduced. This BMI is calculated as weight divided by the square of height with kilograms per square meter (kg/m^2). Due to the BMI, obesity is divided into three severity grades: A BMI of 30–35 is considered as grade I obesity, 35–40 as grade II and a BMI >40 as grade III.

The available therapy programmes, outpatiently or inpatient, only seldomly reach the demanded high-class standards which are necessary for an evidence- based treatment for morbid obesity patients. Beside the available conventional therapy strategies, like psychological consultation, food therapies and diet measures, surgical therapy concepts for morbid obesity have increased during the last years.

Since the availability of minimally invasive access to the abdominal cavity, bariatric surgery has shown to be a safe and effective treatment option with long-term weight loss in the morbidly obese patient. Until now, some different bariatic procedures are available such as the laparoscopic "Roux-en-Y Gastric Bypass", the laparoscopic "Sleeve Gastrectomy", the laparoscopic "Biliopancreatic Diversion with Duodenal Switch" as well as the laparoscopic "Adjustable Gastric Banding".

Especially the Adjustable Gastric Banding (Lap. AGB) has become one of the most popular bariatric procedures in the last decade. Many studies could show that the AGB is a safe procedure which effectively results in a significant weight loss with long-term durability. Another important argument for this procedure has estimated to be its reversibility in case of recurrent increase of weight or postoperative complications such as band migration or intragastric/intraesophageal band erosion. Since the change from the so-called perigastric technique to the "pars flaccida approach", the incidence of those unsatisfactory complications decreased significantly.

The adjustable band is a soft silicon elastomer band that is placed approximately 3 cm caudal to the gastroesophageal junction creating a 10–20 ml gastric pouch above the band. The adjustable band with its elastic ballon then can be inflated through a port system according to the individual weight situation of the patient.

In a recent publication by Buchwald et al., it became evident that until 2003, approximately 25 % of all bariatric operations worldwide have been performed by this technique.

13.2 Operative Indications

13.2.1 Indication for Bariatric Surgery

Basically, a surgical intervention for weight loss stands at the last place of the therapy cascade. A bariatric operation should only be carried out if all available conservative therapies have not led to an effective weight reduction. The selection criterias for bariatric surgery are clearly defined by guidelines of the Nationwide institutes for Health and Clinical

F.A. Granderath (✉)
Department of General and Visceral Surgery, Hospital Neuwerk "Maria von den Aposteln", Mönchengladbach, Germany
e-mail: fagzellamsee@yahoo.com

A. Kirschniak
Department for General, Visceral and Transplant Surgery, University Hospital Tübingen, Tübingen, Germany

H.J. Bonjer (ed.), *Surgical Principles of Minimally Invasive Procedures*, DOI 10.1007/978-3-319-43196-3_13

Excellence (NICE), the American Nationwide Conference of State Legislatures as well as the European association for Endoscopic Surgery (EAES).

According to the EAES clinical practice guidelines on obesity surgery 2005, the following general indication has been determined:

"Obesity surgery should be considered in adult patients with a documented BMI greater than or equal 35 and related comorbidity, or a BMI of at least 40. All patients must fully understand and agree with postoperative care, and must be free of general contraindications. Adults with a BMI between 30 and 35 accompanied by substantial obesity-related comorbidity or after prolonged medical treatment should undergo obesity surgery only in the context of controlled clinical trials."

Based on this precondition the following directives are formulated furthermore by some obesity socities:

1. The age of the patients lies between 18 and 65 years.
2. The patients must have received an intensive medical/conservative treatment for weight loss in an obesity treatment center.
3. The patients should have carried out a conservative therapy carried out under medical control for the weight reduction with all adequate non- surgical therapies for a minimum period of 12 months
4. Patients with an endocrinological cause should be excluded.
5. A general anaesthesia ability should be given in all patients
6. Consciousness of the patients about long-term (if necessary lifelong) follow-up under medical control.
7. Readiness of the patients to change the existing eating habits and way of life.

13.2.2 Absolute Contraindications

As an essential contraindication for a bariatric procedure the following directives are stated by the appropriate national and international professional societies:

1. Abuse of alcohol or drugs
2. Existence of accompanying psychological comorbidities such as schizophrenia, active depressions or personality disorders.
3. Lacking Compliance of the patient with regard to the necessary lifestyle modifications as well as the suitable aftercare under medical care.
4. Manifest malignancies.
5. Manifest esophagogastric diseases (e.g. gastric ulcer)
6. Limited anaesthesia ability of the patient
7. Pregnancy.

13.2.3 Relative Contraindications

1. Large or paraesophageal hiatal hernia
2. Previous upper abdominal laparotomy

13.3 Preoperative Work-Up

The preoperative evaluation primarily should include a thorough documentation of the patients history with all non-surgical attempts for weight loss including psychological examination and dietary counseling.

The required preoperative testings usually depend on the general health condition of the patients and the personal preference and experience of the operating surgeon.

Basically, a complete blood count including thyroid hormones, serum cortisol, serum cholesterol and serum triglycerides should be carried out.

Morbid obesity commonly causes cardiac and pulmonary affections, so thorough cardiovascular and pulmonary assessment is mandatory. This should include a cardiac stress test to exclude any contraindication to anesthesia, an echocardiogram to assess left ventricle ejection fraction, pulmonary function tests and arterial blood gas analysis.

An ultrasound examination of the abdomen should be done routinely to determine concomitant intraabdominal diseases such as cholelithiasis. In case of unclarity, a CT scan or an MRI should be performed.

Due to a rather high incidence of Sleep apnea in morbidly obese patients, all patients should be screened either by anamnesis or by a formal sleep study.

A complete upper gastrointestinal tract is necessary in all patients. This should include an esophagogastroduodenoscopy with biopsies of the gastroesophageal junction and stomach in order to diagnose esophageal mucosal abnormalities (e.g. reflux esophagitis, Barrett's mucosa, esophageal/gastric malignancies). A barium swallow is necessary to search for a hiatal hernia.

The necessity of preoperative esophageal function testing is discussed controversially. However, esophageal manometry with 24 h pH monitoring or multichannel impedance measurement can give helpful information about the presence of gastroesophageal reflux or esophageal boby motility disorders which can adversely affect the postoperative outcome.

13.4 Operating Room

13.4.1 Patient Position

The patient is placed in reverse Trendelenburg position with both legs abducted. Ideally, the patient should be arranged in a half-standing position. To prevent slippage of the patient after positioning or intraoperatively, a device to support the perineum with additional foot rests is necessary. The patients legs optionally can be fixed to the table using adhesive strips (Fig. 13.1).

13.4.2 Positioning of the Operating Team

The operating surgeon stands between the spread legs of the patient. The camera assistant stands on the left side of the patient (Fig. 13.2). When necessary, a further assistant stands on the patients right side, e.g. for liver retraction. The nurse stands at the left foot of the patient. The monitor is located at the upper right –hand side of the patients head.

13.5 Surgical Technique

13.5.1 Trocar Position

Usually, laparoscopic gastric banding is performed with five trocars. After establishing the pneumoperitoneum, the optical trocar (A) is placed approximately 10 cm above the umbilicus depending on the size and thickness of the abdominal wall. The second trocar (B) then is placed 5 cm below the xyphoid. The third trocar (C) for left liver lobe retraction is placed in the mid-clavicular line at a level between the umbilicus and the optical trocar. The fourth trocar (D) for the preparation device is placed subcostal in the mid-clavicular line left and the fifth trocar (E) 5–10 cm below paraumbilically on the left side (Fig. 13.3).

(A) Camera (Assistant)
(B) Grasping device (Surgeons left hand)
(C) Liver Retractor (second assistant or mecjanical retracting device)
(D) Preparation device (e.g. Harmonic scalpel)
(E) Additional retraction or preparation

13.5.2 Exposure

After introduction of the instruments the left lobe of the liver is retracted cephalad and laterally for visualization of the gastroesophageal junction. Liver retraction can be effectively achieved by using a mechanical liver retractor with extracorporal fixation. Liver retraction has to be performed carefully to avoid capsule injury. To optimize the exposure of the hiatal region, the cardia can be retracted down (Fig. 13.4).

13.5.3 Retrogastric Tunnel

At first, the pars flaccida is opened and dissection will be continued to the right diaphragmatic crus. This can be performed with a harmonic scalpel, by hook or by scissors. At this point, a nasogastric tube should be inserted for better

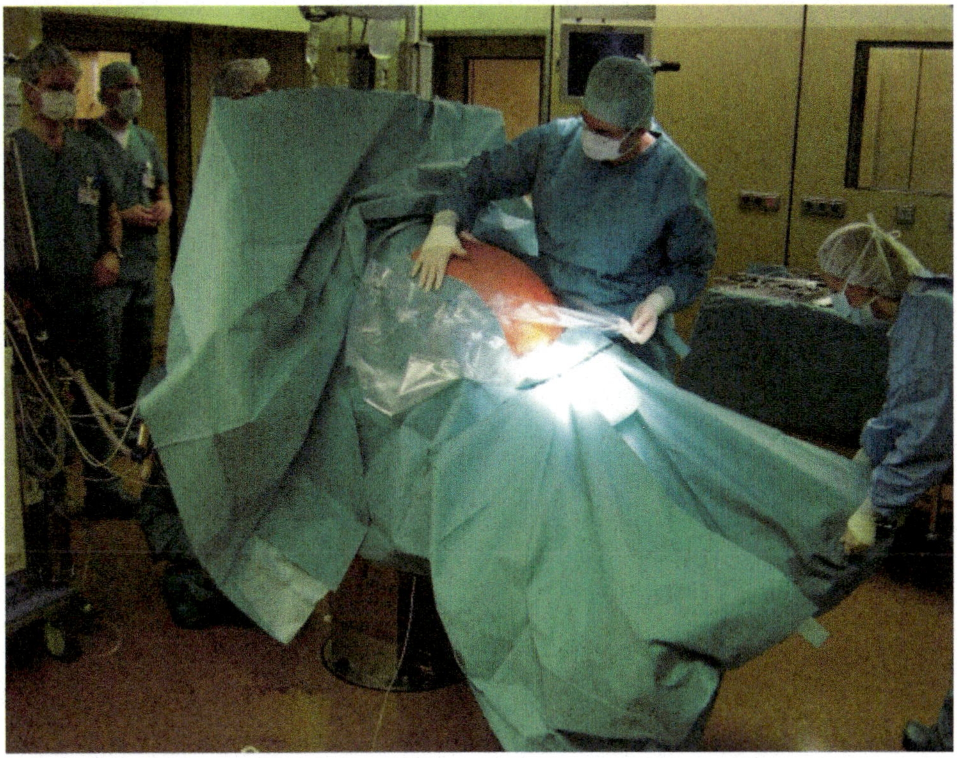

Fig. 13.1 Positioning of the patient

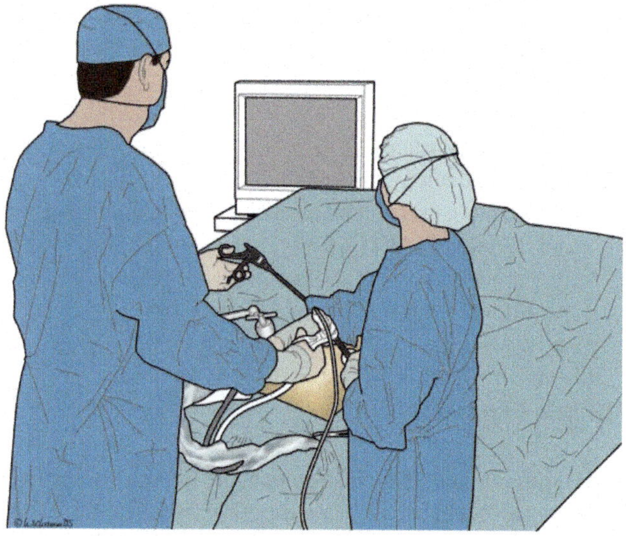

Fig. 13.2 Operating team

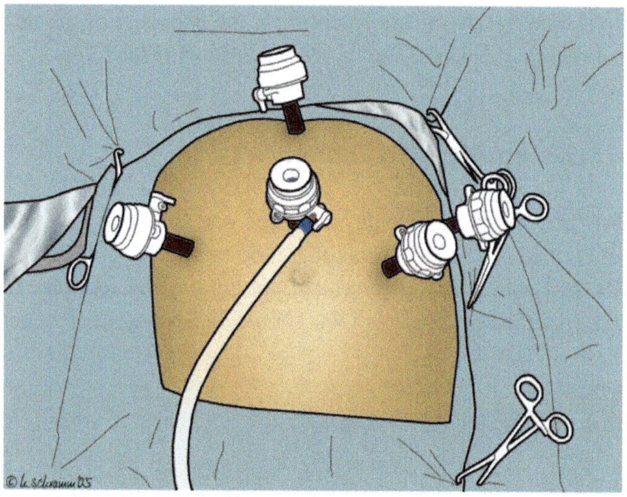

Fig. 13.3 Trocar placement

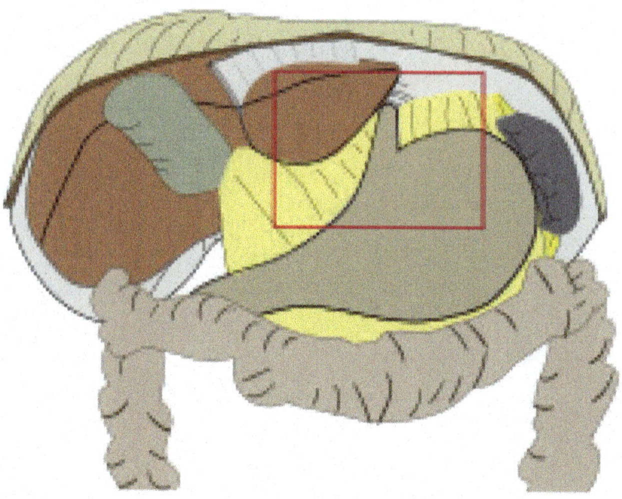

Fig. 13.4 View to the gastroesophageal junction

visualization and identification of the distal esophagus and the gastroesophageal junction. Before the retrogastric tunnel is prepared, the cardia can be gently retracted downwards to the patients left side with an atraumatic grasper. An incision of the gastrophrenic ligament has to be performed at the angle of His with identification of the left crus (Fig. 13.5).

Then the retrogastric passage is performed bluntly from the right to the left crus. This can easily be done by an angled instrument (e.g. Goldfinger). At this point, care has to be taken not to injure the small retrogastric vessels. The retrogastric tunnelling should be performed closely to the hiatal crura to avoid opening of the lesser sac. To find the best dissection plane, a balloon-tipped gastric tube now can be inserted by the anaesthesiologist into the stomach. After inflation to 15–25 ml, the tube is pulled back up to the level of the cardia. Now the retrogastric space can be tunnelled bluntly until the tip of the instrument appears at the angle of His. At this point care has to be taken in order to avoid splenic injury or laceration of the upper short gastric vessels (Fig. 13.6).

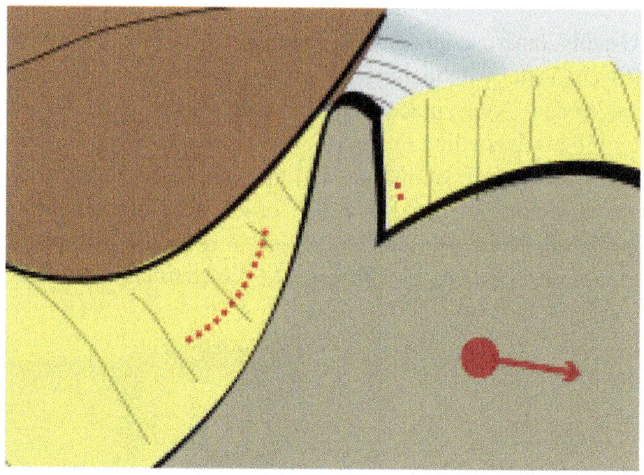

Fig. 13.5 Peritoneal incisions and direction of stomach retraction

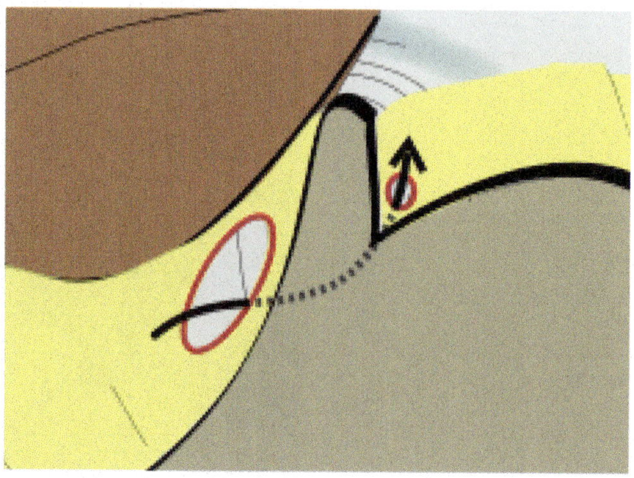

Fig. 13.6 Retrogastric tunnel

13.5.4 Band Placement

After extracorporal preparation of the gastric band and the catheter system, the gastric band now will be introduced into the abdominal cavity. Care has to be taken not to touch the ballon during this manoeuvre to avoid ballon leakage. The band system easily can be introduced via a 15 mm trocar. The gastric band now will be pulled through the retroesophageal tunnel either with the retroesophageal grasping devive or by connecting the band to the Goldfinger. After the band is pulled through with the ballon placed over the complete esophageal circumference, the band can be loosely closed (Fig. 13.7).

For creation of a small gastric pouch above the band, the ballon of the nasogatric tube now has to be inflated again with approximately 15 ml. Now the band will be closed completely below the inflated ballon. To prevent slippage of the band, the fundus will now be fixed with three to four simple sutures to the stomach wall above as well as below the gastric band. The first suture should be fixed at the left crus, the following sutures surround the band completely. At this point it is important to ensure that the gastric fixation is not too tight for subsequent effective filling of the band. The nasogastric tube now can be deflated and removed by the anaesthesiologist (Fig. 13.8).

13.5.5 Port Placement

After thorough revision of the operative field, the band catheter now will be removed from the abdominal cavity through the subxypoidal or the leftmost trocar. The liver retractor as well as the working trocars now can be removed. After extension of the selected trocar incision, the port has to be fixed to the fascia. The reservoir is connected to the catheter and the port will be sutured to the fascia with three to four stitches and positioned subcutaneously. Rotation of the reservoir must be avoided at this point to ensure sufficient punctures postoperatively.

13.6 Postoperative Care

Postoperative care often depends on the surgeons personal experience and standard. The nasogastric tube can be left in place for 1–2 days to prevent gastric dilatation or bloating. During postoperative hospital stay, a upper GI contrast study or cinematographic x-ray with water-soluble contrast should be performed to confirm the correct position of the band and to preclude esophageal or gastric leakage. Afterwards, the patient can return to eating and drinking. For the first postoperative period the patients should be administered to a standard postoperative diet with mixed fluid and solid food. After discharge, the patients can return to normal diet. Usually patients can leave the hospital within the first 4 days after surgery. A standard follow-up should be performed the control weight loss.

13.7 Complications

13.7.1 Infection

Due to the prevention of port or band infection, intravenous antibiotics may be necessary for a maximum of 5 days after surgery. Acute or persistent chronic port infection usually requires surgical reintervention. If the infection is isolated to the port without any signs of band infection or other intraabdominal affections, it should be considered to only explant the port system with preservation of the gastric band. The catheter then can be cutted and clipped and left in the abdominal cavity. After consequent antibiotic therapy with com-

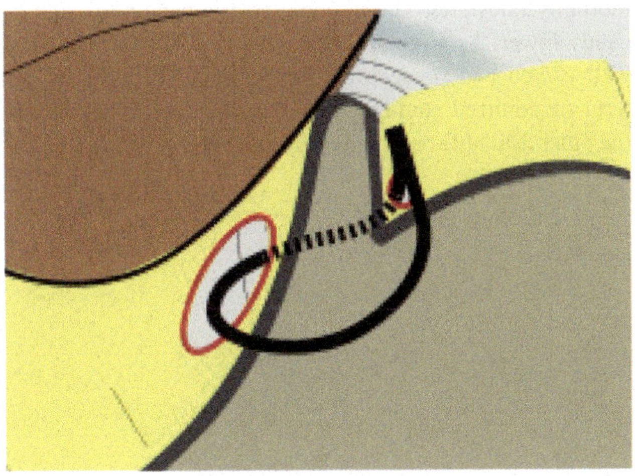

Fig. 13.7 Placement of the band

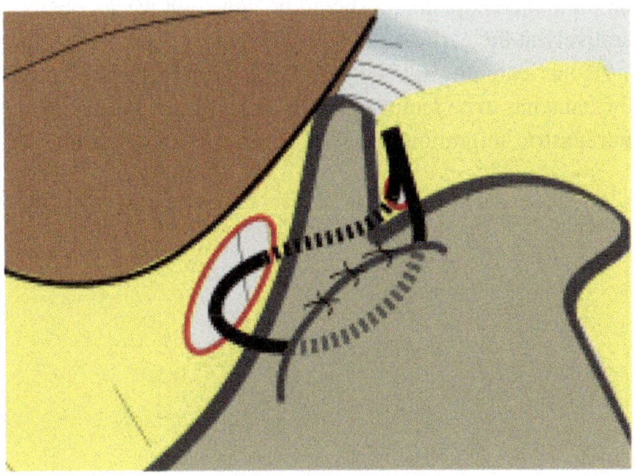

Fig. 13.8 Fundus fixation above the band

plete resolve of the infection, a new port system can be implanted. If there is any evidence of intrabdominal infection, both band and port system have to be removed.

13.7.2 Pouch Dilatation/Slippage

Pouch dilatation commonly occurs in case of a too tight band or when the patient continues to overeat during the short- and mid-term postoperative period. If a too tight band is suspected, a cinematographic x-ray barium swallow can ensure the diagnosis. The too tight band also can lead to a band slippage. This slippage is induced by the increased size of the pouch pushing the gastric band distally. Therefore the band has to be loosened immediately. The location of the slippage somewhat depends on the unique technique of band implantation. Posterior slippage more likely occurs with the perigastric technique, whereas anterior slippage commonly occurs with the pars flaccida approach. Usually, surgical reintervention is necessary according to the morphological situation. In case of cephalad position of the stomach, the fixation sutures have to be divided and the stomach has to be reduced through the band. The band then can be re-positioned and a new gastric fixation be performed.

13.7.3 Band Erosion

Band migration with esophageal or gastric erosion is a rare complication after gastric banding with occurrence rates of 1–3 % in the literature. There is a chacteristic tendency of foreign body to migrate or erode, so every step of band implantation has to be done carefully. To avoid this complication, serosal damage has to be avoided. Furthermore, the band should not be too tight around the gastric wall. All fixation sutures should be done only to approximate the gastric tissue without constriction of the gastric wall. Additionally, the first band adjustment should be done 6–8 weeks postoperatively at the earliest.

If there are any signs of band migration or band erosion, the band has to be removed immediately. In case of complete intragastric migration the band sometimes can be removed endoscopically with laparoscopic surveillance. After band removal with simultaneous repair of the perforation, another bariatric procedure can be performed after complete healing (Fig. 13.9).

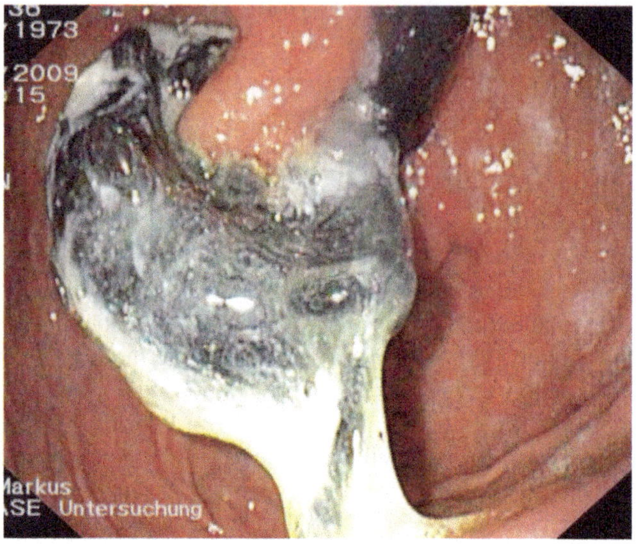

Fig. 13.9 Intragastric band erosion

13.8 Results

Altogether, laparoscopic gastric banding has shown to be a safe and effective bariatric procedure leading to significant weight loss with resolution of obesity related comorbidities such as diabetes, sleep apnea or cardiovascular affections. The reported percentage of weight loss has been reported to be more than 50 % excessive weight loss at 5 years. The average weight loss after alternative procedures such as the Gastric bypass or the biliopancreatic diversion often is higher, however, the peri-and postoperative morbidity and mortality rates after laparoscopic gastric banding is significantly lower. As a result, laparoscopic gastric banding is a well established procedure in bariatric procedures. Long-term randomized studies comparing the gastric banding to the other available procedures are not yet available.

Gastric Bypass

14

Mario Morino and Gitana Scozzari

14.1 Introduction

Gastric bypass is a malabsorptive and restrictive bariatric procedure first described by Mason and Ito in 1967. Their original gastric bypass consisted of a 100–150 ml horizontal pouch anastomosed to a loop of proximal jejunum. In 1977 Griffen introduced the Roux-en-Y gastrojejunostomy in place of the loop gastrojejunostomy, and in 1983 Torres stapled the stomach vertically rather than horizontally, a modification that has become the standard method for constructing the gastric pouch. The laparoscopic approach to gastric bypass has been described by Wittgrove, Clark and Tremblay in 1994. To date, gastric bypass is one of the most applied bariatric procedures. According to a 2008 survey [5] on bariatric surgery, it accounts for 51 % of bariatric procedures in the USA and 49.3 % worldwide.

The gastric bypass involves three main components: creation of a small gastric reservoir resulting in food intake reduction (restrictive component), bypass of the duodenum leading to a change in the secretion of gastrointestinal hormones (hormonal component) and exclusion of a variable length of the absorptive small bowel producing a degree of malabsorption (malabsorptive component).

14.2 Indications and Preoperative Work-Up

Strict indications and a comprehensive preoperative work-up are crucial to obtain good clinical results. We refer to the 2004 EAES Consensus Conference [1] (http://www.eaes.eu/getmedia/65103216-27ef-4de6-9034-1cc447a41b20/Sauerland-Obesity-Surgery-guidelines-EAES-Surg-Endosc-2005-pdf.pdf).

M. Morino, MD (✉) • G. Scozzari, MD
Digestive, Colorectal and Minimal Invasive Surgery, University of Torino, Torino, Italy
e-mail: mario.morino@unito.it

14.3 Operating Room

The operating room must be equipped for laparoscopic bariatric surgery. Notably, the operating table should be able to sustain the weight of the obese patients and capable of being put into reverse Trendelenburg position.

The patient is placed in the lithotomy position in steep reverse Trendelenburg with legs wide apart and arms positioned upwards. The procedure is done under general anesthesia and endotracheal intubation. A Foley catheter and a nasogastric tube are inserted after anesthesia induction. The operating surgeon stands on the patient's right during bowel manipulation, and between the patient's legs during the supramesocolic phase of the procedure; first assistant (camera assistant) stands on the right, and the second one on the left side of the patient. The scrub nurse stands at the level of patient's left foot (Fig. 14.1).

14.4 Surgical Technique

Since its introduction in 1994 [2], laparoscopic gastric bypass has been compared to open surgery in different randomized and non-randomized clinical trials [3]. Published studies showed no difference between the two approaches in regard to excess weight loss, long-term quality of life, or resolution of comorbidities, whereas the laparoscopic approach demonstrated significant advantages in terms of shorter length of stay, lower incisional pain, faster return to daily activities, better aesthetic results and lower complication rates with a markedly decreased rate of wound infection and incisional hernia. Although operative times vary from surgeon to surgeon, with the increased laparoscopic experience to date the mini-invasive and the open approach are more or less equivalent. Costs per procedure are also similar, since the major cost of disposable instruments needed for laparoscopy equals the cost of longer hospital stay for open procedures. Although gastrojejunal

H.J. Bonjer (ed.), *Surgical Principles of Minimally Invasive Procedures*, DOI 10.1007/978-3-319-43196-3_14

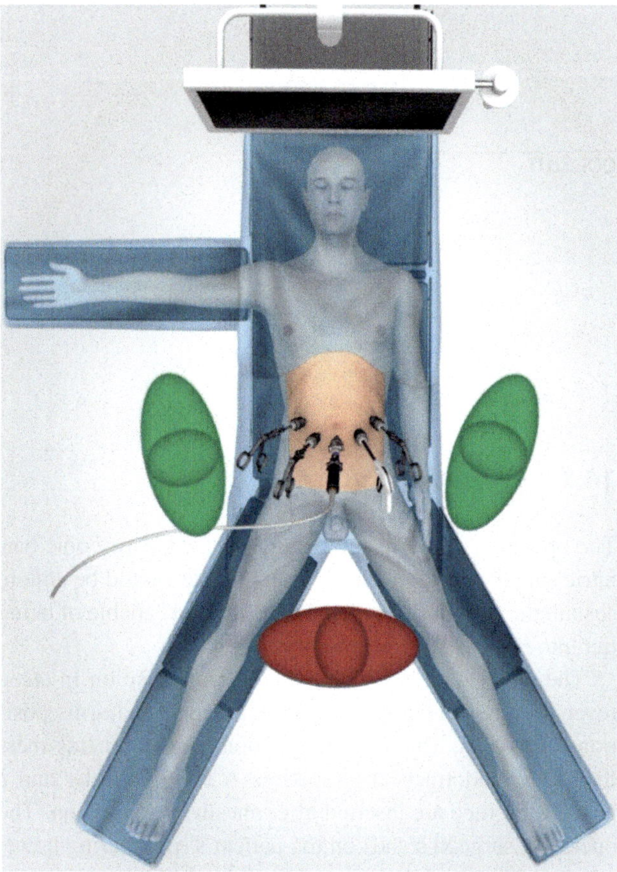

Fig. 14.1 Patient positioning for laparoscopic gastric bypass

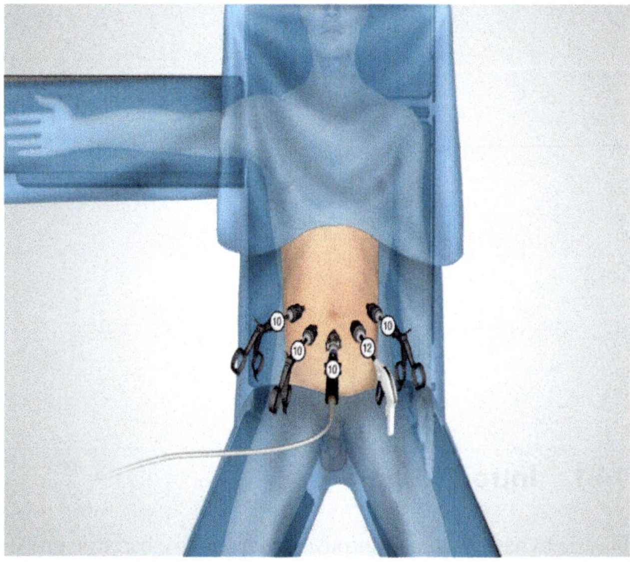

Fig. 14.2 Trocar positioning for laparoscopic gastric bypass

anastomotic strictures have been described more frequently after laparoscopic gastric bypass, other major complications such as anastomotic leak, venous thrombosis, and pneumonia are decreased in laparoscopic approach, which has furthermore demonstrated to reduce overall postoperative mortality.

Therefore, to date laparoscopy is the preferred approach in obese patients, and it must be considered as the gold standard.

14.5 Operative Technique

The pneumoperitoneum is established according to surgeon's preference: using a Veres needle, an Hasson cannula or an optical trocar. Hasson's technique could be quite difficult in severe obese patients. Insufflation to 14–16 mmHg will usually be adequate to achieve correct visualization.

14.6 Position of Trocars

The trocars' positions are shown below in Fig. 14.2.

14.7 Liver Retraction

In obese patients the liver is often very large and can represent an impediment to visualization of the esophagogastric junction and the gastric body. To retract the left lobe of the liver, a Nathanson-type retractor inserted through a epigastric port or a paddle retractor introduced through port just below the xiphoid or laterally in the right hypocondrium are used.

14.8 First Operative Phase: Roux-en-Y Limb Construction

The transverse colon is lifted with an atraumatic grasper and the ligament of Treitz is identified. The jejunum is transected 50 cm distally to Treitz with a linear stapler and the mesentery is transected perpendicularly to the bowel wall using bipolar electrocautery or ultrasound shears. Afterwards, the Roux-en-Y limb is measured, with the aid of two graspers, one of which with a strip placed 10 cm from the tip. Care must be taken when handling the intestinal limbs, always grasping the antimesenteric bowel border.

At the level chosen for the jejunojejunostomy, the biliopancreatic limb is fixed to the alimentary one with a stay suture. The jejunojejunostomy is created with a firing of a 45-mm linear stapler using a white cartridge inserted through two small enterotomies created on the antimesenteric side of the bowel loops. The site of stapler insertion is closed, preferably by hand sewn extramucosal running suture.

The triple-stapled technique for jejunojejunostomy, described by Madan and Frantzides, involves two staple lines fired in opposite directions, with a third staple line closing the common enterotomy. This allows for a large patent anastomosis with a lower risk of stenosis. Closure of all mesenteric defects with interrupted stitches of non-reabsorbable suture should be carefully done in order to decrease the incidence of internal hernia, a postoperative complication that has become more frequent in the laparoscopic era, due to the lack of adhesions after laparoscopic surgery.

14.9 Technical Consideration: Limb Position

The retrocolic-retrogastric, retrocolic-antegastric, and antecolic-antegastric routes all are acceptable for the Roux limb (Fig. 14.3), and while debate continues over the best approach, literature data does not seem to definitively prove the superiority of a technique over another. Antecolic technique is considered to be technically easier, with consequent reduction of operative time, whereas the main concern is that excessive tension may be placed on the gastrojejunal anastomosis causing a potential increased leak rate. If antecolic limb position is chosen, the omentum is divided in the midline down to the colon wall ('omental split') and the Roux limb is brought into the upper abdomen through the defect in the omentum, in order to reduce the distance from the gastric pouch.

In the transmesocolic approach, once the colon is reflected cephalad and the ligament of Treitz is identified, a 2- to 4-cm opening is made above the lower edge of the pancreas in the mesocolon. Afterwards, the end of the Roux limb is placed carefully into the upper abdomen through the mesocolon, behind the stomach (retrocolic-retrogastric way) or anteriorly to this (retrocolic-antegastric way).

14.10 Technical Consideration: Limb Lengths

Several authors have studied the effects of different limb lengths. In patients with BMI below 50 kg/m^2, both retrospective and prospective data failed to show a benefit for longer alimentary limbs. In patients with preoperative BMI above 50 kg/m^2, most authors reported significantly improved excess weight loss with longer limbs, although alimentary limbs longer than 150 cm may increase nutritional complications. Therefore, different authors suggest that Roux limb length should be adapted to patient's preoperative BMI, and should be created so that it measures 75–100 cm in patients with BMI under 50 kg/m^2, and between 100 and 250 cm in case of a higher BMI.

14.11 Second Operative Phase: Gastric Pouch Construction

The gastric pouch is constructed creating a 15- to 30-ml vertical, lesser curve-based, pouch. A window in the gastrohepatic ligament is created using the electrocautery hook, 5–6 cm distally to the gastro-esophageal junction, close to the wall of the lesser curvature of the stomach to decrease blood loss and to preserve vagal nerves. The perigastric dissection proceeds until the space posteriorly to the stomach has been opened, making sure that there are no posterior adhesions. The window must be small (1–1.5 cm) in order to permit the linear stapler passage avoiding vascular injuries to the pouch.

Afterwards, with an endoscopic 45-mm linear stapler, a transverse division of the stomach is created introducing the stapler through the trocar in the right hypochondrium. The level of the division can be chosen simply measuring 5–6 cm from the cardia with a decimetre rule or a marked instrument, or using a calibration balloon inserted into the stomach; generally the line is just below the first vascular arcade. It is very important to remember to remove the nasogastric tube before the stapler is fired.

After the transverse division, sequential transections of the stomach vertically up to the angle of His should result in a 20- to 30-cc pouch (for the longitudinal stapling, the stapler is introduced through the trocar in the left hypochondrium) (Fig. 14.4). We recommend stapling the stomach over a calibrating orogastric boogie, 12-mm in diameter, to allow for a well shaped pouch and to avoid esophageal injuries. For the

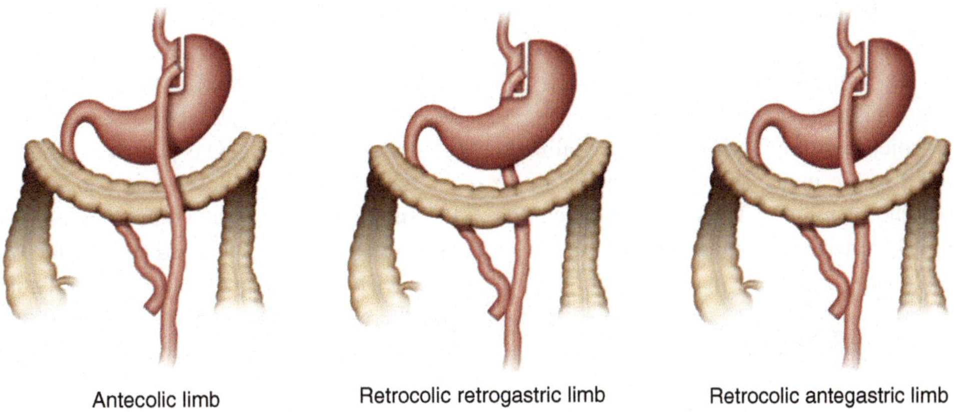

Fig. 14.3 Roux-en-Y limb positions for gastric bypass procedures

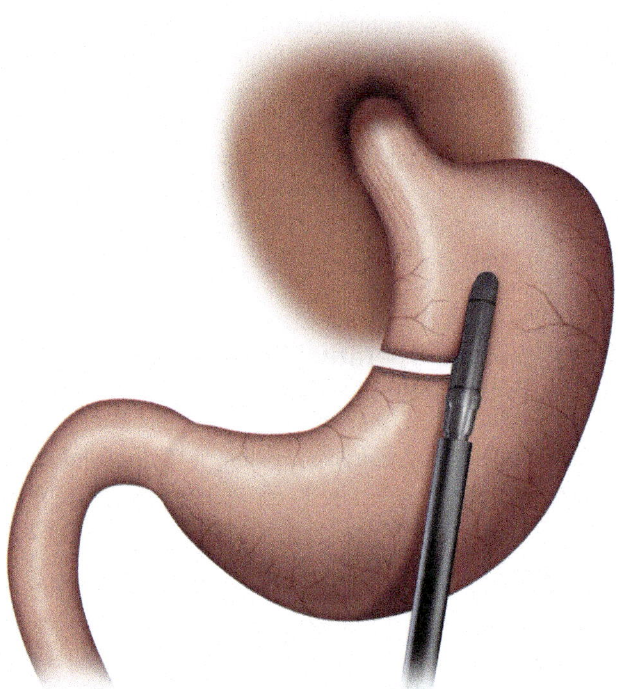

Fig. 14.4 Creation of the gastric pouch

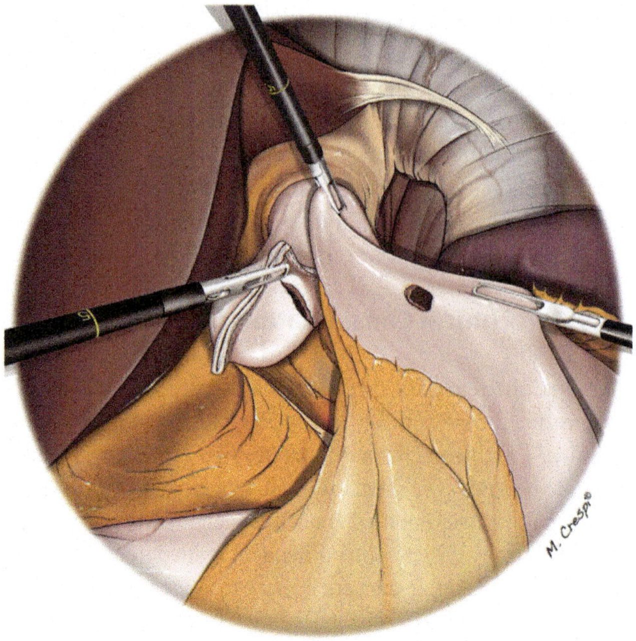

Fig. 14.5 Enterotomies in the gastric pouch and Roux-en-Y limb for placement of lineal stapler. (Reproduced with permission of Prof. Guy-Bernard Cadière, illustrator: Massimiliano Crespi)

transverse and the first longitudinal gastric transection, we suggest to use green cartridge (4.8-mm staples) due to the gastric wall thickness, while in the proximal stomach blue cartridge (3.5-mm staples) can be safely used. To facilitate the upper completion of the pouch, opening the peritoneum over the diaphragmatic muscle at the angle of His with electrocautery hook allows to better visualize the angle of dissection; during the dissection, that must stay close to the left crus, care must be taken to avoid injuries to the spleen.

14.12 Third Operative Phase: Gastrojejunal Anastomosis

The gastrojejunostomy is a critical aspect of the gastric bypass procedure because patients may develop early leaks and/or late stenosis. Moreover, gastrojejunostomy must be carefully calibrated, since a strict passage can lead to dysphagia and vomiting, while a too large anastomosis can result in insufficient weight reduction.

Before the gastrojejunostomy construction, the alimentary limb is brought in the upper abdomen, taking care to avoid any twist on the mesentery. The anastomosis can be hand-sewn or stapled, either linear or circular.

14.12.1 Hand-Sewn Technique

Although the hand-sewn technique is the least expensive option and has the added benefit of decreasing the wound infection rate, it requires advanced laparoscopic skills.

The anastomosis construction begins with a posterior, running layer created between the inferior staple line of the gastric pouch and the antimesenteric side of the Roux limb using 3–0 absorbable suture, incorporating the staple line in the suture. Two enterotomies are made in the gastric pouch and jejunum and a second posterior running, full thickness layer is performed and continued anteriorly beyond the termination of the first posterior suture. Prior to completion of the anastomosis a calibrating bougie is carefully passed through the anastomosis and the two anterior sutures, inner (full thickness) and outer (seromuscular), are completed.

14.12.2 Linear Stapled Technique

The gastric pouch and the jejunal loop can easily be anastomosed by a linear stapler. To facilitate the anastomosis, a stitch is placed between gastric pouch and limb. With the electrocautery hook, two little enterotomies are made in both the Roux limb and pouch (Fig. 14.5). The linear cutter (45 mm, blue cartridges) is placed and fired (Fig. 14.6).

The enterotomy is closed using an hand-sewn absorbable 3–0 suture, or with a second application of the stapler. This gastrojejunostomy can be created either with or without a hand-sewn outer layer. This technique is faster and cheaper than the circular one, and does not require a dilation of the port site for stapler introduction, since the linear stapler can be introduced through a 12 mm trocar. Nevertheless, this technique presents some disadvantages: the anastomosis may not be uniform from case to case, parallel staple lines created may cause segments of gastric necrosis causing a

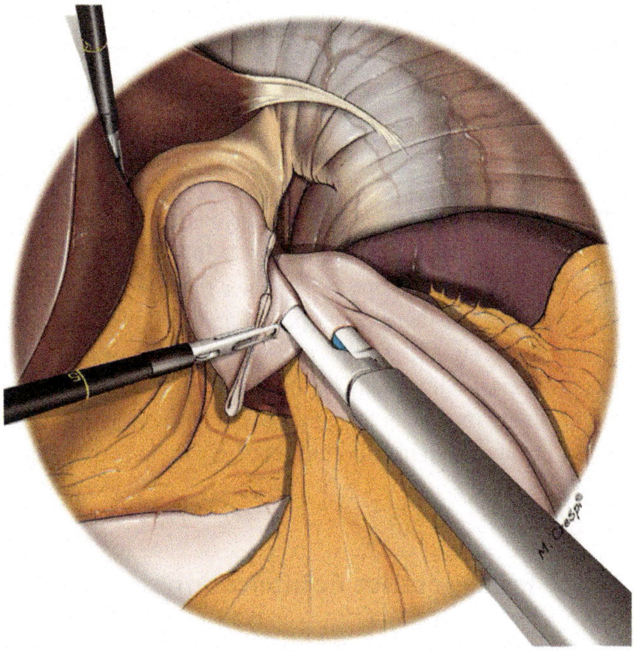

Fig. 14.6 Stapled anastomosis between gastric pouch and Roux-en-Y limb. (Reproduced with permission of Prof. Guy-Bernard Cadière, illustrator: Massimiliano Crespi)

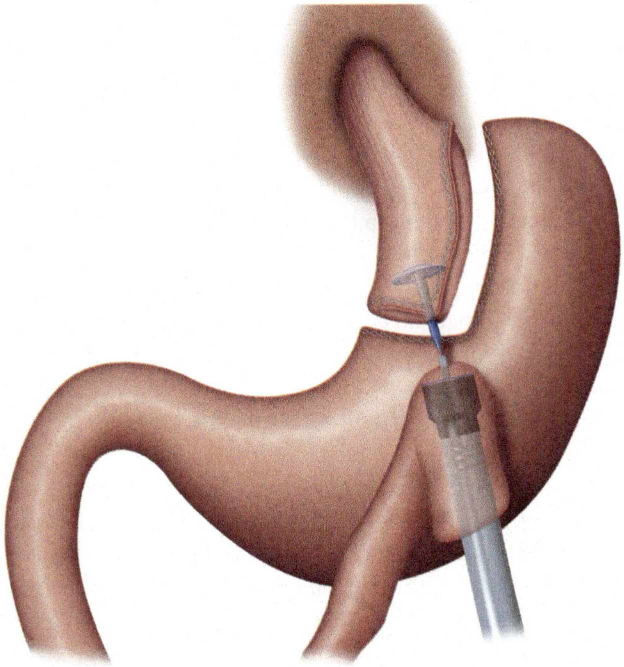

Fig. 14.7 Circular stapled anastomosis between gastric pouch and Roux-en-Y limb

leak, and small pouch size may be compromised as a larger pouch is required to accept the linear stapler.

14.13 Circular Stapled Technique

The circular-stapled anastomosis advantages include shorter operative time and a standardized anastomosis size; from an economic point of view, it is the most expensive technique, since it requires a circular stapler for the anastomosis and a linear one for the pouch construction. Concerning stapler size, published data on randomized and non-randomized comparisons between 21- and 25-mm stapler strongly favoured the latter, due to the lower anastomotic strictures rate. Two common variations involve the way in which the circular anvil is placed in the gastric pouch.

(a) *pulldown.* In the pulldown technique, largely popularized by Michel Gagner, the anvil is fixed to the end of a nasogastric tube (of note, while until recently the anvil had to be angled and fixed manually to a nasogastric tube, to date the anvil is sold ready-to-use from the manufacturer). The anvil is guided into the posterior pharynx orally by the anesthesiologist and then a jaw lift is performed and the anvil drawn gently down into the oesophagus. Catching the nasogastric tube end with a grasp through a small opening of the pouch previously created with the electrocautery hook or the ultrasound dissector, the tube is pulled just to properly position the anvil in the gastric pouch. After the anvil has been correctly positioned, the nasogastric tube is removed from the anvil and take-out from the abdomen through the trocar in left hypochondrium. Technical note: occasionally the anvil will be difficult to pull down: most of the time it is caught at the cricopharyngeal junction and sometimes taking down the balloon of the tracheostomy tube will facilitate its passage.

(b) *intra-abdominal.* The circular stapler can be introduced into the stomach by making an enterotomy on the gastric fundus, far from the pouch suture line, and inserting the anvil in the pouch through the gastric wall prior to completing the vertical division of the stomach. To catch the anvil, we suggest to introduce it into the abdomen after having inserted it in a small portion of a nasogastric tube, with a silk suture passed through the tip; the silk suture will be easily caught with a grasp or a specifically designed instrument, such as in our personal technique. The intra-abdominal technique may take more time to perform, but it has the advantage of significantly reduce the wound infection rate and to avoid the anvil passage through the oesophagus with possible pharyngoesophageal injury, while it leaves an anterior gastric enterotomy to be closed (generally, with a running hand-sewn reasorbable suture).

Once the anvil has been placed in the gastric pouch and the Roux limb has been brought into the upper abdomen, the circular stapler is introduced into the abdomen, usually through the left mid-clavicular port after dilation of the port site. The circular stapler can be wrapped with a plastic cover to protect the abdominal wall incision. The circular stapler is placed into the lumen of the jejunum after a large enterotomy has been made with ultrasound shears, and the needle of the stapler is extruded through the wall of the jejunum, approximately 4 cm from the cut end. The needle is docked to the anvil under direct vision checking that the Roux limb mesentery is not twisted. The stapler is fired and removed, and the Roux limb end is closed with a linear stapler. The blind end of the alimentary loop should not be very long, and undesired excess jejunum can be excised while closing the end of the Roux limb. At the conclusion of the procedure the left mid-clavicular port site is largely irrigated with povidone-iodine and fascial stitches are made (Fig. 14.7).

14.14 Checking for Anastomotic Leak

All gastrojejunal anastomoses, regardless of technique, are checked by obstructing the Roux limb with an atraumatic clamp. The anastomosis can be checked by filling the intra-abdominal field with water and insufflating air into the gastric pouch, or with methylene blue test (150 ml of diluite methylene blue injected through the nasogastric tube). Closure of any leak is done with a transanastomotic hand-sewn suture. Some authors routinely perform an intraoperative upper endoscopy to check the anastomosis.

14.15 Staple-Line Reinforcement Materials

The staple lines can be reinforced by a hand-sewn running suture, or by different materials that have been tested in order to reduce staple-line bleeding and/or leaks, such as bovine pericardial strips and glycolic copolymer sleeve. All these options have never proven to be cost-effective.

14.16 Drains and Tubes

A perianastomotic surgical drain should be placed and removed postoperatively after a radiographic contrast study confirms the integrity of the anastomosis and the patient begins a liquid diet.

The nasogastric tube may be removed at the end of the surgical procedure, or kept in place and removed after the contrast study.

14.17 Postoperative Care

Bariatric patients with minimal comorbidities may be safely transferred from the operating room directly to the ward, whereas patients with cardiac or pulmonary diseases, particularly sleep apnea syndrome, may benefit from a 24–48 h intensive care unit admission. As with other clean-contamined procedures, there is no evidence supporting prophylactic postoperative antibiotics. Considering that deep vein thrombosis with pulmonary embolism is one of the most feared bariatric surgery complications, all patients should receive one or more forms of prophylaxis; these include early ambulation, pneumatic compression devices, low-molecular-weight heparin, and inferior vena cava filter in selected high-risk patients. Careful postoperative pain control is recommendable since it aids in early ambulation, which improves pulmonary mechanics and reduces risk of venous thrombosis. Patients with fever greater than 38.5 °C, tachycardia above 110 heart beats per minute, oliguria, or who "don't look right" should undergo further evaluations, because these findings may be the first indication of leakage. It is critically important to remember that physical examination of the abdomen in a morbidly obese patient is frequently unreliable.

14.18 Postoperative Complications

Reported perioperative (≤30 day) mortality rates range from 0.2 to 1% in most recent published series [4]. The most severe early complications include anastomotic leakage, gastrointestinal tract hemorrhage, internal herniation with or without strangulated bowel obstruction, and perforated marginal ulcer. A severe complication of the gastric bypass is the so-called "bypass obstruction", a diagnosis that includes both paralytic and mechanical ileus involving the bypassed upper digestive tract. Bypass obstruction is the most urgent of all closed segment bowel obstructions because of the large volume of digestive fluids entering the bypassed upper digestive tract, and it implies a great urgency for diagnosis and treatment. Less severe complications include anastomotic stenosis, usually occurring during the first postoperative months, wound infection, and incisional hernia. Long-term gastric bypass complications include stomal stenosis, perianastomotic ulcer, vitamin and mineral deficiencies, internal hernia, dumping syndrome (an adverse event caused by eating refined sugar, symptoms of which include rapid heart rate, nausea, tremor, faint feeling and diarrhoea), and, more rarely, hypoglycaemic symptoms due to hyperinsulinemic state (nesidioblastosis).

14.19 Postoperative Imaging

Although routine postoperative imaging has not been shown to reduce morbidity or mortality after laparoscopic gastric bypass, it is recommendable to perform a contrast study of the gastrojejunostomy with water-soluble contrast on first or second postoperative day, to confirm the integrity and patency of the anastomosis and to compare it if studies will be needed in the follow-up.

Upper GI series are very useful in evaluating the febrile, tachycardic or oliguric patient, since it is considered to be the gold standard for demonstrating leaks from the gastric pouch or proximal anastomosis; unfortunately, it is ineffective in evaluating the distal anastomosis. If a leak is suspected distal to the gastrojejunostomy, immediate return to the operating room should be considered. CT scan can be useful in evaluating the gastric pouch, proximal anastomosis and distal anastomosis. It should be remembered that CO_2 insufflation is generally reabsorbed by 24 h and that free intra-abdominal gas seen after that time should raise the suspicion of a leak. Upper GI-series and CT are not 100 % sensitive, and a negative imaging study should never preclude a return to the operating room if there is clinical suspicion of an intra-abdominal leak.

14.20 Follow-Up

Close, long-term follow-up is recommended for patients after gastric bypass. A typical scheme for follow-up would be at 1 and 4 weeks, followed by quarterly visits during the first year and annually thereafter, to assess weight loss, resolution of comorbidities, long-term complications, and need for continuing education and support.

14.21 Different GBP Techniques

Several variations to the "standard" gastric bypass have been proposed.

14.21.1 Mini-gastric Bypass

The mini-gastric bypass was the first version of the gastric bypass, but it was soon abandoned because of biliary reflux with bile gastritis and esophagitis, and dangers of esophageal cancer. The current laparoscopic mini-gastric bypass, proposed by Rutledge in 2001, is a modification of the classic loop gastric bypass described by Mason and Ito, and consists of a long, narrow, vertical gastric tube along the lesser curvature of the stomach that is end-to-side connected to a loop of small bowel approximately 200 cm from the ligament of Treitz in an antecolic fashion. Despite isolated reports promoting the minigastric bypass as a simpler alternative approach, with shorter operative times and lower cost, the chronic alkaline bile reflux remain a significant concern.

14.21.2 Long-Limb Roux-en-Y Gastric Bypass

Long-limb and very long-limb or distal gastric bypass, are gastric bypasses with a long Roux limb and a long bypassed limb joined together to form a short common channel (150 cm or less) of distal small intestine. This modification was designed by Torres and Oca, and later promoted by Brolin, to enhance the malabsorptive effect in patients previously submitted to standard gastric bypass with failed weight loss.

14.21.3 Banded Gastric Bypass

A prosthetic band can be used to stabilise the gastroenterostomy, preventing late stretching of the opening and improving long term weight control. The bands or rings used in these operations, largely promoted by Fobi and Capella, are various (e.g., linea alba, fascia lata, Gore-Tex, Marlex, Silastic ring, porcine and bovine grafts), although Silastic ring tubing is the most commonly used material. Banded gastric bypass does not seem to result in a significantly different weight loss or comorbidities resolution, and could lead to worse gastrointestinal symptom, such as emesis rate and food intolerance. Furthermore, the presence of a foreign body can lead to complications such as stenosis, erosion, and infection.

14.21.4 Laparoscopic Staged Roux-en-Y Gastric Bypass

In the effort to minimize perioperative morbidity in the super-super obese patient (BMI >60 kg/m^2), the concept of a two-stage laparoscopic gastric bypas has been developed. The staged gastric bypass consists of a modified gastric bypass with construction of a larger gastric pouch and a low gastrojejunal anastomosis. Construction of a large gastric pouch avoids the difficult dissection of the angle of His, while the construction of a low gastrojejunal anastomosis minimizes tension on the anastomosis and hence reduces the chance for leaks. In the second stage, 6–12 months later, the volume of the gastric pouch is reduced by performing a sleeve gastrectomy of the gastric fundus.

References

1. Sauerland S, et al. The EAES clinical practice guidelines on obesity surgery. In: Neugebauer EAM, Sauerland S, Fingerhut A, et al., editors. EAES guidelines for endoscopic surgery. Twelve years evidence-based surgery in Europe. New York: Springer; 2006.
2. Wittgrove AC, Clark GW. Laparoscopic gastric bypass, Roux-en-Y 500 patients: technique and results with 3-60 month follow-up. Obes Surg. 2000;10:233–9.
3. Nguyen NT, Goldman C, Rosenquist J, et al. Laparoscopic versus open gastric bypass: a randomized study of outcomes, quality of life, and costs. Ann Surg. 2001;234:279–91.
4. Podnos YD, Jimenez JC, Wilson SE, et al. Complications after laparoscopic gastric bypass: a review of 3464 cases. Arch Surg. 2003;138:957–61.
5. Buchwald H, Oien DM. Metabolic/bariatric surgery Worldwide 2008. Obes Surg. 2009;19:1605–11.

Sleeve Gastrectomy

15

Konstantinos Albanopoulos and Joanna Papailiou

15.1 Introduction

Sleeve gastrectomy (SG) is a relatively new bariatric procedure that has come to be the most popular choice among metabolic surgeons. It was first published in 1993 by Marceau et al. [1] as part of the duodenal switch malabsorptive operation, in an attempt to improve results of biliopancreatic diversion without performing a distal gastrectomy. Over the years tremendous interest has been shown worldwide by bariatric surgeons. It has been used as a first-step procedure in severely obese patients, as a sole bariatric operation in patients with body mass index (BMI) ranging from 35 to over 65, as a good choice for patients >65 years old, high risk patients, patients with diabetes mellitus type 2 (DM2), in combination with ileal transposition, with Roux-en Y gastric bypass, etc. Evidence have shown that SG reduces ghrelin levels leading to hunger suppression and possibly accelerates gastric emptying, showing that way a physiologic advantage in maintaining weight loss over other restrictive procedures. It can be performed both open and laparoscopically (LSG), with the latter being the preferable approach.

LSG has been proved to have low morbidity and mortality rates, achieves satisfactory excess body weight loss, varying from 51 to 83 % in 1 and 5 years, and requires less postoperative follow-up. Furthermore, it is a procedure where no anastomoses are required, takes 30–45 min to be performed in experienced hands and has a small learning curve, facts that have rendered LSG as the most attractive bariatric procedure among surgeons.

K. Albanopoulos, MD, PhD (✉) • J. Papailiou, MD, MSc, PhD
Department of Propaedeutic Surgery,
Medical School, University of Athens, Athens, Greece
e-mail: albanopoulos_kostis@yahoo.gr

15.2 Indications

Selection criteria include BMI >40 kg/m^2 or BMI >35 kg/m^2 with at least two comorbidities associated with morbid obesity, previously attempted nonsurgical weight-loss treatments and failed to achieve long-term weight loss, patient's personal preference, high-risk patients, older patients, contra-indications for other types of bariatric procedures (inflammatory bowel disease, celiac sprue). Young patients with no other comorbidities may be perfect candidates, since they potentially have a long lifespan without needing to take daily substitutes or medicaments for lifetime. Furthermore, LSG has been shown to be an excellent choice as a first-step bariatric procedure in super-super obese patients with BMI >60 kg/m^2 and can be easily followed by another malabsorptive procedure if patients do not reach a satisfactory weight. Contraindications include substance abuse, patients that had previous upper GI operation (i.e., for perforated ulcer), severe gastric reflux disease, unhealed gastric ulcer and Barret's esophagus.

15.3 Preoperative Work-Up

A multidisciplinary approach of SG candidates is essential. Preoperatively, the patient is evaluated by the bariatric surgeon, a dietitian, a psychologist and an internist or endocrinologist. Patient's eating habits must be evaluated by a trained dietician and more than one visit may be essential so as for the patient to familiarize with the strict postoperative diet and be educated to a new way of consuming food (smaller quantities, good chewing, multiple meals/day). Psychiatric/psychological evaluation should be carried so as to rule out psychocological or neurological disorders associated with boulemia, to estimate patients' postoperative expectations and ensure that the patient has a clear and realistic understanding of the benefits, risks and long-term consequences of this surgical treatment.

H.J. Bonjer (ed.), *Surgical Principles of Minimally Invasive Procedures*, DOI 10.1007/978-3-319-43196-3_15

A preoperative gallbladder ultrasound is performed to evaluate the existence of gallbladder stones, so as to proceed to concomitant cholecystectomy after patient's informed consent. Esophagogastroscopy is required to rule out Barret's esophagus, gastric ulcers or unidentified gastric tumors. Patient is tested for H. pylori and eradication therapy is preoperatively prescribed. Manometry is a prerequisite only in severe preoperative GERD symptoms. In selected cases, further preoperative cardiac, pulmonary, and endocrine evaluation may be needed.

Patient must be fasted at least 12 h before surgery and without per os fluids the last 8 h. Preoperatively, properly sized compression stockings must be applied and the area from the nipples to the pubic symphysis is shaved.

15.4 Operating Room

After induction of anesthesia and endotracheal intubation, the patient is set up in a semilithotomy position with both hands extended (Fig. 15.1). Antisepsia and dressing is carried in a routine manner. The fiberoptic light cable, gas tubing and suction irrigator are usually placed to the head of the patient, while the video monitor is placed on the left side of the head of the patient. The scrub nurse and Mayo instrument tray is positioned toward the right foot of the operating table. The surgeon takes position between the legs and the assistant, on the right side of the table.

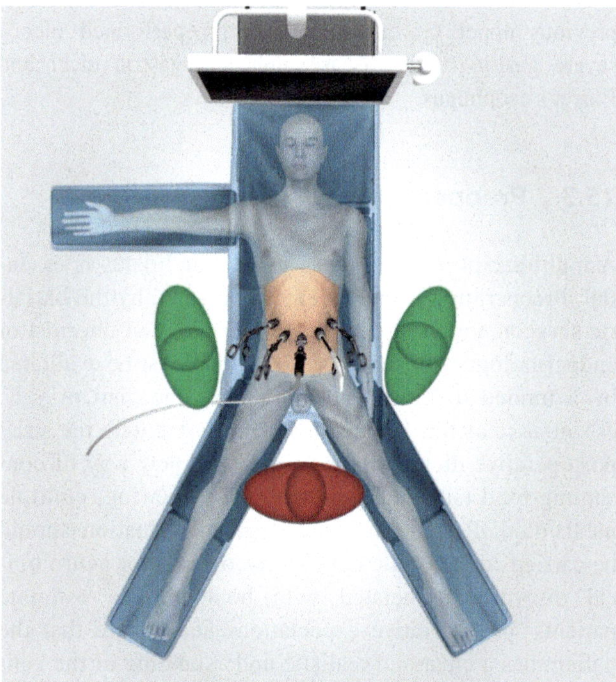

Fig. 15.1 Positioning of the patient for sleeve gastrectomy

15.5 Surgical Technique

An orogastric tube is placed by the anesthesiologist to decompress the stomach before the beginning of the procedure. Usually three to five ports are used, depending on the experience of the surgeon and the intraoperative difficulty (Fig. 15.1). Entering the abdominal cavity is performed with a Veres needle and then a 10 mm trocar or an Optiview™ (Ethicon EndoSurgery, Cincinnati, OH) for the videoscope, approximately 20 cm below the xiphoid process and 2–3 cm to the left, while the patient is still in supine position. We prefer to perform the inscision through the left rectus abdominal muscle, so as to have a better view of the gastroesophageal junction and avoid suturing the midline after the removal of the trocar. If this is very near the umbilicus, the trocar may be placed through the umbilicus. Intraperitoneal space is insufflated with CO_2 at 15 mmHg. Patient is then placed in a steep anti-Trendelenburg position and the rest of the trocars are inserted under direct vision. A 10 mm trocar is placed immediately under the xiphoid process for the liver retractor, a 12 mm port is used for the endoscopic cutting-suturing instrument, placed in the right midsubcostal line 5–6 cm below the level of the videoscope and a 5 or 10 mm port is used for the ultrasonic dissector placed on the left midsubcostal line at the same level as the videoscope (Fig. 15.2). An extra 5 mm port may be placed if additional traction is needed. This can be placed on the left anterior axillary line, again at the same level of the first trocar. A 30° videoscope is inserted in the abdominal cavity and all four quadrants are explored. A flexible fan or loop-shaped liver retractor is induced through the xiphoidal port and the left lobe of the liver is retracted superiorly and medially. In case a liver retractor is unavailable someone can use a spare videoscope as a lever or a grasper that is entered under the liver and

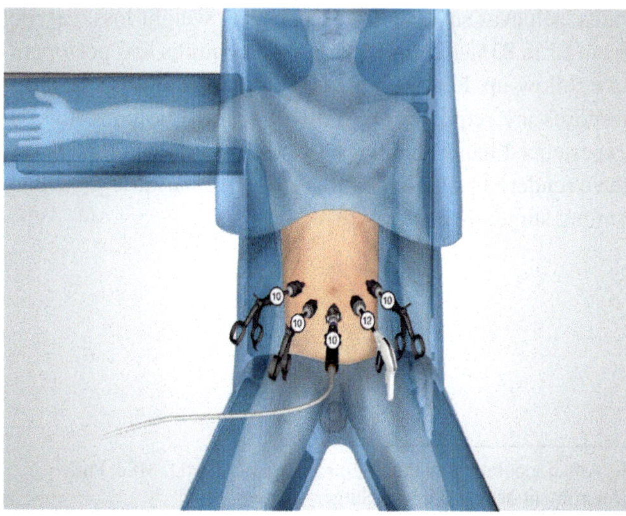

Fig. 15.2 Trocar positioning for sleeve gastrectomy

locked grasping the right crus muscle of the diaphragm, stabilizing the left liver lobe. All trocars are inserted obliquely towards the surgical field.

Exposure, identification and instrumental palpation for confirmation of the pylorus is performed. In general, the surgeon is using the left and right midsubcostal ports for the two instruments and the first assistance handles the videoscope and the liver retractor if needed. In case of five trocars, a second assistant is used. If the left liver lobe and the stomach is relatively small in size and the surgeon is experienced, he can use only three port sites, one for the laparoscope, the 12 mm trocar and the left working trocar. The surgeon can push the left liver lobe with the laparoscope during the stapling for better visualization.

The dissection begins with the surgeon grasping the greater curvature of the stomach with a Babcock clamp, retracting the stomach anteriorly. Many surgeons start dividing the branches of the right gastrepiploic artery from the distal great curvature of the stomach at 6–8 cm proximal to the pylorus (Fig. 15.3). We prefer beginning at 2–3 cm from the pylorus, since it is possible that pylorus after gastric adaptation to SG postoperatively might act as a reservoir (Fig. 15.3). Up to now, no gastric emptying problems have been ever referred by patients. The suitable point is selected and opened with blunt dissection. Ultrasonic dissector begins sequential division of the greater omentum and the short gastric vessels along the greater curvature proximally to the level of the left crus. The surgeon has not worry about any thermal injuries at the surface of the greater curvature of the stomach since this part is going to be removed, though he must always be careful in case of an incidence that will force him to stop the procedure. A slight traction of the stomach caudally and to the right by the assistant's grasper helps stretching the tissues and the gastrosplenic ligament. If the stomach is very large, the second assistant may stretch the omentum laterally via the fifth lateral anterior axillary port. It is important to free all the posterior attachments of the stomach to the pancreas, since they can tear and result in significant bleeding during stapling or prevent the surgeon from making the sleeve "tight".

At the short gastric vessels, surgeon must clearly visualize the tissue grasped by the ultrasonic dissector, especially in its tip, so as to avoid partial dissection of the next short gastric vessel, which would also result in bleeding and distortion of the surgical field. In case of hemorrhage you can put a gaze and tamponade through one of the two working ports. A better visualization of the lesser sac space and the path of the gastrosplenic ligament are obtained if the stomach is grasped along its posterior wall beneath the cut. Short gastric vessels dissection is completed when the spleen is free and the left crus of the diaphragm and esophagus are visualized. Caudal traction helps to identify and expose a possible hiatal hernia. With further Babcock retraction near the top of the great curvature, a few posterior peritoneal adhesions at the back of the stomach may be recognized and divided (Fig. 15.4).

At this point the surgeon asks the anesthesiologist and confirms the removal of the orogastric tube. The anesthesiologist then inserts transorally, with caution, the bougie to the pyloric channel. It is very important that the orogastric tube is removed, because otherwise it may be stapled and incarcerated in the staple line. The surgeon can help directing the bougie to the pylorus with two bowel graspers. A lot of discussion has been done over the size of the bougie that

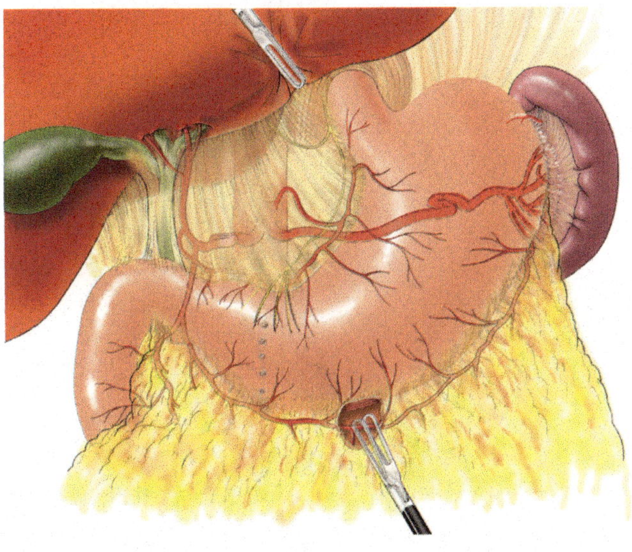

Fig. 15.3 Dividing the branches of the right gastro-epiploic artery. (Reproduced with permission of Prof. Guy-Bernard Cadière, illustrator: Christian Bogaert)

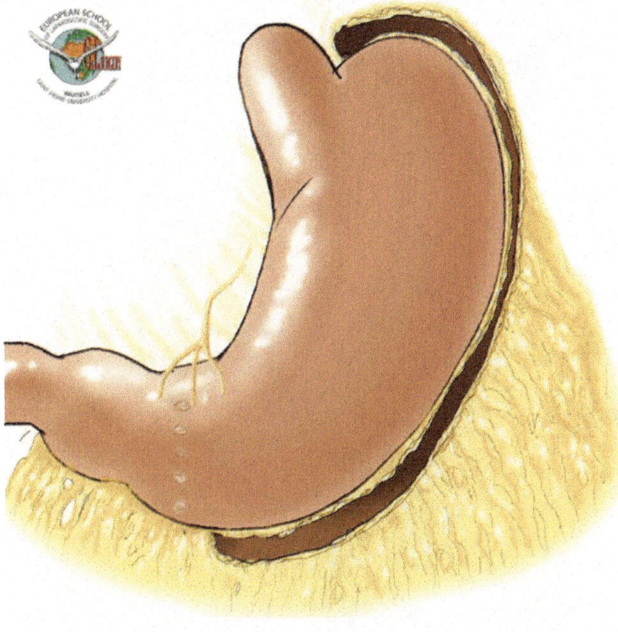

Fig. 15.4 Release greater curvature completed. (Reproduced with permission of Prof. Guy-Bernard Cadière, illustrator: Christian Bogaert)

should be used in LSG, with a number of studies presenting contradictory results. Sizes in literature vary from 32–60 Fr, though most surgeons use a 32–42 Fr bougie, our team prefers the 38 Fr bougie. A linear stapler device is inserted through the 12 mm trocar, tightly suppressed to the bougie and gastric division begins (Fig. 15.5).

At this step it is important that the assistant retracts the body of the stomach caudally for the first firing and laterally for the rest so that no folding of the wall of the stomach will occur inside the stapler. Stapling continuous cranially along the bougie while the surgeon applies the stapler with his left hand, retracting the gastric stunt from the staple line with his right hand. Usually a total of 5–6 firings are enough. Green cartridges are used for the first two firings, in order to secure the staple line at the thickened antral stomach and blue cartridges are suitable for the rest of the staple line. We prefer to have the last firing approximately 1–2 cm away from the gastroesophageal junction in an attempt to reduce the percentage of staple line leakage from that area. Extra caution must be taken not to push the stapler down during applying, something that may result in taking too much tissue from the posterior wall of the stomach and lesser from the anterior. Some surgeons use buttress material in an attempt to reduce staple-line hemorrhage and possibly leak rate. Our team and other investigators too have not seen any differences in leak rates by staple line reinforcement either with buttress materials or with the continuous suture [2]. We do not use it routinely and in cases we have a staple-line hemorrhage we prefer to use an eight figure interrupted suture with a polypropelene nonabsorbable 2/0 suture or a metallic clip. If we decide to oversew the staple line we use a continuous polypropelene nonabsorbable 2/0 suture, though surgeon must keep in mind that he might make the sleeve even "tighter". We always reinforce the staple line in cases of LAGB removal and simultaneous LSG and inform the patient of a higher risk for leak rate (Fig. 15.6).

Having throughout the procedure the bougie in position and pressing it to the lesser curvature with the stapler, helps the surgeon to achieve a smooth shaped sleeve and avoiding formation of hourglass-shaped SG. Moreover, it is mandatory to push down and to maintain the bougie beyond the gastric angulus in order to avoid an excessive narrowing at that spot, that may cause dysphagia and vomiting and a postoperative stricture.

The anesthesiologist then removes the bougie and inserts the nasogastric tube. Pylorus is clamped by compression and the anesthesiologist instills methylene blue mixed with saline through the nasogastric tube (usually 60 cc) to test for any staple line leaks. We prefer to leave the nasogastric tube in place for 24 h postoperatively, since we believe that it helps in releasing the entrapped air and the increased pressures of the gastric tube, mechanisms that might be an additional risk for leak.

The resected stomach is extracted from the right midline port site; a finger dilatation of the anterior and posterior abdominal rectus sheath may be required. No drains are placed. Abdomen is decompressed, all trocars are removed and port sites are injected with local anesthetic. Skin is sutured with endodermal absorbable No3/0 or interrupted plain or vertical mattress No3/0 nonabsorbable sutures.

After the procedure, patients are transferred to the recovery room and then to their room. Only few patients with

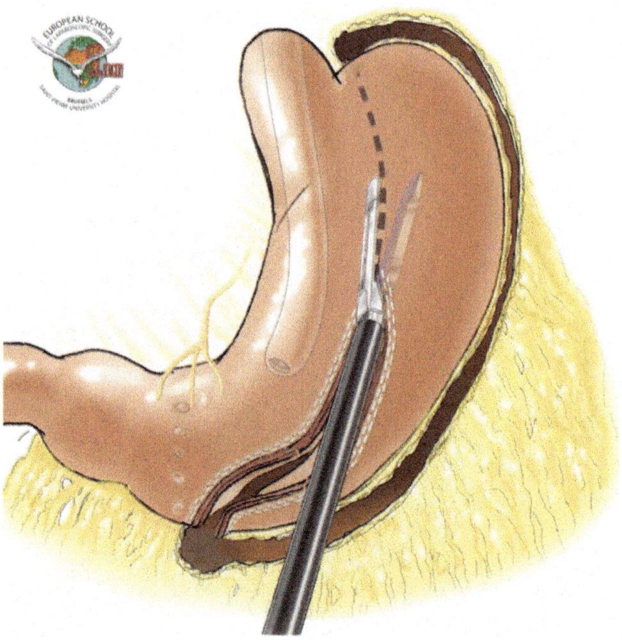

Fig. 15.5 Bougie guides transection of the stomach. (Reproduced with permission of Prof. Guy-Bernard Cadière, illustrator: Christian Bogaert)

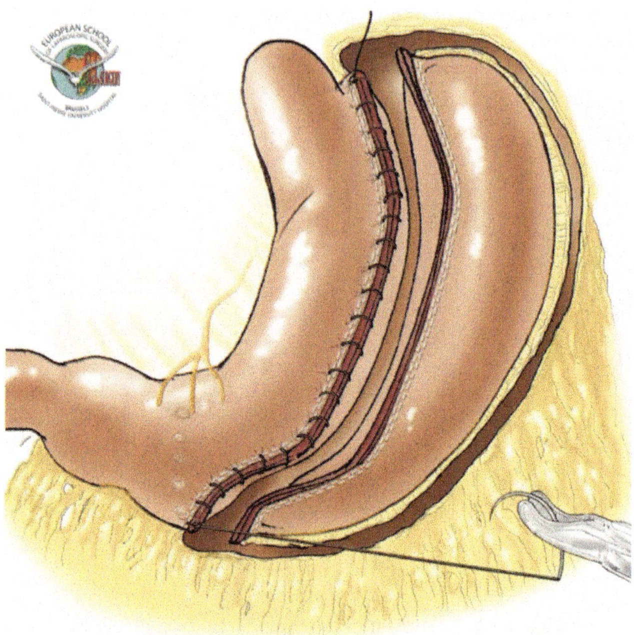

Fig. 15.6 Staple line reinforcement by running suture. (Reproduced with permission of Prof. Guy-Bernard Cadière, illustrator: Christian Bogaert)

serious comorbidities may require intermediate care unit for 24 h.

In single-incision laparoscopic sleeve gastrectomy (SILS-SG), patient is placed again in semilithotomy reverse Trendelenburg position, with the surgeon between the legs and the assistant on the right side of the patient. The specially designed trocar for SILS is placed with open technique through a 2–3 cm umbilical incision. Pneumoperitoneum is produced at 15 mmHg pressure. A 30° video laparoscope is used along with a 5 mm ultrascissor dissector, standard straight graspers and a multiple applications 60-mm stapler (Echelon Flex-Ethicon-Endosurgery). SILS-SG's feasibility depends strongly on the experience of the bariatric surgeon, patient's left liver lobe size and short umbilicus-xiphoid distance (<25 cm). To retract the left liver lobe you can put another trocar under the xiphoid process or put an external suture with straight needle through the abdominal wall, pass it under the left lobe and exit again through the abdominal wall at the right midclavicular line. Furthermore, you can use an external suture for the traction of the greater curvature of the stomach, if needed. The operative steps are similar to standard LSG and the specimen is extracted by the umbilical incision. The fascial defect is closed with a figure of eight absorbable suture No2/0 to avoid postoperative port site hernia. Lately, robotic SG has been referred in the literature [3] involving a higher cost of disposables, without adding any actual benefit to the procedure.

15.6 Postoperative Care

Patient is administered LMWH at prophylactic dose 6 h after the operation and is mobilized the same evening. The nasogastric tube is removed on the first postoperative day. If there is no indication of a complication and his blood tests are normal, the patient starts liquid diet and is released from hospital on the second postoperative day. He is administered LMWH in prophylactic dose for 20 days postoperatively, PPIs in cases of gastroesophageal reflux symptoms, a multivitamin supplement for a month and he is prescribed by the dietician a liquid diet for the first ten posotperative days followed by semiliquid diet for another 10 days. Patients in our clinic are instructed to have a complete blood count and CRP every 2 days until the 15th postoperative day. We have noticed that white blood cell count and CRP increase in the first 24 h and then progressively decrease. If these values continue rising or re-increase or if the patient experiences fever, discomfort, tachycardia, tachypnea, abdominal pain, nausea, vomiting or any other clinical signs suggestive of complication we request the patient to visit the hospital for a physical examination. In case of leak suspicion we perform gastrografin swallow test and dependently an abdomen CT scan.

One of the most serious complications after SG is gastric leak. Leaks are identified as early leaks (first to third postoperative day), intermediate leaks (fourth to seventh postoperative day) and late leaks (>8th postoperative day). The majority of leaks are located near the esophageal junction. Up to now no universal guidelines are issued about its management and every institution has its own protocols, though all surgeons agree that early diagnosis is key to adequate treatment. In our department we have developed a treatment algorithm, according to our experience and the evolving published data. Prolonged hospital length of stay is a common consequence of gastric leak, with an average of 4–6 weeks.

Another not so frequently mentioned complication of SG is stricture of the gastric tube. The patient usually presents with dysphagia, epigastric pain and continuous vomiting and a contrast swallow test reveals the site of the stricture. It is most likely to occur when no bougie is used in the initial operation, or if it is removed before the end of the stappling, by kinking of the gastric tube or during oversewing of the staple line or after a cured leak due to retraction by scarring. Therapeutic esophagogastroduodenoscopy with balloon dilations are used to relieve the stenosis. In case of failure, some surgeons favor therapeutic stenting for bridging the distal gastric stenosis, while others prefer to proceed to laparoscopic stricturoplasty if the length is small or seromyotomy for longer stenosis. After seromyotomy a leak test must be executed to ensure no gastric mucosa perforation is done and myotomy is covered by omentoplasty with interrupted absorbable sutures. If none of these methods provide a satisfactory result and resection and conversion of SG to gastric bypass proximal to the stricture or even total gastrectomy is the remaining solution [4].

Following surgery patients are monitored by the dietician for weight loss, BMI, weist to hip ratio and their nutritional status and habits. Their immediate postoperative diet consists of only fluids for 10 days, blender for the following 10 days and free diet afterwards. Total blood count and CRP are performed Nutritional and metabolic blood Following surgery, patients were monitored for weight loss, BMI and percentage EWL, WHR in 30 days, 3, 6 and 12 months postoperatively. Nutritional and metabolic blood tests are performed on a frequent basis (at 3, 6 and 12 months after surgery and annually thereafter). At 12 months and annually thereafter patients are advised to have a gallbladder ultrasound for possible chololithiasis.

SG is considered to be a technically easier operation compared to gastric bypass and biliopancreatic diversion. It has a small morbidity and mortality rates with satisfactory results in body weight loss even in super-super obese patients. Despite the low rate of complications that range from (0.7–4 %) some of them are potentially fatal. Therefore the surgeon must always be careful in the operating details and alert for their existence and their mechanisms of production will help preventing them and preserving the safety of the technique.

References

1. Marceau P, Biron S, Bourque RA, et al. Biliopancreatic diversion with a new type of gastrectomy. Obes Surg. 1993;3:29–35.
2. Albanopoulos K, Alevizos L, Flessas J, et al. Reinforcing the staple line during laparoscopic sleeve gastrectomy: Prospective randomized clinical study comparing two different techniques. Preliminary results. Obes Surg. 2011;22(1):42–6.
3. Diamantis T, Alexandrou A, Nikiteas N, et al. Initial experience with robotic sleeve gastrectomy for morbid obesity. Obes Surg. 2011;21:1172–9.
4. Zundel N, Hernandez JD, Galvao Neto M, et al. Strictures after laparoscopic sleeve gastrectomy. Surg Laparosc Endosc Percutan Tech. 2010;20:154–8.

16 Laparoscopic Biliopancreatic Diversion with Duodenal Switch

Catalin Copaescu

16.1 Introduction

The biliopancreatic diversion with duodenal switch (BPD-DS) was proposed in 1988 by Hess and Marceau [1], as a modification of the biliopancreatic diversion (BPD) previously described by N. Scopinaro [2], aiming to reduce some of the its complications (marginal ulcers and dumping syndrome). The technique of BPD-DS combines *a pylorus-preserving gastric sleeve resection* with a *duodenal switch,* providing a moderate food intake restriction with a considerable reduction of the fat absorption, as a support for an efficient and durable weight loss. BPD-DS has been shown to have the best results of any bariatric procedure, in terms of magnitude and duration of weight loss as well the co-morbidities control. (Fig. 16.1).

M. Gagner performed the first laparoscopic duodenal switch (LBPD-DS) in 1999 [3]. The procedure is a complex one, associating an important risk of peri-operative morbidity, especially in the super-obese (SO) patients. The advantages of laparoscopic surgery may decrease the surgical trauma, the pulmonary and wound complications.

Moreover, the actually recommended strategy of 2-steps LBPD-DS is likely to increase in popularity for the treatment of morbid obesity, especially with the recent advent of laparoscopic sleeve gastrectomy (LSG) for higher-risk patients [4].

16.2 Indications and Contraindications

16.2.1 Indications

- The obese patients with ***BMI greater than 40 kg/m2***, who have attempted unsuccessful behavioral weight loss therapy are considered good candidates for primary LBPD-DS.
- Also, it is well-known that, in the obese patients with ***BMI greater than 50 kg/m2***, the long-term efficiency of LBPD-DS is superior to any other bariatric operation. On the other hand, the indication for a primary LBPD-DS in this subgroup is limited because of the complexity of the procedure and the relative high morbidity and mortality risk. There for a LBPD-DS performed *as a second stage bariatric procedure* (after LSG) is more appropriate for these cases.
- LBPD-DS is more indicated for the morbidly obese patients with ***severe arthritis*** having a need for a long term therapy in comparison with the high ulcerogenic potential of a gastric bypass (GBP).
- Similar to Scopinaro-BPD, LBPD-DS is very effective on ***metabolic disorders*** (Type II diabetes mellitus, severe dyslipidemia) but associates less complication (no marginal ulcers or dumping syndrome)
- LBPD DS is also often considered as a ***redo procedure after failure of other bariatric procedures*** like open/laparoscopic gastric banding (GB), laparoscopic sleeve gastrectomy (LSG), greater curvature plication (GCP) or vertical banded gastroplasty (VBG). Especially after VBG, LBPD-DS is superior to BPD or GBP as the small bowel would be anastomosed to the duodenum, away from the site of the previous surgery.

16.2.2 Absolute Contraindications

Absolute contraindications would include those patients who are vegetarian, or have inflammatory bowel disease.

16.2.3 Relative Contraindications

Relative contraindications of LBPD-DS include:

- patients with *previous abdominal surgery* especially those who undergone prior open gastrectomy. The gastric dissection may be difficult due to intense adherences.

C. Copaescu, MD, PhD
Minimal Invasive & Bariatric Surgery Department, Ponderas Academic Hospital, Bucharest, Romania
e-mail: catalincopaescu@gmail.com

H.J. Bonjer (ed.), *Surgical Principles of Minimally Invasive Procedures*, DOI 10.1007/978-3-319-43196-3_16

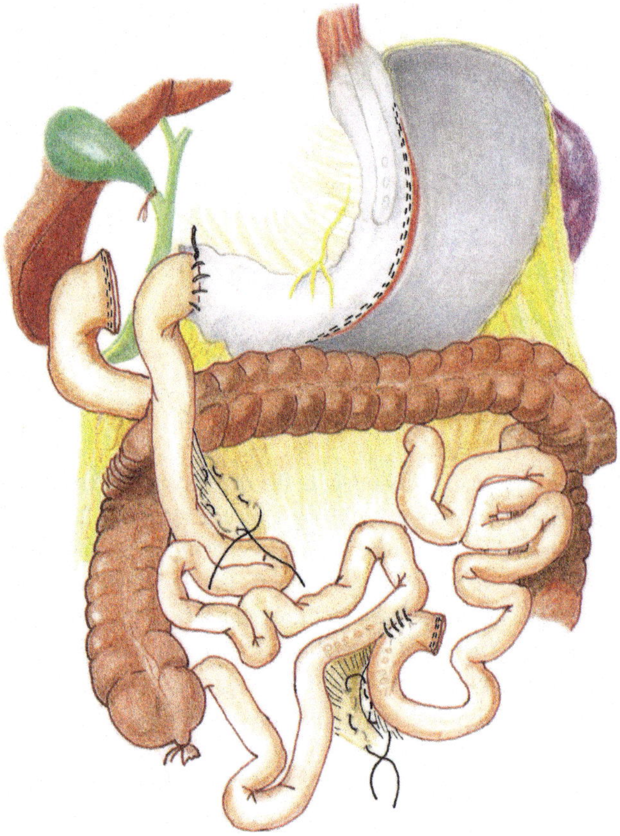

Fig. 16.1 Biliopancreatic diversion with duodenal switch

- patients who have *colon resections* that could affect water reabsorbtion, resulting in uncontrollable diarrhea.
- patients with *proteinuria* (this condition may severely influence on the protein balance).
- patients with severe *gastro esophageal reflux disease.* As the gastric sleeve resection removes the fundus of the stomach it is impossible to perform an anti-reflux procedure (total or partial fundoplications), except for the hiatal closure and/or a cardiopexy (Narbona-Arnau or Lucius Hill like procedure). These patients are probably better served by the Roux-en-Y GBP.
- pathologies requiring a *future retrograde colangio-pancreatography* (ERCP) – because it is virtually impossible to perform it up through the biliopancreatic limb.

16.2.4 Relative Contraindications for One Step LBPD-DS

Relative contraindications for one step LBPD-DS include high risk patients/situations. In these cases a ***LSG*** as a ***first step*** of ***LBPD-DS*** is recommended.:

- patients with BMI over 50 kg/m^2, especially over 60 kg/m^2
- patients presenting severe co-morbidities (liver cirrhosis, respiratory or renal failure, coagulopathies)
- an estimated technically difficult procedure
- surgeon's low level of expertise with LBPD-DS (mentor is necessary)

16.3 Preoperative Evaluation and Work-Up

Due to the complexity of the pathology and of the LBPD-DS procedure it is necessary for all the patients to be included in a *Bariatric Program* run in a certified *Center of Excellence in Bariatric Surgery.*

The preoperative evaluation, including all diagnostic tests, is critical in the screening process of a bariatric patient, as it is the opportunity to identify abnormalities and conditions that must be treated prior to surgery.

The *respiratory tests* are mandatory to evaluate the lung function. Moreover, in a large number of morbidly obese patients *sleep studies* are necessary in order to identify those cases that require continuous positive airway pressure (CPAP) for several weeks before the operation.

Abdominal sonography with vascular Doppler evaluation and sometimes *CT- scan* are necessary to identify other pathologies and the thrombotic risk.

An *upper GI contrast study* and an *esophago-gastro-duodenoscopy* are routinely performed to exclude any gastric or duodenal pathology as well the presence of Helicobacter Pylori (HP). If HP are identified medical therapy is administrated in order to eradicate the bacteria.

Colonoscopy is indicated in the patients with clinical history of an inflammatory bowel disease and in all the patients older than 50 years.

Routinely, the *laboratory tests* include electrolyte and hematology panel.

All the patients are seen by an *anesthesiologist.* The preoperative evaluation of the airway (including the neck girth of the patient) is necessary in order to identify and avoid any potential difficulty.

Each patient undergoes preoperative evaluation by a *psychiatrist* and by a *nutritionist.*

The LBPD-DS patients are admitted to the hospital on the day before surgery and are instructed to take a clear liquid diet. Patients are given an anticoagulant, Fragmine, in the evening of day before operation.

Bowel cleansing with purgatives (Dulcolax-ten tablets) is routinely recommended. As the small bowel is emptied additional space will be obtain and the loops are easier to be manipulated.

All the patients are told to take their antihypertensive medications, including the morning of surgery but to hold any anti-diabetic medication.

16.4 Operating Room and Patient Set-Up

In order to perform the laparoscopic BPD-DS the patients undergo *general anesthesia and endotracheal intubation*. Often the control of these patients is challenging justifying the presence of a very skilled anesthesiologist, familiar with the particularities of a bariatric patient. When the anesthesiologist identifies that an obese patient will be difficult to intubate, the safest approach and the standard of care requires awake *fiber optic intubation*.

During the anesthesia appropriate *vital parameters monitoring* is mandatory. Occasional *central IV line* is required. A *urinary catheter*, an 18 Fr *oro-gastric tube* to decompress the stomach, as well *sequential pneumatic compression boots* are placed on. Prophylactic antibiotic therapy is administrated at the beginning of the procedure.

The procedure is performed using the *French position*: the patient is laying on the operating table with the legs abducted. Initially the surgeon stands between the patient's legs with the assistants on both sides and later on, during the procedure, he will move left laterally (Fig. 16.2).

Operating tables designed for bariatric patients are recommended. A proper placement and fixation of the patient on the operating table is essential to avoid postural complications. Foot plate supports attached to the operating table will properly secure the extremities. Using gel pads may decrease the risk of postural trauma, especially in extreme obese patients and/or estimated long lasting operations.

A *laparoscopic complete equipment* including an high resolution camera is recommended. The image will be displayed on *two separate monitors* able to rotate around the patient, accessible to all the members of the team. A 10 mm

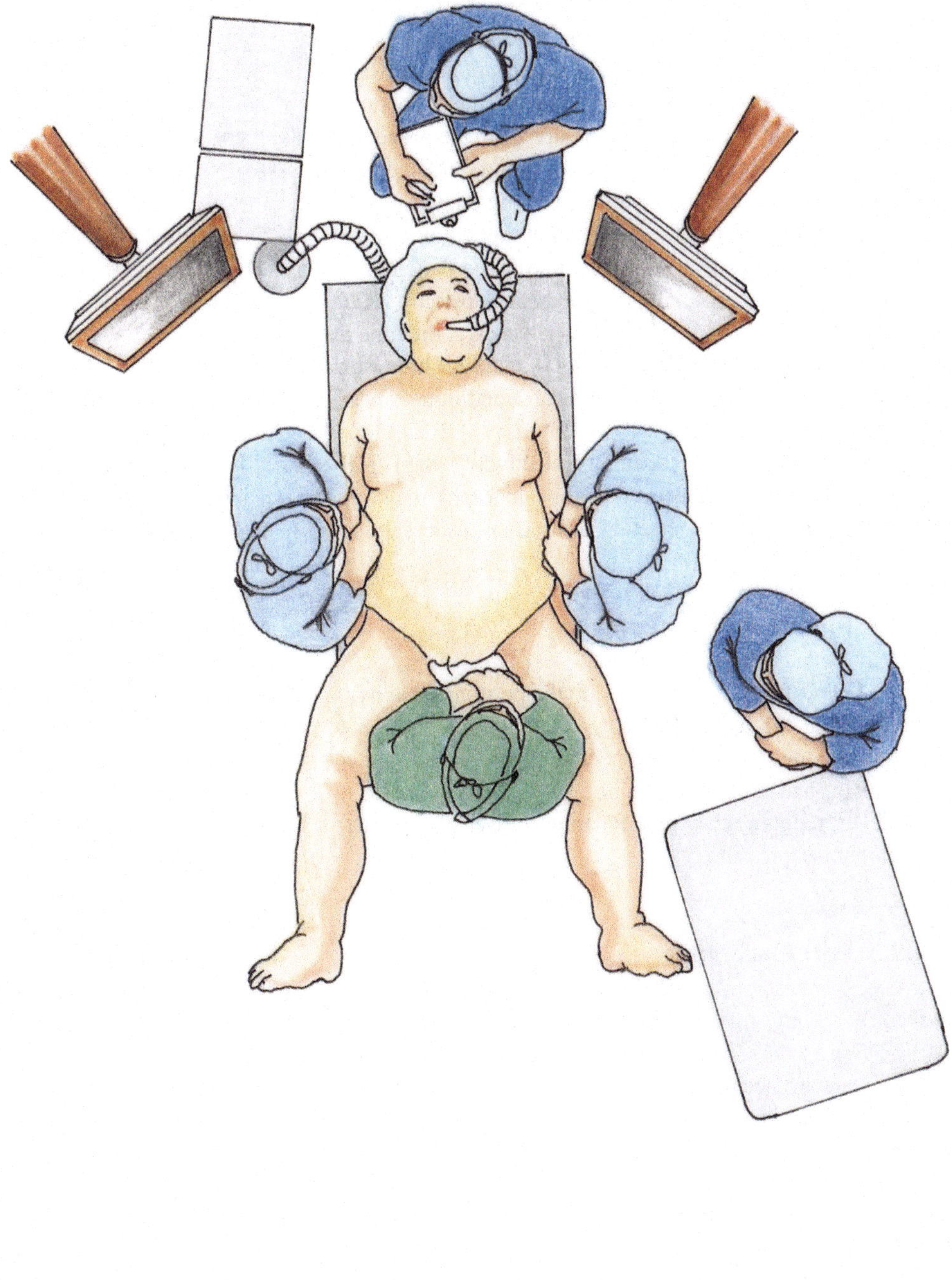

Fig. 16.2 Patient positioning for laparoscopic biliopancreatic diversion with duodenal switch

45° extra-long laparoscope, an adequate liver retractor and long laparoscopic instruments (length greater than 42 cm) are necessary. Endoscopic staplers and efficient energy devices are mandatory.

16.5 Surgical Technique

16.5.1 Surgical Technique Strategy

The laparoscopic BPD-DS involves several steps which include: division of the duodenum, sleeve gastrectomy, measurement of the alimentary limb, creation of a duodenoenterostomy, approximation the common channel and a distal ileoenteric anastomosis. This order of the operative steps is usually respected as well some surgeons prefer to start the procedure with the distal anastomosis (the ileo-ileostomy).

The demonstrated advantages of the *LSG as a first step* of a LBPD-DS in high risk obese patients determined us to consider that is safer to start with the sleeve resection. For example, if the LBPD-DS candidate presents intra-operative arguments for an estimated technically difficult procedure (severe fat infiltration of the viscera, short and retracted mesentery) or he/she is not able to tolerate a long pneumoperitoneum, the operation may be shortened at this point, without compromising the rest of the procedure or the patient. The enteric anastomosis especially the duodeno-ileostomy which is the most challenging one, may be performed at the time of the *second stage*, after at least 6 months and an important weight loss, with improved technical conditions and a decreased anesthetic risk.

Cholecystectomy is performed selectively when gallstones are present. Intraoperative ultrasonography may help in the diagnosis. Routine appendectomy is not necessary.

16.5.2 Pneumoperitoneum

For the LBPD-DS, the first entry into the peritoneal cavity is established at the umbilicus using an open technique or a blind technique. Pneumoperitoneum is initially limited to 12 mmHg and later this value may gradually rise to 15 mmHg, reducing the hemodynamic impact of the intra-abdominal gas pressure.

16.5.3 Port Placement

Seven ports are routinely inserted for the laparoscopic BPD-DS procedure, but up to nine ports may be used. Extra-long trocars are occasionally needed in patients who have a very thick abdominal wall.

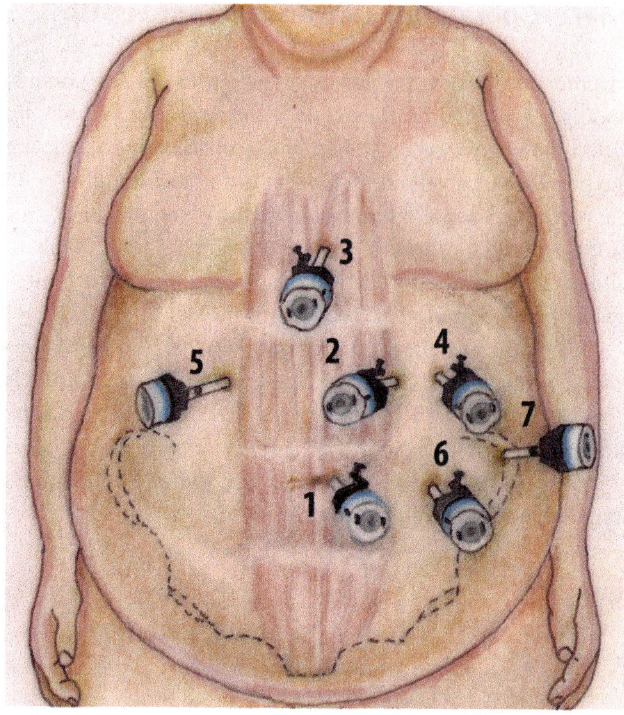

Fig. 16.3 Port positioning for biliopancreatic diversion with duodenal switch

The standard position of the trocars is depicted in Fig. 16.3. Three 10 mm reusable trocars, one 5 mm reusable trocar and three disposable 5–12 or 5–15 mm ports are inserted:

- A 10 mm reusable trocar at the umbilicus – used to introduce the 10 mm 45° laparoscope (Optical trocar 1)
- A 10 mm reusable trocar at the epigastric left paramedian position. This access port is used to introduce the 10 mm 45° laparoscope (Optical trocar 2) facilitating the adequate view of the structures at the time of proximal dissection and resection of the gastric fundus.
- A 10 mm reusable one at the subxifoidian area, slight to the right paramedian position, at the level of the left liver edge. Through this access port the articulated 10 mm liver retractor (Cuschieri Retractor, Karl Storz, Germany) is introduced to elevate the left liver lobe. I prefer the Ternamian reusable cannula (Karl Storz, Germany) which permits a blunt and less traumatic insertion, lowering the hemorrhagic risk at this level.
- A 5–15 mm disposable port is inserted in the left subcostal area, in the midclavicular line. Through this port energy devices, endoscopic staplers as well other laparoscopic instruments (forceps, scissors, needle holder) are introduced into the operative field.
- A 5–15 mm disposable trocar is inserted in the right mid-abdomen, in the right subcostal area, several centimeters above the level of the umbilicus, in the midclavicular line.

- A 5–12 mm disposable trocar is inserted in the left infra-umbilical area, and
- A 5 mm reusable port is placed in the left, lateral position, in the anterior axillary line approximately 3–4 cm below the left costal margin.

Additional disposable or reusable trocars are inserted according to the individual characteristics of the patient.

16.5.4 Gastric Sleeve Resection

The operating table is positioned in reverse-Trendelenburg, slight rotated toward the right side and the surgeon stands between the patient's legs. A 10 mm articulated liver retractor is introduced through the 10 mm xyfodian port to elevate the left lobe and to expose the entire anterior aspect of the stomach. An external arm will hold the retractor for a stabile position during the procedure (Fig. 16.4).

The gastrectomy begins by transecting the gastric vessels of the greater curvature at the level of gastric angle, where entering into the *lesser sac* is facile. Appropriate control of the vascular branches divided towards the His angle or duodenum is obtained only with an opened *lesser sac*.

The short gastric vessels are divided with a long laparoscopic sealing/divider instrument (LigaSure, Medtronic, US.) or an ultrasonic dissector (Harmonic-ACE, Ethicon, US). Care must be taking not to injury the spleen or its vessels during the completion of greater curvature freeing or division of the retro-gastric attachments.

Distally, the dissection is continued along the greater curvature, near the gastric wall, for 2–3 cm beyond the pylorus. At this point, a retroduodenal tunnel is created by gentile dissection maneuvers starting with the inferior duodenal margin. The dissection is carried out very close to the posterior wall of the duodenum, in a plane superior to the gastroduodenal artery (which is often seen posterior). A small supraduodenal window is created medially to the common bile duct and lateral to the hepatic artery, to orientate the transection of the duodenum between these very important structures. The small arterial branches approaching the superior margin of the proximal duodenum are preserved.

The duodenum is usually divided 2–3 cm distal to the pylorus with a 45–3.5 linear stapler which passes gently along the retroduodenal just-created route. Injury to the pancreas, the gastroepiplooic or the gastroduodenal arteries is avoided.

The control of the bleeding on the distal duodenal stump may be realized with a running suture of 2.0 Vircyl. This suture may incorporate periduodenal fat in an attempt to reduce the possible postoperative duodenal leak. Haemostatic clips or buttresss material cannot be used on the proximal duodenal stump when a stapled duodeno-enterostomy is intended.

The sleeve gastrectomy is initiated at 6 cm proximal to the pylorus, with a firing of 4.8 or 3.5 linear stapler inserted through the right sided 5–15 mm disposable port. Next, a 56 French bougie inserted oro-gastrically by the anesthesiologist is *passed* into the distal antrum and aligned medially along the lesser curvature of the stomach.

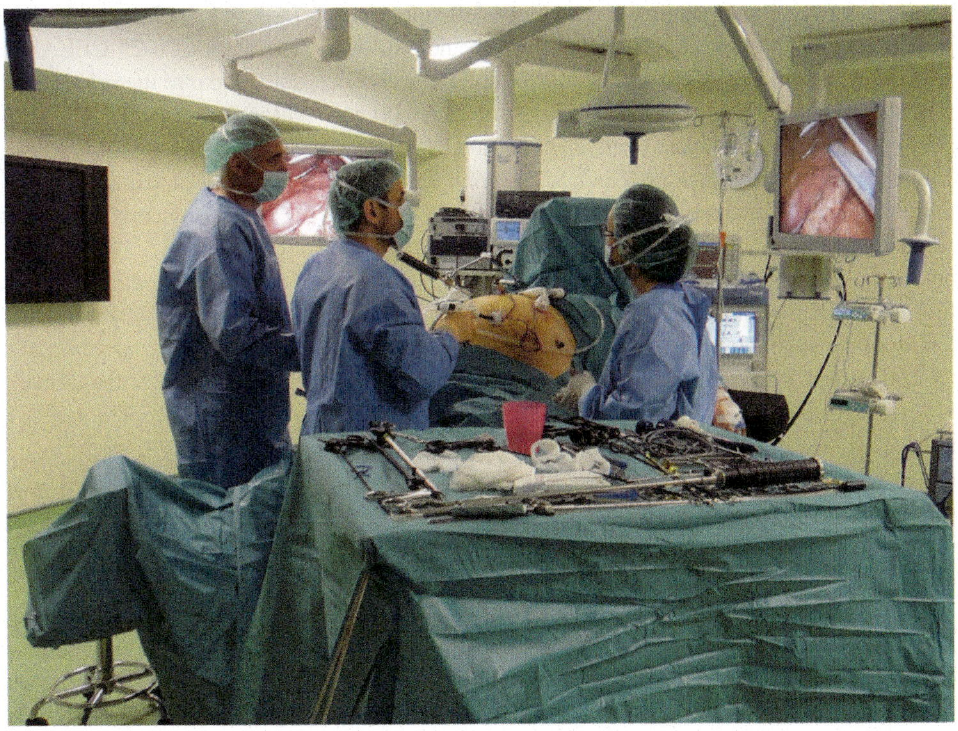

Fig. 16.4 Positioning of the surgical team

The LSG is completed by sequential firings of blue or green 60 mm straight linear staplers, inserted through the left sided 5–15 mm disposable port and oriented parallel to the calibration bougie. Before every firing the stomach is retracted laterally. Careful inspection of its anterior and posterior aspect is necessary in order to ensure enough distance away from the incisura anglaris and lesser curvature, to avoid any ischemic gap along the stapled line, any stenosis or axial twist of the gastric tube. Also we are aware that a too close transaction to the gastroesophageal junction may result in a severe stenosis or leak and a too far transaction may lead to fundus dilatation and weight regain.

Buttress material is often used for sleeve resection: nonresorbable bovine pericardium (Peristrips Veritas, US) or Bioabsorbable Seamguard (Gore, Flagstaff, Arizona, US). This material covers both the anterior and the posterior gastric walls trying to decreased the bleeding and the leakage rate from the staple line.

Looking insistently for bleeding sources on the stapled line after intraoperative rise up of the blood pressure with Neosynephryne is our routine attitude thus significantly reducing the rate of postoperative hemorrhagic complications. Haemostatic clips or stapled line oversewing are used to control the bleeding [5].

The 56-Fr bougie is removed and the resected lateral part of the stomach is extracted in a plastic bag.

16.5.5 Small Bowel Measurement

The operating table is placed in the horizontal position and tilt to the left, while the surgeon moves to the left side of the patient. The small intestine is measured with the help of two previously marked at 5 cm atraumatic double-fenestrated 5 mm graspers starting from the ileocecal valve. A 100 cm common channel is marked with a green stitch. Another 150 cm are proximally measured and, at this point, the proximal end of the alimentary channel is marked with a black stitch. The enteric measurement continues up to the first jejunal loop, evaluating the dimension of the biliopancreatic limb (BPL) and completing the information about the total length of the small bowel.

This information is very important to appreciate if individual adjustments to the above mentioned figures are needed. It was demonstrated that the total length (TL) of the small bowel vary from 4 to 10 m and only a combination of 40 % of TL for the *alimentary channel* with 10 % of TL for the *common channel* provides good long-term results and less complications. An error in this distribution may affect the late outcome of the patient from a severe malabsobtion (the common channel is relatively too short) to inadequate weight loss (the alimentary limb is too long). The limbs are constructed in increments of 25 cm, the final length being the point nearest to the 10 or 40 % of the TL. For example, the common channel (CC) may be 50, 75 or 100 cm while the alimentary channel (AL) may be 250, 275, 300 or more [1].

Beside the importance of this very useful rationale in a large majority of cases the formula 75/100 for CC and 250 cm for AL is appropriate.

Next, at the proximal end of the AL, the ileum is transected with a 45–2.5 linear stapler and its mesentery is divided. The distal end of the transected ileum will be brought up to the duodenum to create the *duodeno-ileal anastomosis*, while the proximal ileal end is anastomosed with distal intestine to form the common channel (CC). The BPL must be coming from the left side of the abdomen while AL and CC are on the right side. There must be no twist of the mesentery and this should been tested prior to both anastomoses.

16.5.6 Duodeno-Ileal Anastomosis

Often, an antecolic end-to side duodenoenterostomy is preferred but sometimes, a transmesocolic route and/or an end-to end variant is chosen. Occasionally, the right colon has to be mobilized and/or the greater omentum divided in order to bring the ileum and its mesentery higher up without tension.

For LBPD-DS, the duodeno-ileal anastomosis can be fashioned in several ways : with a *circular stapler*, a *linear stapler* or manually and all these variants are described below.

16.5.6.1 Circular Stapler

The anvil of a 25-CEEA circular stapler (Covidien, US) is delivered into the proximal duodenal stump using two different ways:

- *Transoral*, using a 25-Orvill® (Covidien, US) or a modified nasogastric tube-anvil apparatus as was proposed by Gagner [3]
- *Transabdominally*: the anvil is introduced through one of the ports and then passed into the duodenum:
  - *via* a *gastrotomy* performed on the area planned to be removed at the sleeve resection or
  - via a *duodenotomy*, closed with a 2.0 purse-string suture.

The end-to site duodeno-enterostomy is created by passing the circular stapler transabdominally, advancing it into the intestinal lumen and attaching it to the anvil. After firing, the circular stapler is removed and the open end of the ileum is closed with a linear stapler. A plastic camera drape, covers the circular stapler and protects the wound during the passage of the contaminated shaft.

16.5.6.2 Linear Stapler

Small enterotomies are done on the inferior margin of the duodenum and on the antimesenteric side of the ileum. Minimal tension between the two is mandatory to prevent the enlargement of the opening after firing. A side-to side duodeno-enterostomy is created by a 30 mm 3.5 linear stapler. The opening is closed with a 2.0 PDO running suture.

16.5.6.3 Manually

The end-to site or end-to end hand sewn duodenoenterostomy may be fashioned in one or, more often, two layers. Two stay-stitches are placed at the superior and inferior borders of the duodenum and ileum. The posterior layer is realized by a 2.0 silk running suture, incorporates the staple line and ensures the opposition of the two. Enterotomies are then performed with the monopolar hook on the duodenum and ileum sites. The second posterior layer is a 2.0 PDO running suture. Next, two other anterior 2.0 running sutures will close the anastomosis (Fig. 16.5).

Finally, a nasogastro-duodenal tube will be placed just before the anastomosis. A methylene blue test is performed with the small bowel distally clamped to confirm the integrity of all staple-lines. The size of the gastric pouch is approximated by the volume of methylene blue required to distend the pouch and usually is around 150 ml.

Apparently the stapled technique is simple but some particularities for the LBPD-DS limit its use:

- The 25 CEEA stapler is often difficult to insert in a relatively small distal ileum,
- The 25 anvil's passage through the pylorus needs dilatation which may favor the dumping syndrome and the postcibal disorders.
- By using of a smaller circular stapler CEEA-21 the risk of stenosis is increased
- Direct insertion of the anvil into a short proximal duodenum needs a purse-string suture which is not easy and time consuming.
- The linear stapler presents a too long inactive tip and sometimes may create ischemic gaps.

In these conditions the manually technique, personally my favorite one, is more and more accepted by the surgeons.

16.5.7 Distal Ileo-Ileal Anastomosis

The proximal end of the transected ileum (the biliopancreatic limb) is anastomosed to the distal ileum, at 75/100 cm proximal to the ileocecal valve, to form a short common channel. This ileo-ileostomy is performed in a standard site-to side fashion with 2.5 linear staplers. Small enterotomies are done on the antimesenteric borders of the two intestinal loops. Each jaw of the linear stapler is inserted into an enterotomy and the instrument is fired (Fig. 16.6). Double stapled technique, with another stapler fired in opposite direction, is more appropriate for this anastomosis as the ileum is often very narrow. The opening is closed with a 2.0 PDO running suture or a linear stapler transversally orientated.

16.5.8 Final Inspection and Mesenteric Defect Closure

All the mesenteric defects, at the ilieo-ileostomy and between the transvers colon mesentery and the ileum mesentery

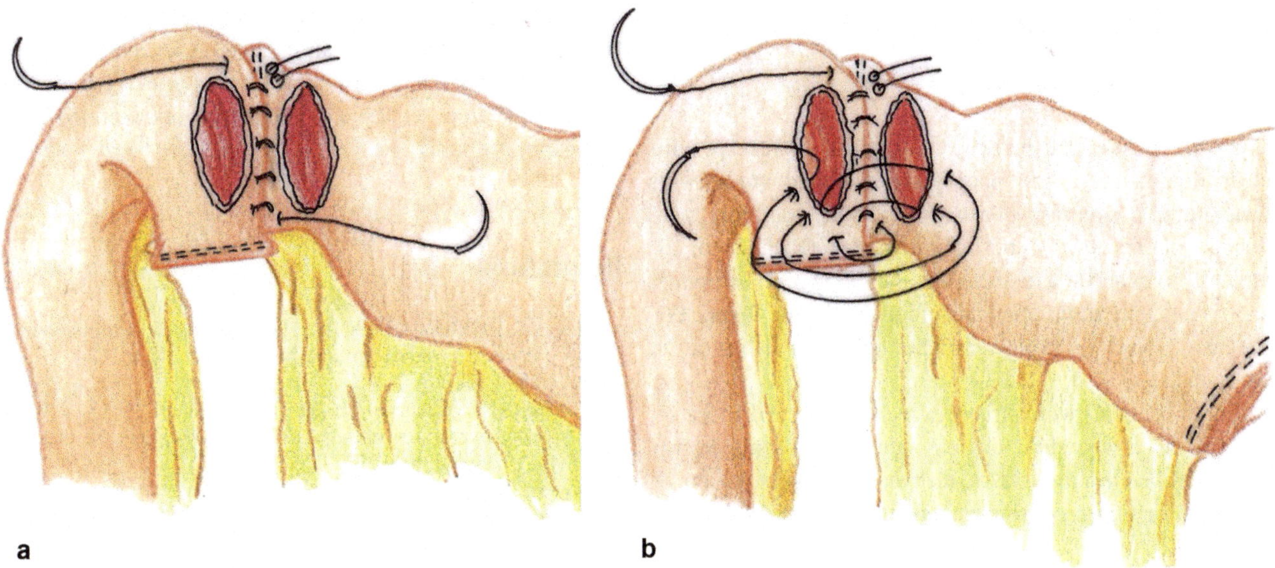

Fig. 16.5 Duodeno-enterostomy

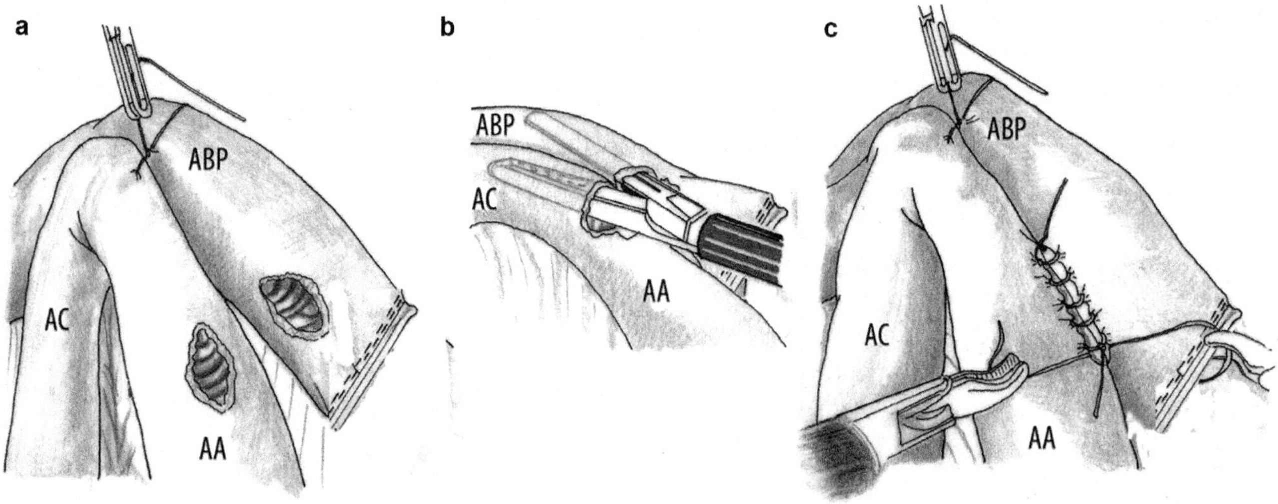

Fig. 16.6 Ileo-ileal anastomosis

should be closed with 2.0 running nonabsorbable stitch. The supracolic retrogastric defect (the defect above the transvers colon) is not closed as the internal hernia may exceptionally occur through it.

Before the end of the procedure, the gastric tube, the two anastomoses are once again inspected, a search for all the bleeding sources is done, the orientation of the limbs is verified.

Next, two suction drains are placed: one near to the proximal anastomosis and duodenal stump, and one over the distal anastomosis.

All trocar sites greater than 10 mm are closed with absorbable sutures using a fascia closure device (Karl Storz, Tutlingen, Germany). The skin is closed with staplers or interrupted 3.0 sutures.

16.6 Postoperative Care

In the *first* postoperative day (POD-1), patients receive only clear liquids diet. An upper gastrointestinal study with water-soluble contrast (Gastrografin®) is routinely performed on the *second* postoperative day (POD-2) in all patients, to evaluate and document the shape of the stomach and its capacity to be filled and emptied into the ileum. For the next 3 weeks a proteinen-riched diet (liquids/puree) is instituted.

For the patients with intraoperatively technical difficulties and for those who show clinical signs of an postoperative complication: *leakage* (fever, tachycardia, leucocytosis) or *stenosis*, the upper gastrointestinal study will be performed in POD-1.

The preoperative medication for comorbidities is continued and later may be adjusted. Oral analgesics are recommended for the next postoperative days. Proton pomp inhibitors (ex. Es-omeprasole) and low molecular heparin are administrated for at least 3 weeks.

Before hospital discharge all the drains are removed.

Follow-up appointments are scheduled for 4 weeks, 3, 6, 12 months and annually thereafter.

All patients receive follow-up nutritional counseling for proteinen-riched diet and are given daily multivitamins, oral supplements with calcium, iron and fat-soluble vitamins (A, D, E, K). Patients with intact gallbladders are prescribed 500 mg/day of ursodeoxicolic acid for a 6 months gallstone prophylaxis.

Laboratory evaluation for nutritional deficiencies is performed at each visit beginning with 3 months. This includes electrolyte and hematology panel as well iron, ferritin, B12, folate, albumin, protein, PTH, calcium, phosphorus, alkaline phosphatase, zinc, selenium, manganese, cholesterol profile, triglycerides, occasional Vitamin D and A levels.

An upper GI Endoscopy is performed at every 6 months or any time imposed by a clinical sign (ex.alterated food tolerance).

References

1. Hess DS, Hess DW, Oakley RS. The biliopancreatic diversion with the duodenal switch: results beyond 10 years. Obes Surg. 2005;15(3):408–16.
2. Scopinaro N, Gianetta E, Civalleri D, Bonalumi U, Bachi V. Biliopancreatic bypass for obesity: II. Initial experience in man. Br J Surg. 1979;66(9):618–20.
3. Gagner M, Matteotti R. Laparoscopic biliopancreatic diversion with duodenal switch. Surg Clin North Am. 2005;85(1):141–9, x–xi.
4. Gagner M, Gumbs AA, Milone L, Yung E, Goldenberg L, Pomp A. Laparoscopic sleeve gastrectomy for the super-super-obese (body mass index >60 kg/m(2)). Surg Today. 2008;38(5):399–403.
5. Copaescu C. Laparoscopic sleeve gastrectomy for morbid obesity. Chirurgia (Bucur). 2009;104(1):79–85.

17 Revisional Procedures for Failed Bariatric Operations

Jacques Himpens and Ramon Vilallonga

17.1 Introduction

The exponential growth in numbers of laparoscopic bariatric procedures is logically followed by a significant number of revisional procedures, either for complications or for outright failures. These failures may be due to technical issues linked with the surgical technique, to a wrong choice of initial procedure's type, to poor compliance from the patient, or to poor follow-up on the surgeon's part. Obviously, the latter two conditions should be addressed by non-surgical means. The former two conditions, however, may benefit from a surgical (laparoscopic) approach.

The decision as to how to surgically correct a bariatric procedure should take into account how the failure actually occurred. The pathogenesis of the failure should lead to the cure.

Unfortunately, corrective procedures, for whatever reason performed, are characterized by a greater incidence of complications than primary procedures. Therefore, when correcting an existing procedure, priority should be given not to endanger the patient. In this frame of mind, several attempts have recently been made to find endoscopic solutions for an ailing bariatric construction because they are considered less invasive. Even so, endoscopic procedures should take into account the pathophysiology of the initial failure as well. If not, outcome will be poor as demonstrated by the several attempts at endoscopically reducing stoma sizes after Roux-en-Y gastric bypass (RYGB), that have not generated the anticipated clinical results.

J. Himpens, MD, PhD (✉)
Obesity Department, AZ Sint Blasius, Brussels, Belgium
e-mail: Jacques_himpens@hotmail.com

R. Vilallonga, MD, PhD
Endocrine-Metabolic and Bariatric Surgery Unit, Robotic Surgery, EAC-BS Center of Excellence, Vall d'Hebron Hospital, Universitat Autònoma de Barcelona, Barcelona, Spain

17.2 Addressing Technical Issues/Flaws

The anatomical alterations caused by a bariatric procedure aim at creating a surgical system consisting of three elements: a gastric pouch, connected cranially to the esophagus through an "inlet", and to the distal structure through an "outlet"(the distal structure can be the stomach itself, as in adjustable gastric band (AGB), or vertical banded gastroplasty (VBG), or the antrum-pyloric system, as in sleeve gastrectomy (SG), or the anastomosed small bowel, as in RYGB) (Fig. 17.1).

The gastric pouch at the center of the system is obtained by the actual transversal (as in RYGB) or vertical (as in VBG or SG), or virtual (as in AGB) transection of the stomach. When reduction of caloric intake is searched for, the pouch should be small, and both inlet and outlet should be rather tight to be effective in terms of weight loss. When any of the compartment elements fails, the procedure will become ineffective.

17.2.1 Inlet Failure

Typically, the inlet is constituted by the gastro-esophageal (GE) junction and its lower esophageal sphincter (LES). When the latter fails, the pouch compartment will inevitably expand towards the esophagus and reflux and weight (re) gain will ensue (Fig. 17.2).

Similarly, in case of pre-existing hiatal hernia (HH), an effective bariatric system cannot be obtained without correcting this situation. Consequently, an essential part in avoiding recurrent weight issues, is to correct any HH at the time of the initial surgery. Because the diagnosis of HH is not reliably obtained by the usual diagnostic means such as endoscopy or barium swallow, a full dissection of the hiatal region is advised, even during the first procedure. This strategy may reduce the incidence of de novo HH that is remarkably high, as described by Higa (Fig. 17.3).

H.J. Bonjer (ed.), *Surgical Principles of Minimally Invasive Procedures*, DOI 10.1007/978-3-319-43196-3_17

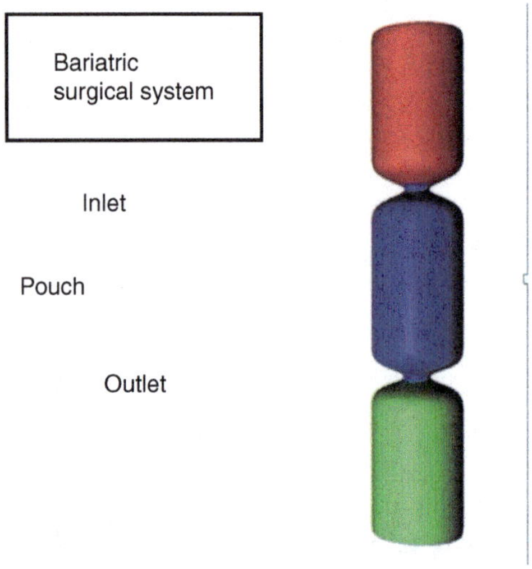

Fig. 17.1 The three components of the “bariatric surgical system”

The cure of a HH is best performed through a thorough dissection, and should imply a **posterior repair**, carried out with non-resorbable suture material.

Anterior stitches, often advocated for simplicity sake, should be avoided, because they do not allow for the anterior angulation of the GE junction, which is part of the anti-reflux mechanism (Fig. 17.4). Conversely, there is no evidence that the correction of a HH should be accompanied by the placement of prosthetic material, because of the risk of erosion into the gastric pouch.

An ingenious technique to reinforce the LES after RYGB was described by Kawahara. With this technique, the remnant is mobilized in its apical fundic part, and this part of the remnant is wrapped around the proximal end of the gastric pouch, much as in Nissen’s fundoplication (Fig. 17.5). This “passive wrap” might reinforce the pressures in the distal esophagus and help reconstitute a continent “inlet”.

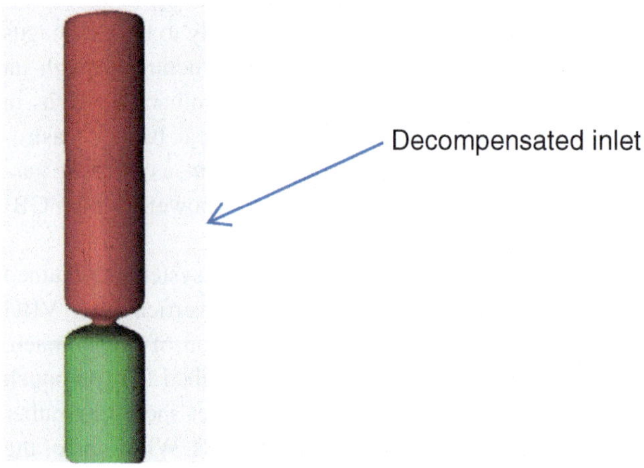

Fig. 17.2 Decompensation of the “inlet” results in the abolition of the bariatric system

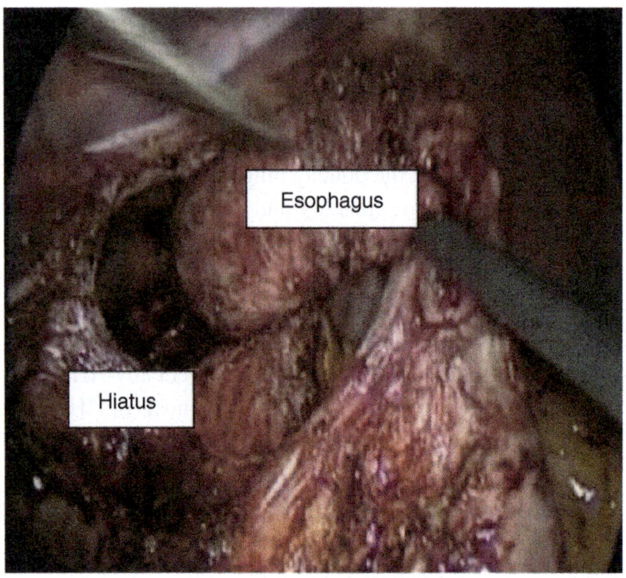

Fig. 17.3 Typical aspect of a hiatus in a redo case. Despite a normal endoscopy and Barium Swallow there is a clear diastasis of the hiatal crura causing herniation

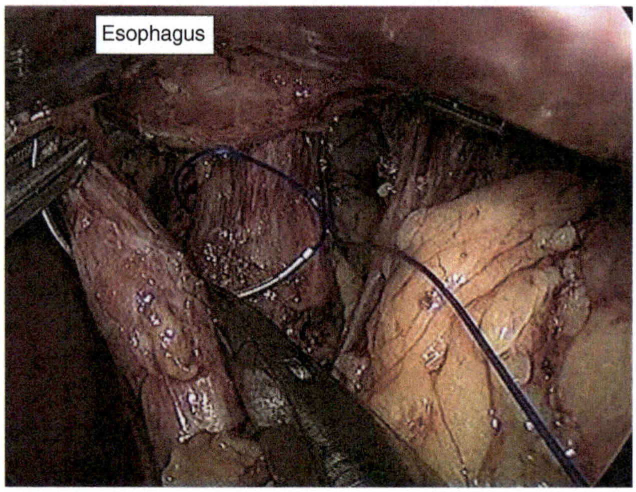

Fig. 17.4 Typical aspect of a cure of a HH with a posterior repair, carried out with non-resorbable suture material

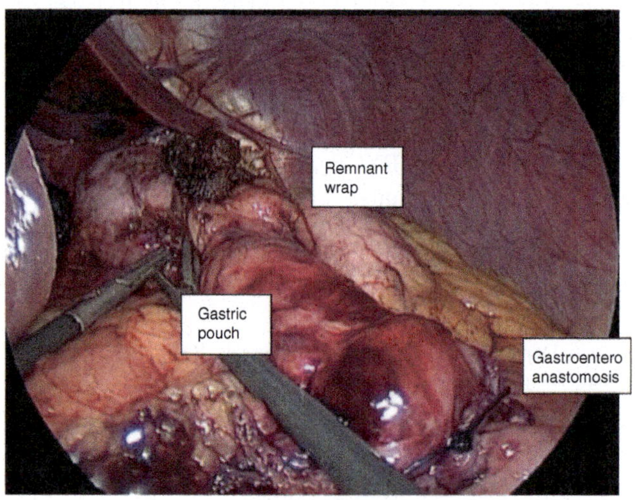

Fig. 17.5 Remnant’s fundus to wrap around the proximal gastric pouch, mimicking a Nissen’s fundoplication. In the inferior part we observe the gastroentero anastomosis

17.2.2 Pouch Failure

Because of the relative obstruction generated by the outlet, and according to Laplace's law, the pouch will have a tendency to dilate, and to accommodate larger volumes of food. Obviously, when pouch dilation occurs together with inlet failure, the food volumes will substantially increase and possibly lead to weight (re)gain (Fig. 17.6).

For AGB, pouch dilation has been described extensively. The pouch volume can be corrected by laparoscopically replacing the band in a more proximal position. There is however hardly a consensus in the literature concerning this strategy, possibly because of the lack of addressing the inlet at the same time.

For VBG, pouch failure usually is caused by the breakdown of the staple line, most likely in consequence of exaggerated intracavitary pressure caused by over-eating. With this etiology, repeat stapling is considered senseless.

For RYGB, it appears that isolated attempts at reducing the volume of the pouch (either endoscopically or laparoscopically) have not been effective on the long term. Consequently, most efforts after RYGB have focused on the outlet (the gastro-enterostomy), see below.

For SG, there is no clear evidence that a larger volume of the stomach is linked with weight regain. Whereas some authors claim good outcomes with re-sleeving the stomach, there is growing evidence that ancillary procedures like a duodenal switch (DS) carry better and longer lasting results. Conversely, when part of the stomach clearly has decompensated secondary to the high pressure system generated by the tubular shape of the stomach, trimming this part of the stomach might be useful. A plausible explanation to this outcome is that part of the body of the stomach constitutes a weak point for the intraluminal high pressure.

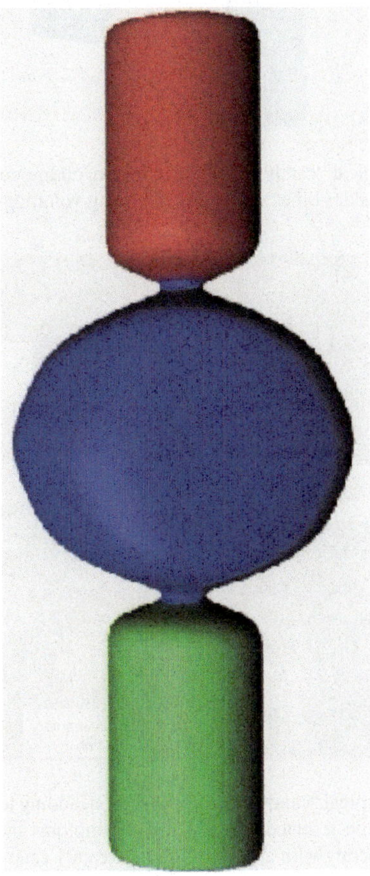

Fig. 17.6 Isolated pouch failure results in larger food volumes

17.2.3 Outlet Failure

When the outlet fails, the pressure gradient between the pouch and the efferent system drops, and both the pouch and the efferent system behave as one system, hence with very limited volume limitation. We mentioned above that too tight an outlet may cause a dilation of the pouch, hence the importance of obtaining an ideal outlet size (Fig. 17.7).

For AGB, the ideal band volume corresponds to the "green" zone described by the manufacturer, and is characterized for the patient by a feeling of restriction without dysphagia. Increasing the volume will bring the patient into the "red" zone where dysphagia will occur, which may lead to wrong food choices. Conversely, too little volume in the band will lead to the disappearance of the outlet barrier and failure of the system (Fig. 17.8).

Another typical condition encountered in AGB is band erosion. In a recent survey of our patients, close to one third of the patients suffered this complication, but many of the patients did not suffer any symptoms. Therefore, the relatively low incidence of erosion reported in the literature probably underestimates the actual incidence of intragastric band migration, because most authors did not actively look for this condition by systematical endoscopy. Treatment of band erosion is quite controversial. Some authors (e.g. Niville) do not hesitate to replace a new band after a lag time

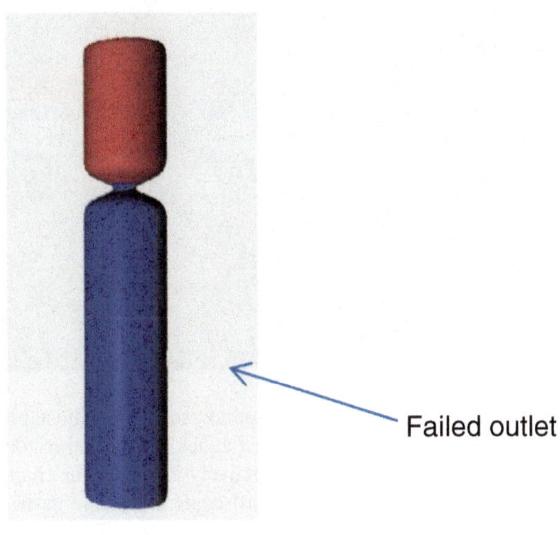

Fig. 17.7 When the outlet fails, the pouch is no longer limited by its outlet, which translates into a considerable increase of functional pouch volume

of a few months. Conversely, Weiner and Allé consider the zone of erosion as a no-go territory and prefer to proceed with biliopancreatic diversion (BPD) and transect the stomach well distal to the diseased area. Most authors, however, rely on the lag time after band removal to allow for the tissues to heal and to permit the safe placement of staples. RYGB is their favorite corrective procedure, while SG, on the other hand, is usually not performed after band erosion.

For VBG, outlet stenosis has been described extensively. Whereas treatment seems obvious (transection of the band), the disappearance of all restriction at the level of the outlet invariably causes massive weight regain. Hence, all procedures addressing the banded outlet in VBG should be complemented by another type of operation, either malabsorptive (BPD), or hybrid (RYGB).

For RYGB, outlet failure results in an extension of the pouch and the efferent system into becoming one system that, because of Laplace's law has the tendency to dilate. Efforts to reduce the volume of this new entity consist of longitudinally transecting pouch, anastomosis and alimentary limb, as proposed by Gagner, or of plicating these elements, as we have done. Unfortunately, these efforts have proven to be vain on the long term, except when one of the elements has evolved to become a large reservoir, as in the candy cane deformity of the blind end of the alimentary limb (Figs. 17.9 and 17.10).

Additionally, in RYGB dilation of the outlet will result in accelerated emptying of the pouch and premature delivery of the food stuffs into the efferent system, a condition that may lead to exaggerated dumping and hypoglycemia, and, subsequently, weight gain. Correcting the outlet for this condition can be achieved by reducing the anastomosis (either endoscopically or laparoscopically), or by the placement of an external restricting system, either non-adjustable (Fobi-ring), or adjustable (an AGB). In our experience, the use of an artificial band has created a significant number of complications, including erosions in a great number of patients.

For SG, the outlet, constituted by the antrum-pylorus unit, is responsible for a number of recurrent weight issues. Whereas the sleeve itself rarely dilates, the antrum will dilate when initial resection has been too parsimonious. There are very few reports on selective antral re-resections, partly because of

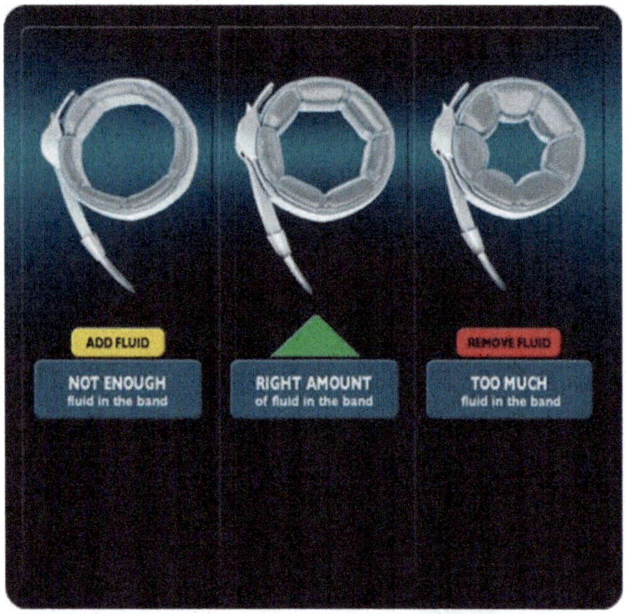

Fig. 17.8 Importance of correct outlet adjustment in adjustable band gastroplasty. The *yellow, green* and *red* zones correspond to too little, adequate or too much restriction, respectively. Zones can be changed by varying the filling volume of the laparoscopic adjustable gastric band (Source: internet shareware)

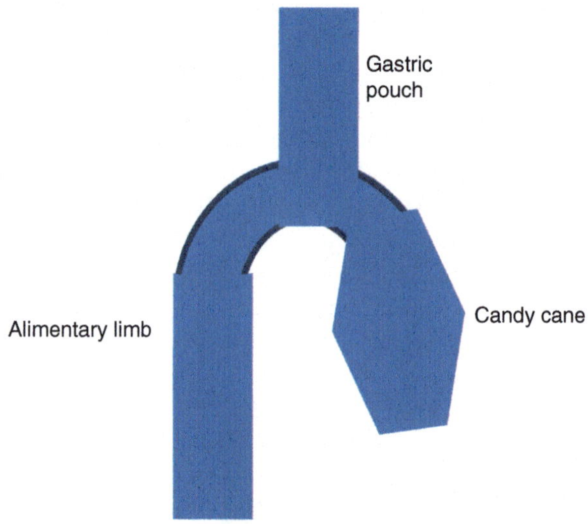

Fig. 17.9 Typical "candy cane" deformation, adding to the volume of the system (besides other symptoms including vomiting)

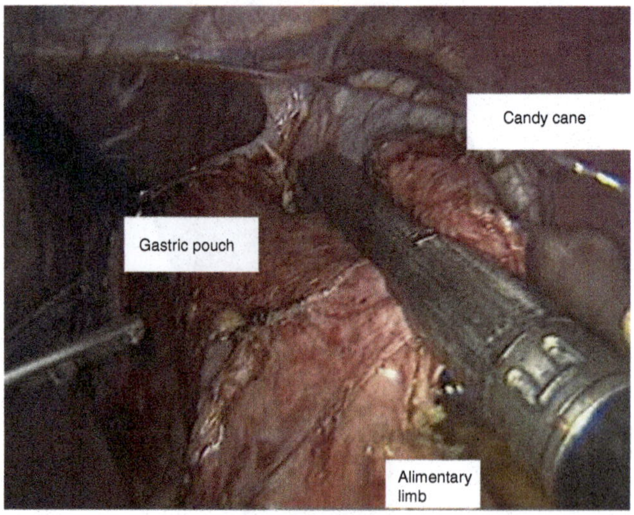

Fig. 17.10 Typical "candy cane" deformation, adding to the volume of the system while resected (besides other symptoms including vomiting). Here resecting with an endostapler the candy cane

fears for interference with the gastric emptying, a condition that might be of significant importance for the secretion of gastro-intestinal hormones including GLP1 and GIP.

17.3 Choice of Secondary Procedure (Conversion)

When all obvious technical flaws have been ruled out, the history of the patient suffering weight (re)gain should be closely analyzed. There is a substantial difference between weight loss failure and weight regain. Whereas the former seems to indicate that the procedure probably did not match the patient's profile from the beginning (hence that a different type of procedure should be performed), the latter might be caused by adjustment of the patient to the procedure, most likely by adaptation of the eating pattern. Adaptation on the patient's part should preferably be addressed by behavioral and dietary counseling. Conversely, in this section we will focus on operations that might be salutary after the outright failure of a bariatric procedure.

Bariatric procedures obtain their goal by reducing the amount of calories made available to the patient's metabolism. Caloric reduction is obtained either by restricting the intake (i.e. the number of calories making it to the digestive tract), or by limiting the uptake (i.e. the number of calories being absorbed through the digestive tract). Some operations will take advantage of the two main mechanisms. As a general rule, failed restrictive operations will be addressed by a malabsorptive construction, and vice-versa.

17.3.1 The AGB

The AGB procedure is considered purely restrictive, because there appears to be no interference with the secretion pattern of the gastro-intestinal hormones. A relevant hormone in the bariatric domain is Ghrelin, an orexogenic peptide that influences glucose metabolism through a decrease of insulin production. This hormone is not influenced by AGB. Since sleeve gastrectomy, unlike AGB, typically is followed by a sharp decline in Ghrelin, transforming an AGB into a SG may appear attractive. There are however practical issues that plead against this choice. First, the incidence of proximal leaks after SG does appear to be higher in redo surgery, and there is sufficient evidence that such leaks are extremely difficult to handle. Second, we have demonstrated that a substantial number of patients develop gastro-esophageal reflux (GERD) after AGB, and that GERD is a frequent and undesired side effect after SG as well. Hence, because of fears for surgical complications and for GERD we are reluctant to convert an AGB into a SG. Alternatively, the typically restrictive AGB might be transformed into a malabsorptive procedure, such as Duodenal Switch (DS). As mentioned above, however, we are concerned to perform a SG in a band patient, and since the SG is an inherent part of the DS, we rather will not perform a DS in a band patient.

Typically, a failed AGB will be converted to a RYGB. We and others have shown that weight loss improves significantly after conversion of AGB to RYGB, be it at the cost of more complications. Some authors prefer to convert AGB to RYGB in two stages. In our practice, removal of the band and performing the RYGB are routinely performed in one stage because the band is used as a landmark as well as a retraction tool. It is important to perform a thorough dissection of the hiatus, to detect any hidden pouch dilation, and to rule out a hiatal hernia, a condition that has proven to appear de novo after AGB. As a routine, we thoroughly dissect the hiatus and perform a posterior hiatal closure. Another important technical detail in our practice is our strategy of systematically resecting the fundus. There is some evidence that resecting the fundus improves weight loss figures, probably because of Ghrelin issues, but more importantly, we feel that resecting the fundus reduces the incidence of post-AGB gastro-gastric fistula, which constitutes a therapeutic challenge. Finally, we routinely transversally incise the pseudo-capsule induced by the band, to avoid dysphagia after the RYGB (Fig. 17.11).

17.3.2 The VBG

Most vertical banded gastroplasties will have been performed by laparotomy and constitute a real challenge for the laparoscopic surgeon. Laparoscopic conversion of a VBG to another construction remains a hazardous endeavor, and the prevalence of complications should dictate our attitude in choosing an alternative procedure. Transforming a VBG into a SG is fraught with a significant number of complications, including substantial mortality and should be avoided. Consequently, reconversion into a DS is hardly advisable as well.

Our attitude after failed VBG is to perform RYGB. The two major hazards after VBG consist of the vertical staple line and the stoma-reinforcing band. The latter often is made of knitted polypropylene, a material that causes very dense adhesions. Removal of the band is often impossible; therefore, some surgeons prefer to transversally incise the band and to perform the gastro-enterostomy a few cm proximal or distal to the band, while others, including us, prefer to resect the portion of the stomach together with the band. Concerning the vertical staple line, care must be taken not to staple to the left of the staple line, because this will result in a lymphocele between the two staple lines. We lost one of our patients who suffered a blow-out of such a lymphocele, several weeks after the procedure. Consequently we favor the policy to resect the VBG-staple line together with the fundus to the left of the staple line, to avoid a blind space between the

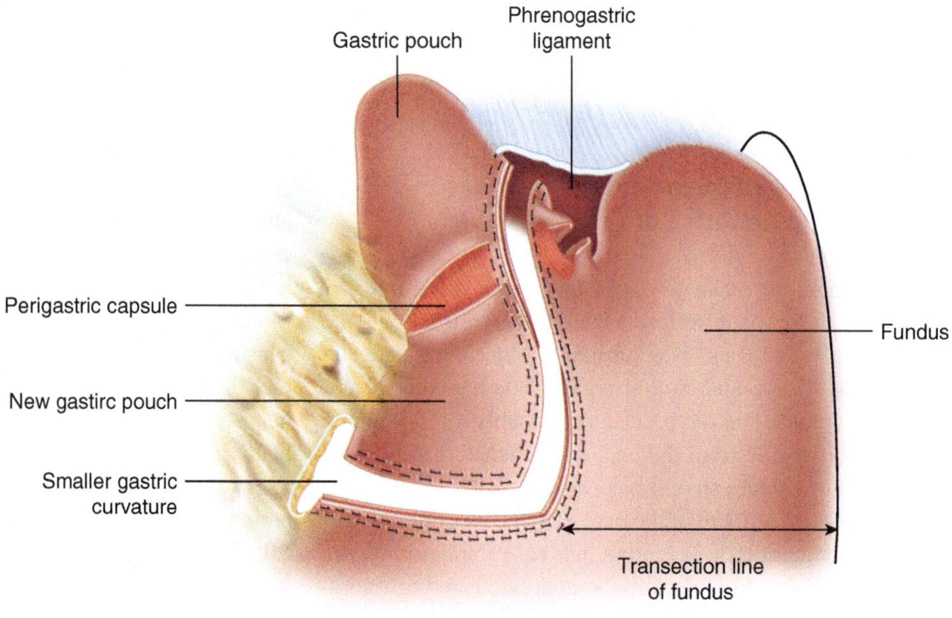

Fig. 17.11 Specific strategy for transforming adjustable band into Roux-en-Y gastric bypass (From: Cadière et al., with permission)

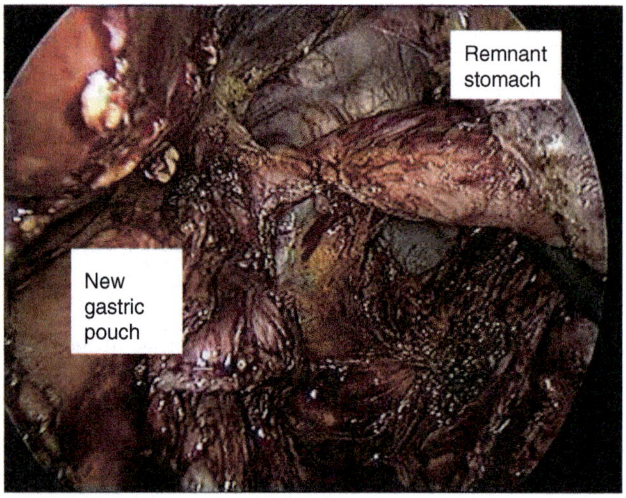

Fig. 17.12 Transection line of fundus. The remnant stomach will be removed through a 12 mm trocar. Adding this resection, avoids possible gastro gastric fistulas formation

staple lines and to prevent the formation of a gastro-gastric fistula (Fig. 17.12).

17.3.3 The RYGB

The RYGB is a "hybrid restrictive-malabsorptive" procedure. Besides manipulating restriction, as with a band, malabsorption may be addressed as well. Christou and Mac Lean demonstrated some time ago that lengthening the alimentary limb after RYGB did not significantly influence long term weight loss. Buchwald and, separately, Brolin, induced extreme malabsorption after RYGB by conversion to a "distal bypass". Typically, a distal bypass consists of a long alimentary limb and of a common limb of some 75 cm. Such a construction however exposes the patient to excessive loss of calories because of the existing volume-restriction with on top of this marked fat malabsorption, and the concomitant loss of fat soluble vitamins. Morbidity and mortality after such a "distal bypass" were considerable and the procedure was abandoned as such. A "softer" version of the distal bypass consists of constructing an alimentary limb and a common limb of 150 cm each. In our experience, weight loss with this type of distal bypass reached 100 % of the excess weight, but still a significant number of patients required re-conversion to a more proximal bypass because of unbearable side-effects. We therefore are no longer keen on this type of procedures, and try to obtain malabsorption by reversal of the bypass to normal anatomy, followed by conversion to a DS. With this strategy, the ill effects of the quite pronounced gastric restriction are avoided, and we can offer the patient a well-known and – documented procedure that has proven to be effective and safe, provided patient compliance with vitamin- and mineral supplementation is good (Fig. 17.13).

17.3.4 The LSG

Except for the rather rare cases where a saccular dilation of the proximal part of the gastric sleeve indicates a loss of the pressure inside the stomach, re-resection of the stomach will usually not be followed by satisfactory weight loss.

Converting the restriction created by the gastrectomy to another weight loss mechanism can be obtained by changing the construction into a RYGB or into a DS. The gastric bypass is perhaps the best (and only) option in case of significant GERD, because conversion into a DS will not significantly influence this condition. In terms of weight loss, however, outcomes after RYGB post-SG are usually rather modest. Conversely, a truly malabsorptive operation such as DS carries excellent results as far as weight loss is concerned. Initially, the SG was considered as an inherent part of a DS construction and only recently did the SG obtain right of existence on its own. Since a significant percentage of patients will experience weight regain after SG they will become natural candidates for DS. The fact that the DS is thus split into two stages improves the morbidity and apparently does not influence the final weight loss. Moreover, staging a procedure with considerable metabolic implications as the DS may add to the safety by allowing to spot and eliminate poorly compliant bariatric candidates. There is no consensus as to the ideal time for a DS after a SG. In our experience, patients request a revisional procedure between the first and the fifth year after the initial procedure, with a median after 3 years (Fig. 17.14).

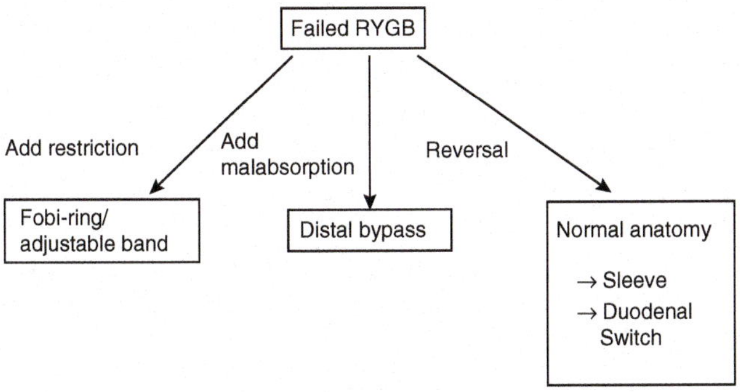

Fig. 17.13 Algorithm for failed Roux-en-Y gastric bypass

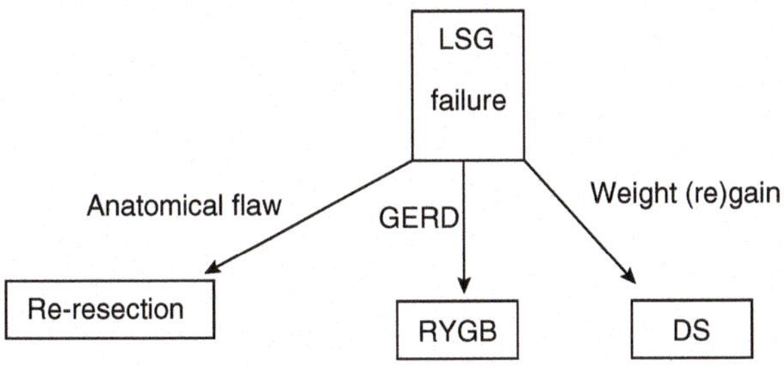

Fig. 17.14 Algorithm for failed sleeve gastrectomy

17.3.5 The DS

Some patients experience problems of insufficient weight loss even after DS. Moreover, the patients may experience unwanted side effects including diarrhea and protein malnutrition concomitantly with weight (re)gain. Obviously, dietary counseling with re-education of the patient in terms of choosing for protein-rich food stuffs rather than carbohydrates is the most important treatment for this condition. As for surgical correction, thanks to the laparoscopic approach, reconstructing the alimentary, biliary and common limb and changing their length for influencing the degree of malabsorption has become quite realizable. As a rule of thumb, therapy-resistant diarrhea (in fact steatorrhea) can be managed by increasing the length of the common limb. In case of severe diarrhea, lengthening the common limb to some 150 cm is advisable (Fig. 17.15).

Since lengthening the common limb will be followed by additional weight gain, because of the increased absorption of fat, two options remain: concomitant shortening of the alimentary limb (Fig. 17.16), or reduction of caloric intake (by reducing the stomach volume).

Fig. 17.15 Lengthening of the common limb at the cost of the biliary. The common loop is lengthened without shortening of the alimenta

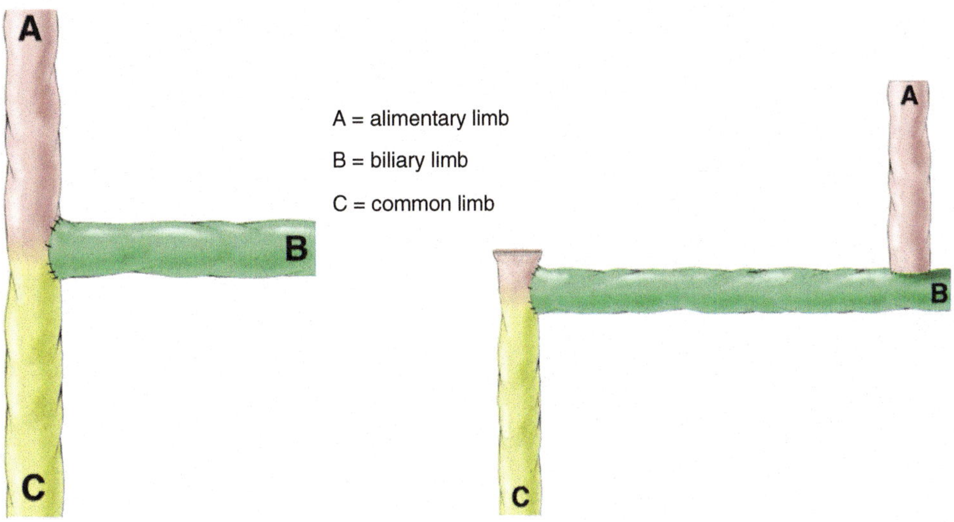

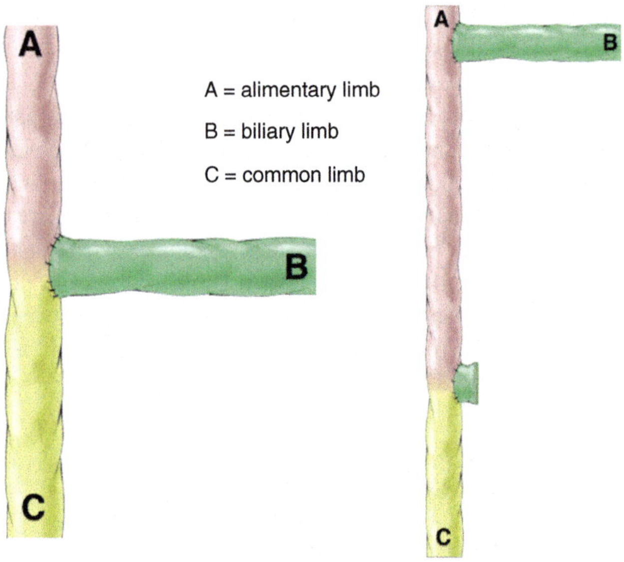

Fig. 17.16 Lengthening of the common limb at the cost of the alimentary. Since the alimentary limb is shortened, protein malnutrition may become an issuery

If shortening the alimentary limb is chosen, care must be taken not to decrease the total "active" bowel length (alimentary + common) below 300 cm, because hypoproteinemia will invariable follow, as demonstrated by Scopinaro. In our practice, we usually will prefer to reduce the volume of the stomach, preferably by radicalizing the resection at the level of the distal stomach, where the risk for fistulas is less.

Conclusion

Thanks to the laparoscopic approach, revisional procedures become less of a challenge. On one hand, adhesions caused at the first laparoscopic procedure are limited, while on the other hand trauma to the patient is less significant during the revisional procedure. Nevertheless, complications are more prevalent in revisional surgery and conservative measures should, as a rule, be attempted first. When conservative measures fail, analysis of the reason why the procedure did not succeed should indicate how to surgically correct the existing construction. The three elements of the bariatric surgical system (inlet, pouch and outlet) must be evaluated and addressed if needed. Alternatively, the ailing mode of action (restriction versus malabsorption) may be altered by laparoscopically converting the procedure to a different type.

Bibliography

1. Himpens J, Cadière GB, Bazi M, Vouche M, Cadière B, Dapri G. Long-term outcomes of laparoscopic adjustable gastric banding. Arch Surg. 2011;146:802–7.
2. Himpens J, Coromina L, Verbrugghe A, Cadière GB. Outcomes of revisional procedures for insufficient weight loss or weight regain after Roux-en-Y gastric bypass. Obes Surg. 2012;22:1746–54.
3. Cadière GB, Himpens J, Bazi M, Cadière B, Vouche M, Capelluto E, Dapri G. Are laparoscopic gastric bypass after gastroplasty and primary laparoscopic gastric bypass similar in terms of results? Obes Surg. 2011;21:692–8.
4. Himpens J, Dobbeleir J, Peeters G. Long-term results of laparoscopic sleeve gastrectomy for obesity. Ann Surg. 2010;252:319–24.
5. Scopinaro N. Thirty-five years of biliopancreatic diversion: notes on gastrointestinal physiology to complete the published information useful for a better understanding and clinical use of the operation. Obes Surg. 2012;22:427–32.

Part VI

Liver

Laparoscopic Liver Resection

18

Giulio Belli, Corrado Fantini, Alberto D'Agostino, Luigi Cioffi, Gianluca Russo, Andrea Belli, and Paolo Limongelli

18.1 Introduction

In the 1990s laparoscopic liver surgery was considered an innovative, promising but very demanding technique reserved for benign lesions or selected cases where the malignant tumour could be removed by minor and superficial resection. Subsequently the widespread introduction of laparoscopic hepatectomy in the surgical community, due to improvements in laparoscopic techniques, technological advances in laparoscopic devices and even to increasing patient' awareness and demand for these procedures, showed it was a safe, successful and well-tolerated treatment for a range of benign and neoplastic hepatic diseases. In fact, after the first laparoscopic partial hepatectomy, reported in 1992, the minimally invasive approach has been used increasingly in the management of hepatic diseases showing that despite several technical challenges, can obtain reduced operative blood loss, fewer early postoperative complications and shorter hospital stay with oncologic clearance and a survival rate similar to open surgery [1].

Therefore, the place of laparoscopy in liver surgery is increasing, and many types of liver resections, including major hepatectomies, are now performed by laparoscopy in specialized centres.

Even in cirrhotic patients laparoscopic hepatectomy is an effective treatment for hepatocellular carcinoma when orthotopic liver transplantation is not feasible due to the age of the patients and the lack of donors [2].

G. Belli, MD (✉) • C. Fantini, MD • A. D'Agostino, MD
L. Cioffi, MD • G. Russo, MD • P. Limongelli, MD, PhD
Department of General and Hepato-Pancreato-Biliary Surgery, S.M. Loreto Nuovo Hospital, Naples, Italy
e-mail: chirurgia.loretonuovo@tin.it

A. Belli, MD
Department of Abdominal Oncology, Division of Surgical Oncology, Istituto Nazionale Tumori Fondazione G. Pascale – Istituto Di Ricovero e Cura a Carattere Scientifico, Naples, Italy

Laparoscopy, by decreasing the abdominal wall injury and probably the parenchymal injury, seems to additionally improve the postoperative course. In fact, advantages of laparoscopic approach seems to be greater in cirrhotic patients in whom postoperative ascites and abdominal wall complications are decreased compared to laparotomy.

In 2008, leaders in the field comprising also our senior author (G.B), met to discuss the current status of laparoscopic liver surgery. The Louisville Statement agreed on three procedural definitions: pure laparoscopy, hand-assisted laparoscopy and hybrid [3] Pure laparoscopy involves complete mobilization and resection via laparoscopic ports, with an incision for specimen extraction. Hand-assisted laparoscopy involves the elective placement of a hand-port for mobilization or resection, which is then used for specimen extraction. Hybrid refers to a procedure where the resection and extraction are performed through a mini-laparotomy, though laparoscopy with or without hand-assistance is utilized for mobilization. Nevertheless, about 75 % of all mini-invasive laparoscopic liver resection are today performed by a pure laparoscopic technique.

Following the Louisville Consensus Conference laparoscopic hepatectomy should be reserved to surgeons with huge experience in both open and advanced laparoscopic surgery.

18.2 Indication

The indication for laparoscopic resection should not be varied from open resection. Lesion size and location are the most important determinants of when laparoscopic resection is appropriate.

The most favourable indications for laparoscopic resection is a solitary lesions, 5 cm or less, located in peripheral liver segments 2–6 (laparoscopic segments).

Left lateral sectionectomy (segments 2–3), anterior segmentectomies or wedge resections are the most widely applied procedures. Left lateral sectionectomy should be

H.J. Bonjer (ed.), *Surgical Principles of Minimally Invasive Procedures*, DOI 10.1007/978-3-319-43196-3_18

considered the standard of care in experienced hands. Lesions located in posterior segments (1, 7, and 8), can be managed by laparoscopy, but this is rarely performed, and it is not universally accepted.

Major liver resections (ie, right or left hemihepatectomies) have been shown feasible but remain difficult procedures which should be reserved to experienced surgeons already facile with more limited laparoscopic resections.

Tumors larger than 5 cm, central, multiple, bilateral or with connections with the liver hilum, major hepatic veins or the IVC are considered relative contraindications in most centers.

However, in some, very experienced centers, even these lesions in selected patients are addressed laparoscopically. At last, laparoscopic redo surgery is an other safe and feasible indications with advantages for patients and good results [4].

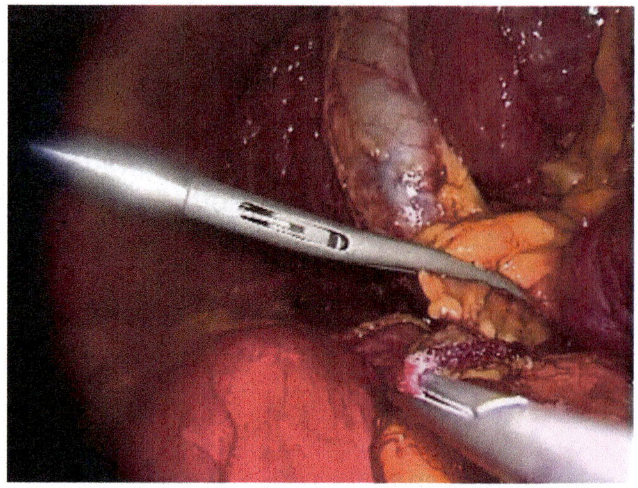

Fig. 18.1 Pringle maneuver by a curved esophageal retractor, passed through the foramen of Winslow, around the porta hepatis, with the vascular tape inserted in its open tip

18.2.1 Patient Position and Set-Up

18.2.1.1 Segments II-III-IV-V

The patient is placed in supine position, with the primary surgeon standing between the patient's legs, with one assistant on each side. With an open laparoscopy technique, continuous CO2 pneumoperitoneum is induced at a pressure of 12 mmHg to prevent the risk of gas embolism.

Once resection has been decided, the lesser omentum is checked to verify the presence of a left hepatic artery and then sectioned close to the Arantius groove.

18.2.2 Segments VI-VII

The patient is placed in a left lateral positioning (right-side up), in mild reverse-Trendelenburg position, with the operating surgeon and the assistant standing by the patient's left flank and facing the abdomen. Four trocars typically are used in this procedure.

18.2.3 Pringle Manoeuvre Preparation

After incision of the pars lucida of the lesser omentum the hepato-gastric ligament is opened and the porta hepatis is surrounded by a tape passed through a 16-Fr rubber drain, used as a tourniquet to perform Pringle's maneuver, if necessary. A second option is to employ a curved esophageal retractor, passed through the foramen of Winslow, around the porta hepatis, with the vascular tape inserted in its open tip (Fig. 18.1). It simply surrounds and subsequently ties the hepatoduodenal pedicle to hang it and facilitate the Pringle manoeuvre, if necessary. Alternatively a vascular clamp can be inserted through an additional trocar.

18.2.4 Exploration and IOUS

A standard diagnostic and staging laparoscopy is performed in all cases to assess the stage of the disease using laparoscopic ultrasonography to confirm the extension of the lesion and its relationships to the vasculature, and to visualize its medial margin inside the parenchyma.

18.2.5 Parenchymal Transection

The extension of resection is identified by the use of intraoperative ultrasonography (IOUS), and the area is marked by monopolar electrocautery. Specifically, a margin distance between the lesion of interest and the cut line on the surface of the liver is precisely measured by IOUS: the scored capsule appears as a hypoechoic linear shadow perpendicular to the ultrasound probe and is used to verify the surgical margin's position and width from the lesion before starting the parenchymal transection. Even during parenchymal transection, ultrasound is employed repeatedly to guide the transection plane away from the tumor margin.

The hepatic transection is performed with a no-touch technique (no tumor manipulation) by sectioning Glisson's capsule with the harmonic scalpel, which is able to secure vascular and biliary structures up to 3 mm; minor bleeding is managed by bipolar electrocautery forceps simultaneously employed with the ultrasonic dissector to provide liver retraction and improve hemostasis. Intraparenchimal control of major vessels may be achieved with surgical clips or devices such as harmonic scalpel or Vessel Sealing System. A linear stapler (vascular cartridge type) may be also employed with or without surrounding the vessels.

Laparoscopic CUSA can be useful to skeletonize the vascular structure and electively *ligate* them. The thickness of the parenchyma is progressively reduced: small structures are clipped and sectioned. Bipolar forceps can be used to control small bleeding and oozing from the transection line.

Argon Beam coagulator can be applied to control blood oozing from the transection plane providing the abdominal pressure (<15 mmHg) is carefully monitored to prevent the risk of gas embolism. Resection bed surfaces may be treated with biologic fibrin glue or hemostatic gel to minimize the risk of biliary leak and to ensure haemostasis. Drain may be inserted next to the site of resection. Desufflation of CO2 is performed before trocars are removed under direct vision.

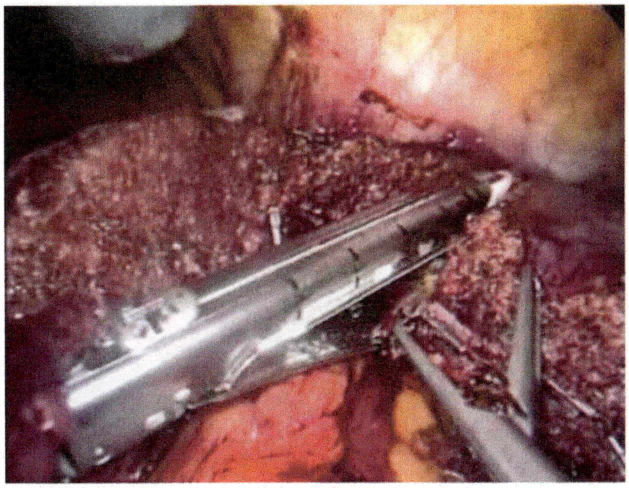

Fig. 18.2 Left hepatic vein sectioned by an endoGIA

18.2.6 Wedge Resection

The patient's position depends of lesion's site. The extension of resection is identified by the use of ultrasonography, and the area is marked by monopolar electrocautery. Specifically, a margin distance between the lesion of interest and the cut line on the surface of the liver is precisely measured by ultrasonography. The ultrasonography is employed repeatedly to guide the transection plane away from the tumor margin. The parenchimal transaction is performed as previously described.

18.2.7 Left Lateral Sectionectomy

Pringle maneuver is only disposed and is usually not performed unless severe bleeding appears. Furthermore, reduction of the blood pressure by up to 25–30 % in the portal region during laparoscopic surgery is well proved. The falciform ligament is then sectioned with endoshears, with mono or bipolar coagulation, or with a harmonic scalpel up to the hepatic veins. In this way, the liver does not fall downward or forward, facilitating the parenchymal transection. We do not section the round ligament, either to save the umbilical vein, as we usually do in cirrhotic patients, or to leave the liver attached to the abdominal wall, so allowing better work with the harmonic scalpel. In addition, in this position, the instrument is located just in front of the section line. The hepatic resection is then performed with a no-touch technique (no tumor manipulation) and with the harmonic scalpel, which is able to secure vascular and biliary structures up to 3 mm; minor bleeding is managed by electrocoagulation, and larger structures are secured with clips. The dissection of Rex's recessus exposes the portal triad of segment III, which can now be divided between clips, or alternatively with a linear stapler without surrounding it. The margin of hepatectomy runs 1 cm to the left side of the falciform ligament and the hepatic transection is continued with the harmonic scalpel on the inferior side of the liver. This maneuver allows us to reduce the thickness of the parenchyma and to identify the vascular and biliary elements of segment II, which are clipped and cut, or alternatively sectioned with a second stapling device, without exposing them. The resection is continued up to the left hepatic vein, which is sectioned by an endoGIA (Fig. 18.2). Only at this moment are the left triangular and coronary ligaments divided, using the harmonic scalpel introduced through the trocar located on the left of the patient. The dissection from the left side is continued up to liver usually does not require additional coagulation, but it can be treated with an argon beam coagulator or sealed with fibrin glue.

18.2.8 Segment VI Resection

After incision of the *pars lucida* of the lesser omentum, a curved esophageal retractor is passed through the foramen of Winslow around the *porta hepatis* with a vascular tape inserted in its open tip. The tape can simply surround the hepatoduodenal pedicle and then be passed through a 16 F rubber drain used as a tourniquet to enable the Pringle maneuver, if necessary. At this point, the mobilization of the liver can begin; the right lateral hepatic attachment and the triangular ligament are divided using Ultracision or Ligasure devices while the round and falciform ligaments are preserved. This dissection is typically carried up to the diaphragm, allowing a more effective mobilization of the liver.

The extension of resection is identified by the use of ultrasonography, and the area is marked by monopolar electrocautery. Specifically, a margin distance between the lesion of

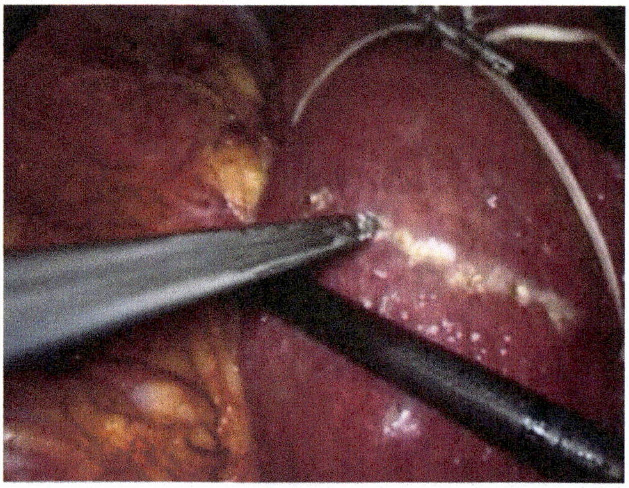

Fig. 18.3 Lifting and handling of the segment VI by an umbilical tape

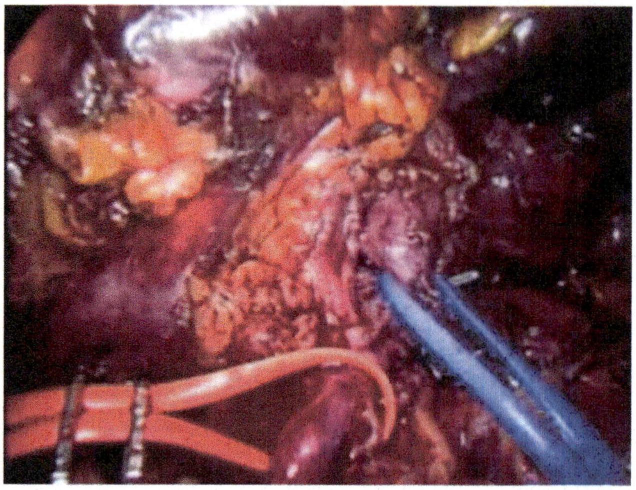

Fig. 18.4 Left arterial and portal branches dissected and isolated on vessel loops

interest and the cut line on the surface of the liver is precisely measured by ultrasonography. It is helpful to pass an umbilical tape, controlled by a grasping instrument inserted in the medial port, around the right mobilized liver to facilitate the lifting and the handling of the segment VI (Fig. 18.3). The hepatic transection is then started by sectioning Glisson's capsule with the harmonic scalpel to secure vascular and biliary structures up to 3 mm; minor bleeding is managed by bipolar electrocautery forceps simultaneously employed with the ultrasonic dissector to provide liver retraction and improve hemostasis.

18.2.9 Left Hemihepatectomy

Control of vascular inflow is the first step of the procedure. The liver is lifted upwards by two forceps, one on the stump of the round ligament and the other on the gallbladder. The left portal pedicle is dissected extraparenchymally.

The peritoneum of the hepatic pedicle is incised in its left aspect and left arterial and portal branches are dissected and isolated on vessel loops (Fig. 18.4). The left hepatic artery is then secured between clips and divided (Fig. 18.5). The left portal branch is separated from the surrounding lymphatic tissue upwards and then downwards to better identify the portal bifurcation. The left portal branch is then managed by two endoclips applied proximally and one distally, and then divided. The left hepatic duct is also exposed outside the liver parenchyma, by division of the hilar plate. The peritoneum of the left part of the hilar plate is incised along the inferior surface of segment IV, and the upper border of the left hepatic duct is smoothly separated from the liver parenchyma. The tissue behind the hepatic duct is dissected and the duct individualized. A tape is placed around the duct in its left

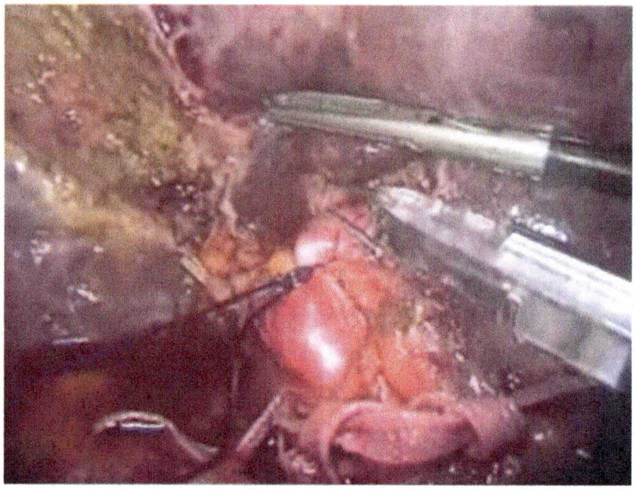

Fig. 18.5 Left hepatic artery secured and divided between clips

portion close to the round ligament, and the left hepatic duct is then obstructed by absorbable clips and divided.

18.2.10 Right Hepatectomy

The patient is placed in supine position with his legs spread with the surgeon placed between the legs.

The falciform ligament is dissected while the round ligament can either sectioned and used as an handle during the parenchymal transection in order to open and expose the transection line, or spared in case of resection in cirrhotic patients in order to preserve the umbilical vein. The liver is then fully mobilized (coronary and triangular ligaments section) and freed from the diaphragm. Cholecystectomy is performed. The gallbladder can be externalized or left attached to the liver bed and used as an handle to retract the right liver lobe. The

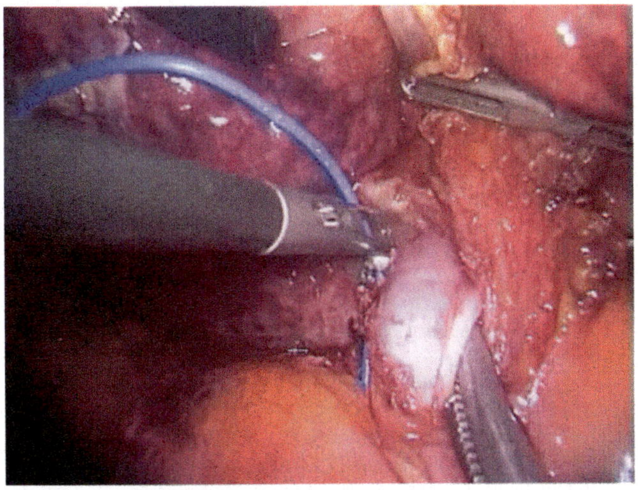

Fig. 18.6 Posterior right side of peritoneum and the stump of the cystic duct used to open the space where the portal trunk runs

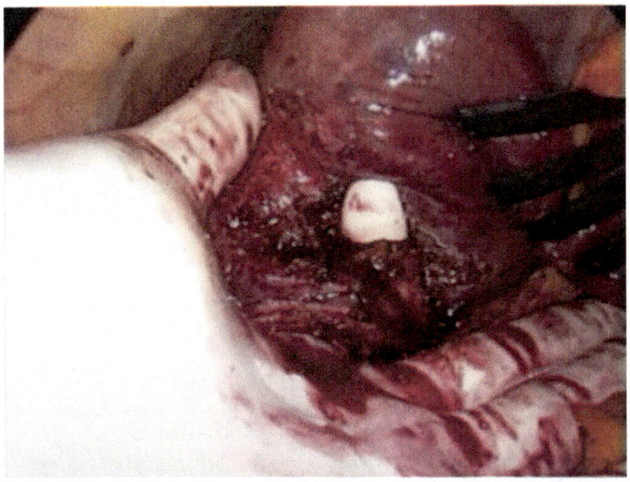

Fig. 18.7 Use of an hand port can be useful in case of large tumors and difficult mobilization of the right liver

peritoneum of the hepatic pedicle is incised longitudinally at its posterior right side and the stump of the cystic duct can be used to open the space where the portal trunk runs (Fig. 18.6). An accessory right hepatic artery is identified and sectioned between clips if present. The right portal branch (RPB) is identified (the portal bifurcation and the origin of the left portal branch must be exposed before occlusion of the RPB. The lymphatic tissue on the anterior side of the RPB is then dissected to expose the right branch of the hepatic artery which is dissected ligated and divided. The right hepatic duct is also identified. It can be ligated at this stage or later on intraparenchimally. At this point the RPB is taped on a vessel loop and ligated between absorbable clips or sectioned by the use of an endo-GIA if there is enough space for its placement. Ischemic demarcation of the transection line is observed on the liver surface and marked with monopolar electrocautery on the Glisson' s capsule. In case of anterior approach parenchymal transection starts and control of the right hepatic vein (RHV) is postponed. The vena cava is dissected by tunnelling below the live using harmonic shears . Accessory small retrohepatic veins are identified and sectioned between clips. Hepato-caval ligament is also divided . The RHV is isolated extraparenchimally and taped with a vessel loop, an endo-GIA with vascular cartridge is then used to section it After incision of the liver capsule the parenchymal transection can be carried out by the use of different devices as previously described.

Particular care is taken to identify and ligate electively the hepatic veins draining segments 5 and 8 toward the middle hepatic vein. Lesion of one of this structures is the main cause of bleeding during parenchymal transection and can cause an important impairment of laparoscopic view. Multiple firing of Endo-GIA can be also used to progress during parenchymal transection but an adequate bite of parenchyma (not too thick) and an adequate vision of the tip of the stapler must be warranted.

The use of an hand port can be useful in case of large tumors and difficult mobilization of the right liver [5] (Fig. 18.7). The handport is usually introduced in the right flank as shown in Fig. 18.2 in line with an hypothetic right subcostal incision that can be used in case of conversion to laparotomy. When the use of the handport is decided and the tumor to be resected is not close to the hilum an intraoperative ultrasound (IOUS) guided intrahepatic approach can be used to transect en-bloc the right hepatic triad (Fig. 18.8). The hilar plate is gently lowered on the back of Segment IV and by the assistance of IOUS two hepatotomies (one on medial and transverse aspect of the gallbladder fossa and the other across the caudate process are created. The right main pedicle, usually running 1–2 cm in depth from the inferior surface of the liver, is then isolated digitally and sectioned by a single firing of Endo-GIA. This technique allow to skip the hilum dissection, thus saving time and can be considered as a technical choice or as a bridge to a total laparoscopic right hepatectomy.

18.2.11 Conversion

Conversion should not be viewed as a complication of laparoscopic surgery, and should be performed for lack of case progress and or patient safety. In emergent situations, efforts should be made to control the bleeding prior to converting, as significant time and blood loss can otherwise occur during the process of conversion. Conversion to a hand assisted approach is more orderly and controlled than conversion to a full chevron or midline incision potentially reducing the risk of further major hemorrhage and hemodynamic instability. Anyway, major vascular injuries, although exceptional, may not allow time for conversion and require a surgeon with extensive laparoscopic training.

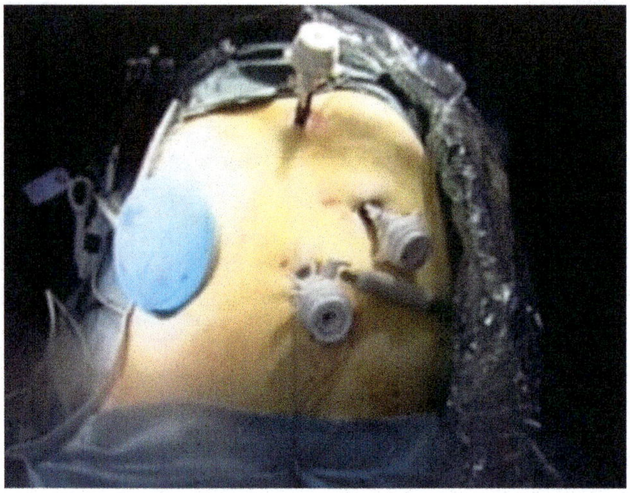

Fig. 18.8 Trocar and handport placement

18.2.11.1 Specimen Retrieval

In the virgin abdomen, specimens are removed through a 5–8 cm Pfannenstiel incision. Regardless of the chosen incision, the abdominal wall is incised to the fascia and the specimen retained under direct laparoscopic vision by hand or large specimen retrieval bag (endopouch).

The specimen is then retracted against the fascia, and the fascia and peritoneum are opened only as much as necessary for retrieval.

The fascial layers are reapproximated and the pneumoperitoneum reintroduced. The operative site is lavaged and examined for hemostasis and biliary tract integrity.

References

1. Cherqui D, Husson E, Hammoud R, Malassagne B, Stéphan F, Bensaid S, Rotman N, Fagniez PL. Laparoscopic liver resections: a feasibility study in 30 patients. Ann Surg. 2000;232(6):753–62.
2. Belli G, Limongelli P, Fantini C, D'Agostino A, Cioffi L, Belli A, Russo G. Laparoscopic and open treatment of hepatocellular carcinoma in patients with cirrhosis. Br J Surg. 2009;96(9):1041–8.
3. Buell JF, Cherqui D, Geller DA, O'Rourke N, Iannitti D, Dagher I, Koffron AJ, Thomas M, Gayet B, Han HS, Wakabayashi G, Belli G, Kaneko H, Ker CG, Scatton O, Laurent A, Abdalla EK, Chaudhury P, Dutson E, Gamblin C, D'Angelica M, Nagorney D, Testa G, Labow D, Manas D, Poon RT, Nelson H, Martin R, Clary B, Pinson WC, Martinie J, Vauthey JN, Goldstein R, Roayaie S, Barlet D, Espat J, Abecassis M, Rees M, Fong Y, McMasters KM, Broelsch C, Busuttil R, Belghiti J, Strasberg S, Chari RS, World Consensus Conference on Laparoscopic Surgery. The international position on laparoscopic liver surgery: the Louisville Statement, 2008. Ann Surg. 2009;250(5):825–30.
4. Belli G, Cioffi L, Fantini C, D'Agostino A, Russo G, Limongelli P, Belli A. Laparoscopic redo surgery for recurrent hepatocellular carcinoma in cirrhotic patients: feasibility, safety, and results. Surg Endosc. 2009;23(8):1807–11.
5. Belli G, D'Agostino A, Fantini C, Belli A, Cioffi L, Limongelli P, Belli A. Laparoscopic hand-assisted right hemihepatectomy by ultrasound-directed intrahepatic approach. J Hepatobiliary Pancreat Surg. 2009;16(6):781–5.

19 Non-resection: Radiofrequency Ablation, Cryo, Microwave

Roberto Santambrogio, Matteo Barabino, and Enrico Opocher

19.1 Introduction

Radiofrequency ablation (RFA) is most commonly performed in the radiology department through a percutaneous approach [1], however, there is a sub-group of patients who may benefit from a laparoscopic approach (LRFA) [2]. The rationale of this technique was to combine the advantages of an improved staging allowed by the intracorporeal ultrasound examination [3] with a safe approach to liver lesions difficult or impossible to be treated percutaneously.

Microwave ablation (MWA) has an important advantage compared to RFA, which is that treatment efficacy is less affected by vessels located in the proximity of the tumor. Cryoablation had now limited application: the complication rate is not negligible, particularly because of the risk for "cryoshock", a life threatening condition resulting in multi-organ failure, severe coagulopathy and disseminated intravascular coagulation following cryoablation.

19.2 Indications

The prerequisite of the success of the procedure is the appropriate multidisciplinary selection of the patient a priori, according to tumor's features, liver function and co-morbidities.

Relative contraindications for LRFA ablation are:

- Tumour located adjacent to main biliary duct (due to risk of delayed stenosis of the main biliary tract)
- Intrahepatic bile duct dilation
- Bilioenteric anastomosis
- Untreatable/unmanageable coagulopathy

R. Santambrogio, MD (✉)
Chirurgia Epato-Bilio-Pancreatica e Digestiva, San Paolo Hospital, University of Milan, Milan, Italy
e-mail: rsantambrogio@mclink.it

M. Barabino, MD • E. Opocher, MD
Chirurgia Epato-bilio-pancreatica e Digestiva, A.O. San Paolo, Università degli Studi di Milano, Milan, Italy

19.2.1 Hepatocellular Carcinoma (HCC)

Barcelona Clinic Liver Cancer (BCLC) group (and further AASLD updates) proposed a staging/treatment classification, based on the authors' synthesis of several studies including variables related relating to the tumor, liver function and physical status [4]. The BCLC group recommended liver resection as the first therapeutic option only for stage A1 patients (single tumor less than 5 cm, Child class A, no portal hypertension, and normal bilirubin), while for patients at the other A stages RFA and/or OLT have been suggested.

If percutaneous RFA should not be accomplished, a LRFA could be indicated in patients that had at least one of the following criteria:

(a) severe impairment of the coagulation tests (platelets < 40,000 and/or International Normalized Ratio (INR) > 1.20);
(b) large tumors (but with a diameter inferior to 5 cm) or multiple lesions requiring repeated punctures;
(c) superficial lesions adjacent to visceral structures which could be displaced by laparoscopic maneuvers: colon appears to be at greater risk than the stomach or small bowel for thermally mediated perforation;
(d) lesions close to intra-hepatic structures: the laparoscopic approach guarantees a lower risk of biliary thermal injuries either performing a "cooling technique" for these lesions or associating a cholecystectomy for lesions close to gallbladder;
(e) deep-sited lesions with a very difficult or impossible percutaneous approach;
(f) short-term recurrence of HCC following liver surgery, ethanol injection or TACE.

19.2.2 Liver Metastases (LM)

Surgical resection represents the gold standard for the management of LM. Unfortunately, only 10–25 % of patients are

H.J. Bonjer (ed.), *Surgical Principles of Minimally Invasive Procedures*, DOI 10.1007/978-3-319-43196-3_19

amenable to liver resection due to the characteristics of either hepatic lesions (location, number, remnant liver volume) or patients (co-morbidities, chemotherapic toxicity, performance status). In this setting of unresectable patients, RFA could represent a good indication. The number of lesions should not be considered an absolute contraindication to RFA: nevertheless, most centres preferentially treat patients with five or fewer lesions. The target tumour should not exceed 3 cm in longest axis to achieve best rates of complete ablation with most of the currently available devices. MWA had the potential to result in less local recurrence because, compared with RFA, MWA shows several advantages such as an improved convection profile, higher intratumoural temperatures, faster ablation, larger ablation volume, and less susceptible to 'heat-sink effect'.

19.3 Preoperative Work-Up

All patients considered for image-guided therapy of their hepatic tumors should undergo high-quality CT or MRI studies. These allow determination of the number and size of lesions, evidence of extrahepatic spread, and the tumor's relationship with contiguous structures such as blood vessels, bile ducts, gallbladder, diaphragm, and bowel. We also perform a pre-ablation planning ultrasound to determine optimal patient positioning and approach.

Laboratory examens including serum chemistry panel with liver function tests and appropriate tumor markers such as alphafetoprotein (AFP) for HCC and carcinoembryonic antigen (CEA) for LM, electrocardiogram and chest x-ray should be performed in all patients.

19.3.1 Hepatocellular Carcinoma (HCC)

The diagnosis and staging of HCC is based on the appropriate imaging studies including triple-phase CT scan and/or MRI according to the AASLD guidelines, and histological assessment only when required [4]. The residual liver function is evaluated using the Child-Pugh classification.

The presence of preoperative portal hypertension is assessed: direct measurement of venous pressure is not performed routinely, and portal hypertension is arbitrarily defined as esophageal varices detectable at endoscopy or splenomegaly (major diameter: >12 cm) with a platelet count <100,000/mm^3 [4].

19.3.2 Liver Metastases (LM)

The pre-operative imaging assessment includes CT, MRI and, in selected cases, positron emission tomography with 18FDG (PET-CT). MRI shows higher sensibility detection after chemotherapy and PET-CT is indicated as complementary exam in front of patients with high risk of extra-hepatic disseminated disease.

19.4 Operating Room

A proper table that allows the patient to be placed in both full Trendelemburg and reverse Trendelemburg positions during operation is essential. The optimal situation is to have the ultrasound monitor in the same line of vision as the monitor for the laparoscopic telescope. A convenient way to visualize both laparoscopic and ultrasound images simultaneously is to employ a screen-splitting device for a single monitor: a picture-in-picture visualization is particularly helpful during LRFA procedure. Generally, the ultrasound unit is located on the right side of the patient adjacent to the armboard with the laparoscopic equipment off the right shoulder of the patient: the surgeon goes to the right side of the patient. Also the RFA/MW machine is positioned on the patient's right side.

An equipment checklist is necessary to ensure that all items are available:

- Laparoscopic equipment (generally housed in a cart on wheels):
  - Monitor: flat panel monitor has better resolution and it is more mobile than the than traditional monitor;
  - Insufflator: we recommend a high-flow insufflator capable of delivering flow rates up to 30 L/min;
  - Camera – processor unit: Laparoscopic camera can be either of single chip or three chip. This has high-quality colour reproduction and highest degree of fidelity;
  - Light source: a high intensity light source is a requisite for a satisfactorily bright laparoscopic image.
- Laparoscopic optics: a 30° or 45° laparoscope is preferable for close-up viewing of the surface architecture of the liver and for providing guidance to the electrode under direct vision. In addition, by rotation of the telescope, it allows different angles of inspection during the electrode infission.
- Energy sources for coagulation and cutting: standard unipolar or bipolar electrocautery can be used for hemostasis and dividing tissue. For cirrhotic patients with extremely vascular tissue such as adhesions, alternative energy sources such as ultrasonic coagulation may be more suitable.
- Ultrasound equipment: we used an ultrasound machine connected to a laparoscopic ultrasound (LUS) probe with a flexible tip, 10 mm in diameter and 50 cm in length. A 5–7.5 MHz linear-array transducer was side-mounted near the tip of the shaft. The length of the transducer surface was 38 mm, which produced an image footprint of approximately 4 cm in length and 6 cm in depth. Recently we also used a micro-convex probe that permits the appli-

cation of intravenous ultrasound contrast agents during LUS of the liver: the addition of contrast enhancement during the intra-operative ultrasound will improve image conspicuity, correct diagnosis of new malignant nodules, ablation efficacy in hepatic tumors and oncologic margin outcomes (Fig. 19.1);
- Suction irrigator;
- Table with small retractors for umbilical incision, trocar cannulae (size and number depend on the planned operation) and laparoscopic instruments (atraumatic gaspers, bowel grasping forceps, coagulated hook and scissors);
- 18G tru-cut biopsy needle: it is useful to use a cutting needle with an automatic trigger mechanism in order to hold the probe with one hand and the needle with the other. Because of the presence of pneumoperitoneum which separates the surface of the liver from the abdominal wall, the use of longer needles (25–27 cm) could be necessary for lesions localized in the posterior segments or in the highest part of the liver (segments IVa and VIII).
- RFA/MWA machine and electrode/antenna: actually we used a dual ablation system which in the same hardware has both a microwave and a RFA energy generator. For RFA technology, we prefer a 17G internally cooled electrode with an exposed tip length of 3 cm and shaft length of 250 mm. For MWA technology, we use a 14G interstitial antenna with a shaft length of 270 mm.

19.5 Surgical Technique

LRFA is performed under general endotracheal anesthesia. A Foley catheter is useful only for cirrhotic patients for monitoring postoperative urinary output. A nasogastric tube is sometimes useful to deflate the stomach before the procedure. If RFA equipment is used, at least two large surface area grounding pads must be used.

Patient positioning is dependent on the location of the hepatic lesions to be treated (Fig. 19.2). Generally, position of the patient is supine on the operating room with the left arm extended: the surgeon stands either on the right side or between the legs of the patient (Fig. 19.2a, b). Patients with tumors in segments VI and VII can be placed in either a oblique position with the right side elevated up to 45° or left decubitis position with the right arm elevated and across the chest and the surgeon stands at either the right or the left side of the patient (Fig. 19.2c, d).

The location of introduction of LUS probe is limited by the location of the trocars: first, the umbilical port can be made for laparoscopic exploration, and the second trocar site for LUS can be selected depending both the preoperative imaging evaluation and the intraoperative conditions as determined by laparoscopy.

Exploration of the liver parenchyma can be usually performed with a direct contact technique: however, the dome of the liver may be difficult to examine because of the lack of adequate contact between the probe and the convex liver surface: this can be overcome by instilling saline solution and scanning the highest part of the organ through the fluid (water-immersion method) (Fig. 19.3). Furthermore, in some instances, it should be useful to low to 6–8 mmHg the pneumoperitoneum favoring a correct angle of transducer contact with the liver surface.

The whole liver is initially screened and each tumor is measured in size by LUS and described according to the Couinaud classification of liver anatomy. After the lesions have been identified, the therapeutic electrode can be accurately inserted into the tumor.

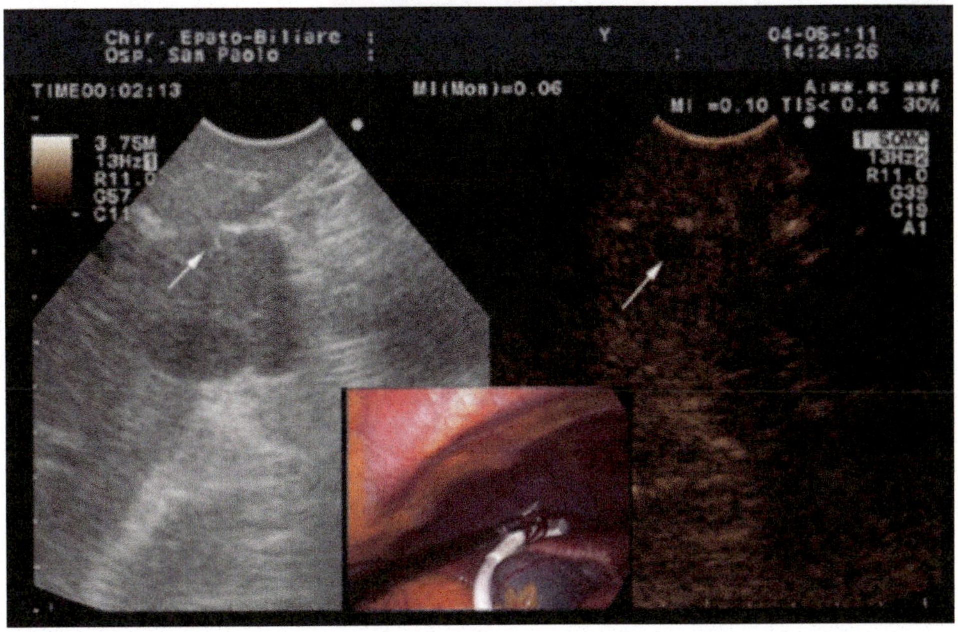

Fig. 19.1 A microconvex transducer is introduced in the peritoneal cavity through a 3-cm access. It permits the application of intravenous ultrasound contrast agent to improve nodule characterization in comparison with unenhanced ultrasound

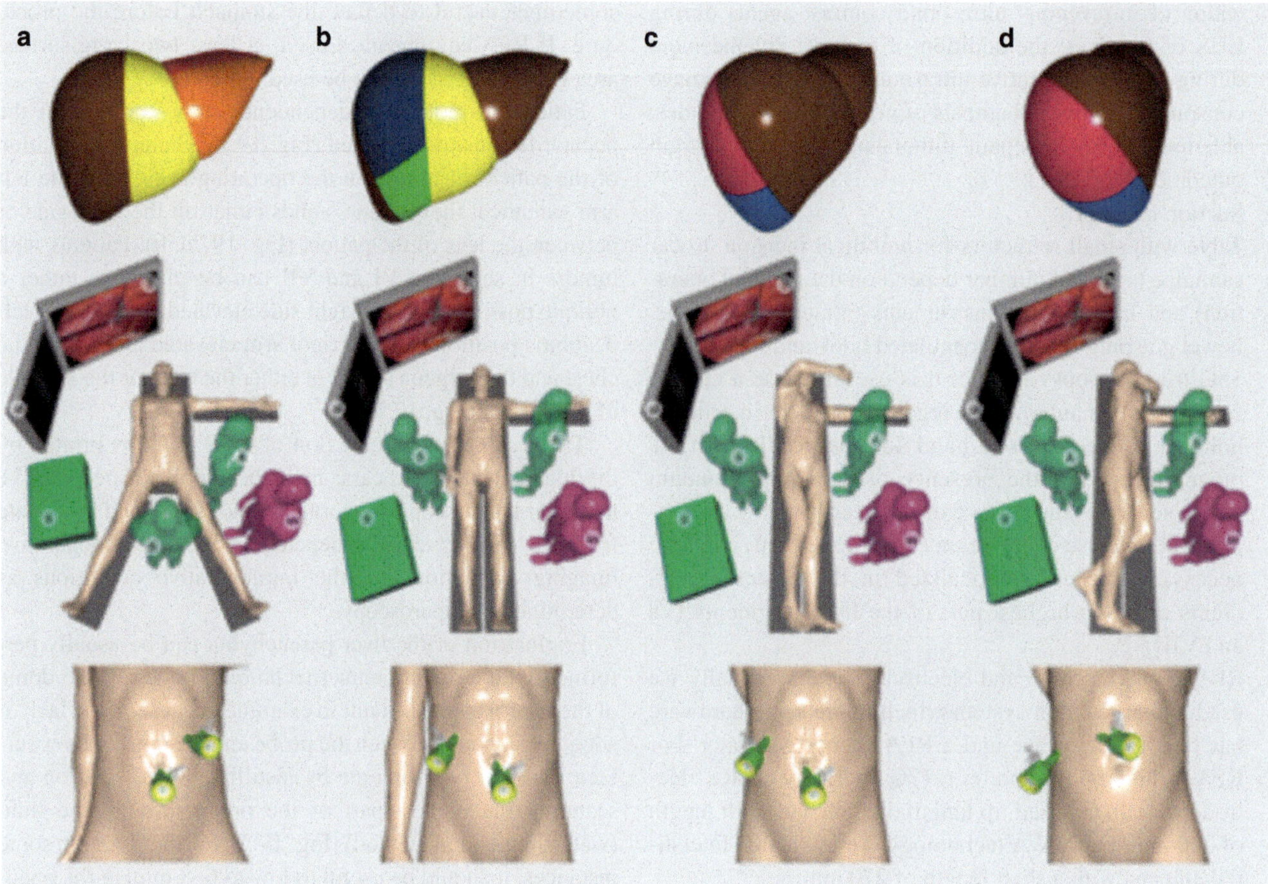

Fig. 19.2 Patient and operating room positions for LRFA. (**a**) supine position with legs abducted (surgeon stands between the legs) for lesions in segments 2,3 and 4; (**b**) supine position with legs adducted (surgeon stands on the patient's right side) for lesions in segments 4, 5 and 8; (**c**) oblique position with the right side elevated up to 45° or (**d**) left decubitis position with the right arm elevated and across the chest (surgeon stands at the left side of the patient) for lesions in segments 6 and 7

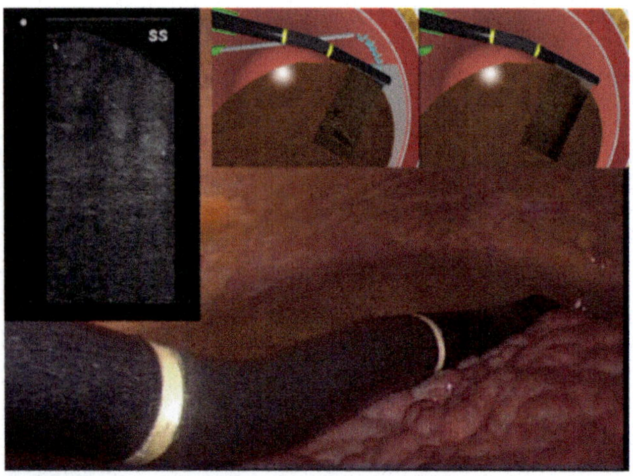

Fig. 19.3 The dome of the liver may be more easily examined by instilling saline solution (SS) and scanning this part of the organ through the fluid which creates an acoustic window

When dealing with lesions localised in segment 1 or in the posterior segments of an enlarged liver, a longer laparoscopic electrode could be necessary (27 cm). A LUS-guided interventional procedure can be successfully performed if the following ideal working conditions are fulfilled: (1) the lesion has to be well visible: the ultrasound probe must be oriented on the liver surface to display the largest diameter of the entire lesion; (2) the electrode must be positioned near the transducer of the LUS probe in order to introduce it slightly oblique to the transducer and with an acute angle to the axis of the LUS probe (Fig. 19.4). In fact, after inserting the electrode into the liver parenchyma, slight rotation of the probe can identify the mark of the electrode and guide its tip into the lesion. For lesions located at posterior segments, it is necessary to insert the electrode on the liver surface further than the lesion: in this case, the transducer can not visualize contemporary the tumor and the electrode tip

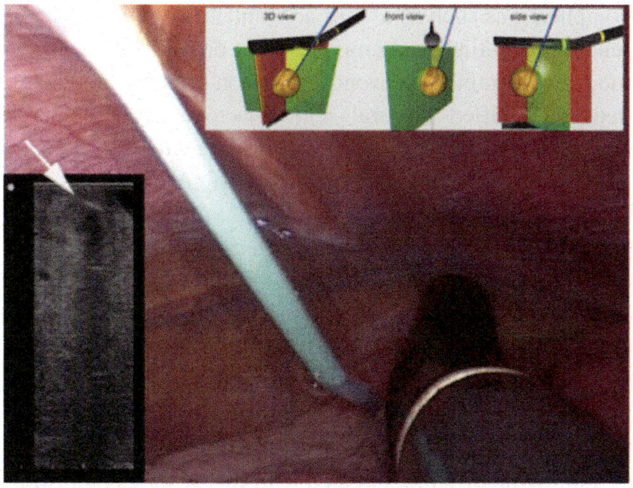

Fig. 19.4 In order to centre exactly the lesion, it is important to evaluate both the angles of the electrode incidence respect to the LUS image of the lesion

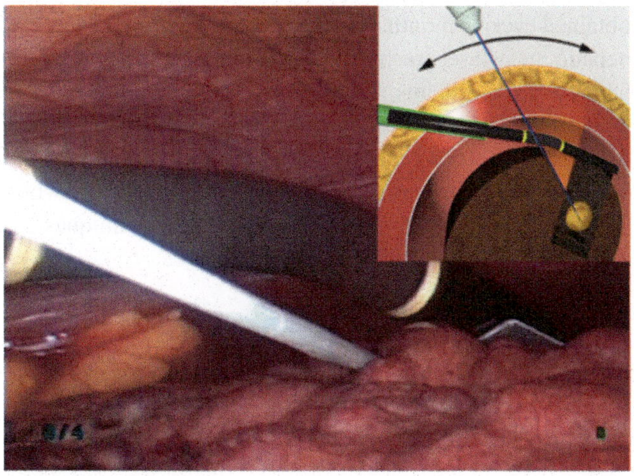

Fig. 19.5 If the lesion is situated into the posterior segments, the electrode must be inserted more fore into the liver (blind zone of insertion) to reach a deep-located tumor (7 segment, i.e.)

(Fig. 19.5). On the other hand, because any LUS-guided interventional procedure is totally free-hand, a puncture adapter has been proposed: the incorporation of the biopsy channel into the shaft of the ultrasound probe permits accurate placement of the electrode only in lesions seated in some areas of the liver.

For lesions that required multiple overlapping ablations, the zones farthest the LUS transducer were ablated first so that the ultrasound artefacts of dissolved nitrogen did not obscure electrode placement for subsequent ablations.

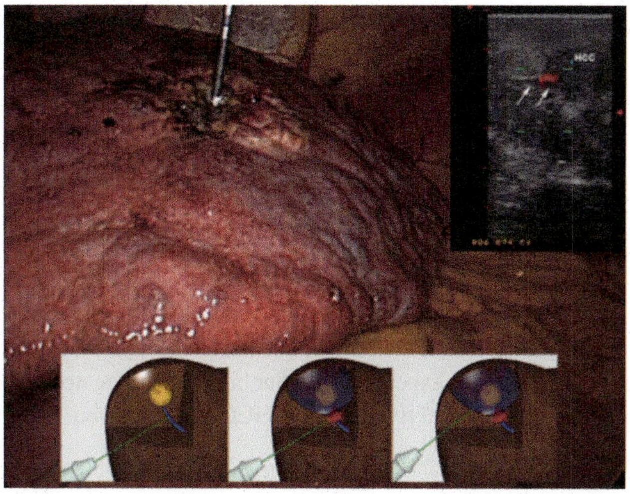

Fig. 19.6 The primary vessel of the lesion was identified by color doppler imaging: using LUS guidance, the electrode was directed towards this area with direct puncture of the nearby blood vessel and the ablation cycle lasted 2–4 min: a discolored area on the liver surface can be visualized. Then, the lesion was treated with the insertion of the electrode in the usual way

19.5.1 Technical Variants: Intra-hepatic Vascular Occlusion

This approach determines an ischemic area surrounding the lesion increasing the necrosis volume [5]. This effect could reduce the risk of immediate therapy failure (partial ablation) and of local recurrences. In order to obtain a selective intrahepatic portal venous occlusion, the primary vessel of the lesion was identified by color doppler imaging: using ultrasonographic guidance, the electrode was directed towards this area with direct puncture of the nearby blood vessel and the ablation cycle lasted either 2–4 min using RFA or 60–90 s using MWA. Another evaluation with color doppler imaging was performed to confirm a coagulative ablation of the vascular area: a discolored area on the liver surface can be also visualized (Fig. 19.6). Then, the lesion was treated with the insertion of the electrode in the usual way.

19.5.2 Technical Variants: Cooling Technique

If the tumor is located in the hepatic hilar region, RFA may cause bile duct stenosis due to physical or heat damage to the bile duct.

It is possible to prevent this biliary damage producing an intraductal cooling of the main bile ducts during laparoscopic RFA: a tube can be inserted in the main biliary duct either through the cystic duct (cholecystectomy must be performed) or through a direct incision of the main bile duct (choledochotomy). However, these procedures could be very difficult in cirrhotic patients.

We prefer a less invasive approach. We insert some gauzes in the peritoneal cavity and we place them around the hepatoduodenal ligament. Then, an irrigator with cold saline solution infuses them: cold vascular flow in the portal and arterial systems protects the bile ducts from the thermal effects of RFA by dissipating the heat generated in the ablated area.

The possible "heat sink" effect of central bile duct cooling might also affect the efficacy of RFA in terms of local recurrences, but in our experience neither biliary damage nor partial ablation or local recurrence of HCC was observed.

19.5.3 Technical Variants: Adhesions for Previous Surgical Operations

Adhesions between the liver and the abdominal wall and viscera are taken down using ultrasonic coagulator and bipolar forceps. In the event of prior right upper quadrant surgery (hepatic resections, i.e.), two/three 10-mm ports are placed in the left upper quadrant if the patient has tumors in segments VI and VII: in this case patient can be placed in a oblique position with the right side elevated up to 45° and the surgeon stands at the left side of the patient. Sometimes, it is also necessary to divide the falciform ligament in order to go from the left lobe to the right. In the other cases, it can be useful to place the patient in the low lithotomy position and the surgeon operates between the patient's legs (see Fig. 19.2).

19.6 Postoperative Care

In the immediate postoperative period, slight pain and nausea are the two most likely effects of image-guided RFA. Administration of an intravenous antiemetic and analgesic agents immediately postablation may be necessary, but subsequent symptoms usually can be controlled with oral drugs. Fever up to 102 °F may occur as part of a postablation syndrome but generally subsides within 5 days. With any of the ablation techniques, liver abscess is a rare but potentially life-threatening complication.

Patients with cirrhosis require careful consideration with regards to intravenous crystalloid administration. Crystalloids that have high-sodium content should be avoided to prevent complications such as ascites accumulation. Potassium canrenoate is routinely administered at a dosage depending on the urinary output. Intravenous infusion of potassium canrenoate is shifted to oral spironolactone (100 mg/day). Furosemide is given if water tended to be retained or if potassium canrenoate alone is ineffective in controlling ascites. The dosage of furosemide is started at a ratio of 20 mg of furosemide per 100 mg of potassium canrenoate. In presence of ascites and hypoalbuminemia, low-salt albumin infusion should begin to maintain a normal oncotic pressure.

LRFA is usually a fast-recovery procedure and patients are discharged from the hospital stay area within 2–3 days after the procedure. For elderly patients and those with other medical conditions (cirrhosis i.e.), recovery may be slower.

Follow-up of tumors treated with LRFA varies by institution. Our current protocol is to perform spiral CT scans after 1 month, followed by additional scans at 4 months and then every 6 months to evaluate for local recurrence, remote intrahepatic recurrence, and extrahepatic disease. In addition to imaging studies, alpha-fetoprotein and CEA levels should be obtained every 6 months in patients with HCC and colorectal hepatic metastases, respectively. As long as sufficient viable hepatic tissue remains, there is no accepted upper limit for how often tumor recurrence may be reablated. However, if extrahepatic spread occurs or extensive intrahepatic LM disease develops, systemic therapy may be preferable, while TACE may be preferred over other ablative techniques for extensive intrahepatic HCC recurrence.

References

1. Livraghi T, Meloni F, Di Stasi M, Rolle E, Solbiati L, Tinelli C, Rossi S. Sustained complete response and complications rates after radiofrequency ablation of very early hepatocellular carcinoma in cirrhosis: is resection still the treatment of choice? Hepatology. 2008;47:82–9.
2. Santambrogio R, Opocher E, Costa M, Cappellani A, Montorsi M. Survival and intra-hepatic recurrences after laparoscopic radiofrequency of hepatocellular carcinoma in patients with liver cirrhosis. J Surg Oncol. 2005;89:218–26.
3. Santambrogio R, Opocher E, Pisani Ceretti A, Barabino M, Costa M, Leone S, Montorsi M. Impact of intraoperative ultrasonography in laparoscopic liver surgery. Surg Endosc. 2007;21:181–8.
4. Bruix J, Sherman M. Management of hepatocellular carcinoma: un update. Hepatology. 2011;53:1020–2.
5. Santambrogio R, Costa M, Barabino M, Opocher E. Laparoscopic radiofrequency of hepatocellular carcinoma using ultrasound-guided selective intra-hepatic vascular occlusion. Surg Endosc. 2008;22:2051–5.

Part VII

Galbladder and Biliary Ducts

Cholecystectomy

20

Jack J. Jakimowicz and Johannes F. Smulders

20.1 Introduction

Laparoscopic cholecystectomy became the procedure of choice for treatment of symptomatic gall stone disease, and nowadays it is considered to be the gold standard. In the United Stated 90 % of cholecystectomies are performed laparoscopically. In spite of improvement of instrumentation, surgical techniques and growing experience of surgeons in laparoscopic procedures the morbidity rate, due to major biliary tract injuries remains relatively high (0.3–0.5 %) [1, 2].This not only has a dramatic impact on the wellbeing of patients but also generates high costs of treatment and leads to medical legal litigation driving up health care costs. Salvader et al. estimated that laparoscopic cholecystectomy-related bile duct injuries were associated with an additional 50,000 US Dollars in costs, 32 days of inpatient hospitalization, 378 days of chronic biliary intubation, and 4 % mortality per case [3]. Adopting the concept of a "standardized operative procedures (SOP)" approach is of paramount importance to assure safety and quality of performance. Breaking up a procedure in component tasks and executing these tasks meticulously can undoubtedly reduce risks of complications in any kind of surgical procedure and certainly in laparoscopic cholecystectomy.

20.2 Indications and Contra-indications

The main indications for laparoscopic cholecystectomy are symptomatic cholecystolithiasis and acute cholecystitis. It is also indicated in patients with calcified (porcelain) and sclera-atrophic gallbladders, because of the theoretical risk of the progression of cancer. Asymptomatic cholecystolithiasis, in general, does not warrant cholecystectomy at all.

J.J. Jakimowicz, MD, PhD, FRCS, Ed (✉) • J.F. Smulders, MD
Department of Research and Education, Catharina Hospital, Eindhoven, 5602 ZA, The Netherlands
e-mail: jakimowi@planet.nl

Absolute contra-indications for laparoscopic cholecystectomy are lack of equipment, lack of surgeon expertise and septic shock from cholangitis. Other main contra-indications for cholecystectomy are generalized peritonitis, septic shock from cholangitis, severe acute pancreatitis, cirrhosis with portal hypertension, severe coagulopathy that is not corrected and known dense adhesions in the upper abdomen. Extreme caution should be taken in groups of patients with severe associated cardiorespiratory diseases, previous upper abdominal surgery, symptomatic cholecystolithiasis in the second trimester of pregnancy.

20.3 Laparoscopic Cholecystectomy Component Tasks of Procedure

20.3.1 Preparation of the Procedure

Several steps have to be taken in preparation of the procedures. Firstly the following instruments have to be set up: a laparoscopic stack, 30 degrees or 0 degree optics 10 or 5 mm, traumatic and atraumatic graspers, curved dissector forceps, straight dissector forceps, laparoscopic scissors, suction and irrigation system and electro surgery unit or other energized instruments for haemostasis and dissection. The patient is positioned is a supine position with legs together and both arms out (Fig. 20.1).

Pneumoperitoneum is established through an open introduction or with a Veres needle. After inserting the first trocar for the laparoscope, the patient is placed in head up position with slight tilt towards the left. The surgeons stands at the left side of the patient, the assistant at the right side. If a second assistant operates the camera, he/she should stand at the left side of the patient, left of the surgeon. In case the scrub nurse operates the camera he/she takes place at the right side of the assistant at the right side of the patient (see Fig. 20.1). This is the so-called "American position". The alternative is the so-called "French position", where the surgeon stands between the patient's legs. Here the assistant stands at the

H.J. Bonjer (ed.), *Surgical Principles of Minimally Invasive Procedures*, DOI 10.1007/978-3-319-43196-3_20

left side of the patient, as well as the camera person, if present. Monitors (minimal two) are place ergonomically in front of the surgeon and assistant at the distance, twice diagonal of monitor, and allowing observation with a gaze down of 10 up to 15 degrees. Nasogastric tube is placed for the duration of the procedure, and is removed before the patient leaves the OR. Antibiotic prophylaxis is not indicated for elective procedure. Use of antibiotics should be considered on indication.

Access and placement/position of trocars. It is up to the surgeon's preference in which way access to the peritoneum is established. Open introduction can be performed at the umbilical area just caudally to or transumbilically. In case a Veres-needle is used to create the pneumoperitoneum it should be inserted not at the umbilicus, but in the left upper abdominal quadrant just below the costal margin (Palmers' point). The use of four trocars to perform a laparoscopic cholecystectomy is strongly recommended, and for safe performance of the procedure almost mandatory. Before placing the trocars local anaesthetics is injected at the incision spot, infiltration the abdominal wall at the place of insertion. The first trocar, the so-called optical one, through which the laparoscope will be introduced, is placed at the umbilicus. In obese patients where the xiphoid-umbilical distance is long, supra-umbilical insertion should be considered. While placing the first trocar to create a pneumoperitoneum use of a so-called optical trocar system allowing introduction of trocar under direct visual control of a laparoscope should be considered. It is recommended to place the second, 5 mm trocar at or above the level of the umbilicus in the anterior axillary line. After inserting an atraumatic grasper the fundus of the gallbladder is grasped and pushed cephalic (cranially). In this way the position of the two remaining working ports can be optimized. The third trocar is a 5 mm one in the midclavicular line for the surgeons left hand and the fourth one for the surgeon's right hand (10 mm) is placed up to 3 cm caudally to the xyphoid to the right of the midline (linea alba), i.e. to the right of the ligamentum tereshepatis. One should be aware of the superior epigastric artery and vein running a few centimetres laterally to the linea alba. For location of the trocars, see Fig. 20.2.

One has to bear in mind that introduction of trocars has to take place after creating adequate pneumoperitoneum, and under visual control. Only after creating peritoneum the choice of location of ports can be correctly assessed, and optimal ergonomic setting achieved, taking in account correct manipulation and elevation angles and the distance to the target area: the gallbladder.

20.3.2 Exploration of the Abdomen and the Operation Area

The exploration of the abdomen is mostly focused on the upper abdomen, providing no other reasons indicate need for extensive exploration of the whole abdominal space. The operation area should be thoroughly assessed for the presence of adhesions, liver pathology, cirrhosis. To determine surgical strategy thorough evaluation of the condition of the gallbladder, presence of post-cholecystitis fibrosis, shrunken gallbladder, or presence of cholecystitis (edema or even necrosis of the wall) as well as presence of fragile thin wall gallbladder is mandatory. Each of the mentioned conditions

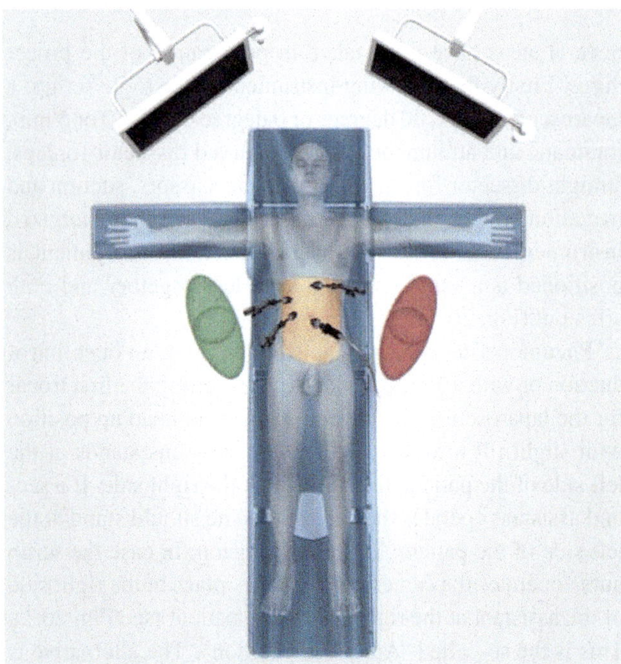

Fig. 20.1 Patient positioning for laparoscopic cholecystectomy

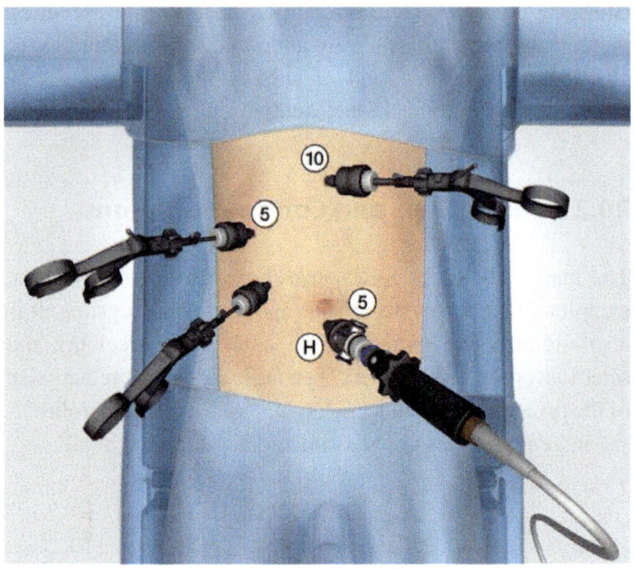

Fig. 20.2 Trocar positioning for laparoscopic cholecystectomy

necessitate correct choice of instruments to be used and determines the way of handling tissue to be able to perform the procedure efficiently and safely. When inspecting the operation area identification of the sulcus of Rouvière, located to the right of the gallbladder between the segment V and VI of the liver, allows determining the dorsal border of dissection. There are, however, some exceptions: vital structures of the hepatoduodenal ligament can also be located above (ventrally) the level of the sulcus.

20.3.3 Dissection of the Anatomic Structures of the Triangle of Calot Area, i.e. the Cystic Duct and Artery: Achieving Critical View of Safety (CVS)

To enable safe dissection of the cystic duct and artery, adequate retraction of the gallbladder to expose the area of Calot's triangle is mandatory. Two atraumatic graspers are used to retract and manipulate the gallbladder. One is retracting the gallbladder and the right liver lobe, grasping the fundus of the gallbladder, and pushing/pulling the gallbladder cranially almost over the liver. This instrument is held by the assistant, static traction holding the gallbladder in position. The second grasper is placed at the infundibulum area of the gallbladder. This instrument is handled by the surgeon himself, and is used to retract the infundibulum anterolaterally and slightly caudally (Fig. 20.3). Correct retraction brings the cystic duct in position, perpendicular towards the common bile duct (CBD), and provides optimal exposure of Calot's triangle.

Exposure is enhanced by dynamic retractions, using flag movements to visualize posterior and anterior aspect of the peritoneal envelope of Calot's area. Dissection starts at the infundibulum of the gallbladder and is performed from front (anterior) and back (posterior) of the triangle of Calot. Dissecting the posterior sheath of the peritoneal envelope enhances the retraction and enables gaining more length of the cystic duct. For the purpose of dissection the use of a curved or straight dissecting forceps is advised. The use of electrosurgical hook counter for dissecting the structure of Calot's triangle is risky and should be abandoned. Dissection, using dissector forceps, consist of picking up a small volume of peritoneum, fatty or fibrotic tissue, and stripping it of from the underlying structures. The use of cautery should be restricted to short burst of 2 up to 3 seconds to minimize thermal spread to surrounding structures. Power settings of the generator, smaller or equal to 20/40 Watt are recommended. Blunt dissection, spreading tissue along the cystic duct and artery allows easy clearing fatty and fibrotic tissue from the structures. In the same way the gallbladder infundibulum is separated from the liver and cystic plate (gallbladder bed is this way brought in sight). One quarter to one third of the gallbladder length should be separated from the cystic plate. Both cystic duct and cystic artery should be circumferentially cleared over a length enabling safe placing of clips or ligatures to control both structures. Once this is achieved there will be two and only two structures left entering the gallbladder. Two broad windows are created, one between the cystic duct and cystic artery, the other between the cystic artery and the infundibulum of the gallbladder and liver. At this point the dissection of Calot's triangle is accomplished and critical view of safety is achieved (Fig. 20.4). A critical view of safety is not a dissection technique, but identification technique to allow safe control and division of cystic artery and cystic duct [1, 4, 5]. Only after achieving CVS one may proceed with division of structures and separate and remove the gallbladder.

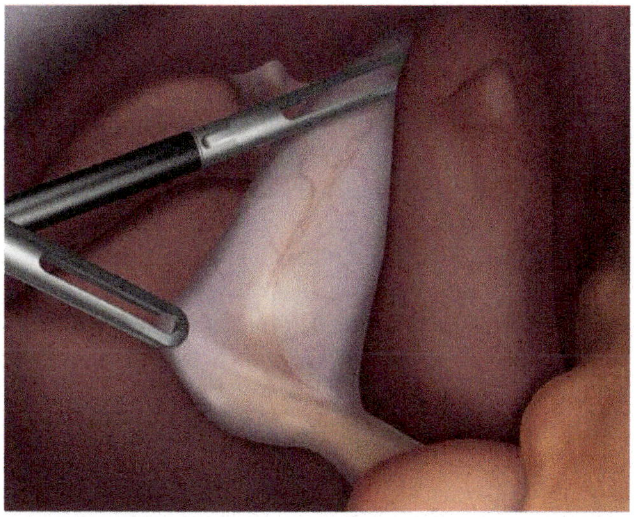

Fig. 20.3 Retraction of the gallbladder exposing Calot's triangle

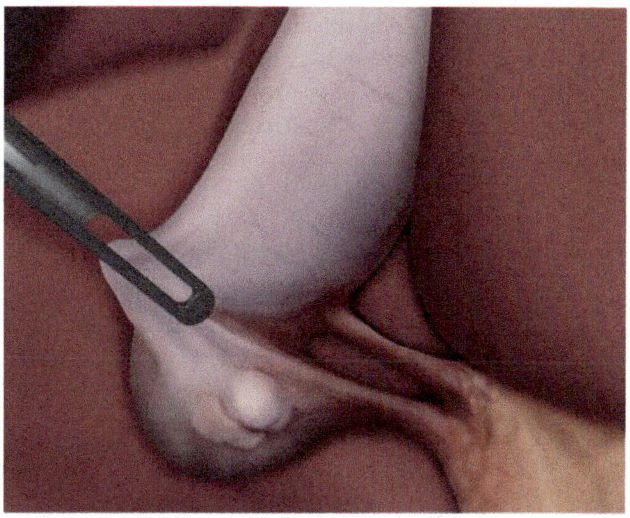

Fig. 20.4 Critical view of safety in laparoscopic cholecystectomy

20.3.4 Intraoperative Diagnostic Procedures: Intraoperative Cholangiography (IOC) and/or Intraoperative Ultrasonography (IOUS)

Routine intraoperative cholangiography in course of laparoscopic cholecystectomy is recommended for verification of anatomy and prevention of CBD-lesions, although it seems not to be a general practice in the Netherlands. The discussion regarding the role of cholangiography is ongoing and is evoked by a new recently recent published cohort study of 92,932 patients which concluded that there was no statistically significant association between intraoperative cholangiography and common duct injury [6]. In some countries, not performing IOC may be seen as negligence if CBD-lesion occurs. A viable alternative for IOC is laparoscopic intraoperative ultrasonography (LIOU). In experienced hands ultrasonography provides both adequate information on anatomy and pathology, as IOC does [7]. In case of obscured anatomy, if CVS is not accomplished, an intraoperative diagnostic procedure should be performed. Emerging new technologies such as near-infrared fluorescent cholangiography may in the near future become a substitute of IOC or ultrasonography

20.3.5 Control of Cystic Artery and Cystic Duct and Division of Both Structures

The most clearly applied method of securing the cystic artery and duct is the use of clips. Two clips should be placed centrally and one peripherally on each of these structures. The distance between central and peripheral clips should be large enough to allow safe division of the structure leaving adequate cuff of tissue, minimally one mm away from the clip (Fig. 20.5).

It is advisable to divide first the artery and then the cystic duct, although it is dependent on the existing access to these structures and judgement of the surgeon (Fig. 20.6) [5]. The sequence of division may be altered depending on specific anatomic situation up to the judgment of the surgeon.

20.3.6 Separation of the Gallbladder from the Liver

Dissecting the gallbladder from the liver/cystic plate consists of sharp or blunt dissection. Instruments, as scissors, cautery spatula, cautery hook, and blunt dissection are mostly used. Taking down and transection of the peritoneum at the edge of the gallbladder, step by step, allows preservation of the cystic plate and avoids bleeding from damaged liver tissue.

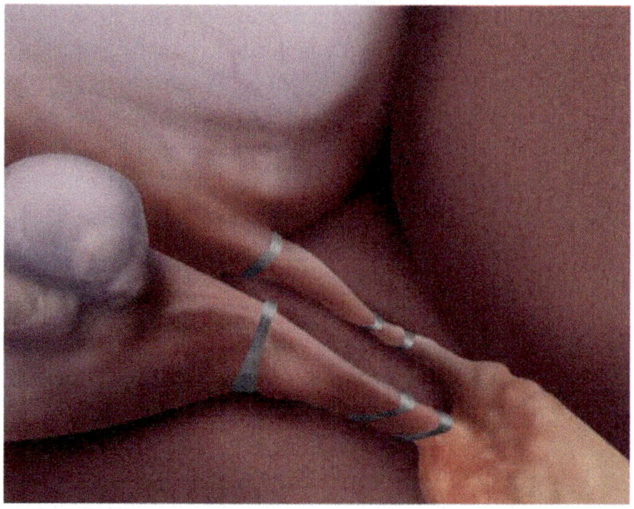

Fig. 20.5 Placement of clips on cystic duct and cystic artery

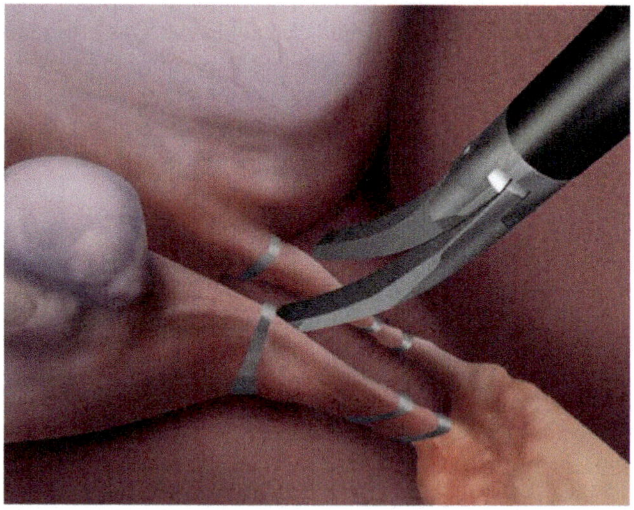

Fig. 20.6 Cutting cystic artery

20.3.7 Inspection of Operation Field and Removal of the Gallbladder

After thorough inspection of the operative field for bleeding or presence of bile, rinsing of the operation field with warm saline to remove tissue debris and blood is performed. The gallbladder can be removed through the subxyphoidal trocar site or through the umbilicus. In the latter, the laparoscope is changed to the subxyphoidal trocar and the gallbladder is removed through the umbilical access wound. When using a 5 mm laparoscope and a 5 mm trocar at the umbilicus it makes sense to remove the gallbladder through the 10–12 mm trocar site at the subxyphoidal place.

In case of multiple or large stones the infundibulum of the gallbladder is pulled out through the chosen trocar site and, after opening the gallbladder small stones are removed and easy extraction of the gallbladder than is possible, preferably using a retrieval bag. Use of retrieval bag may prevent spillage of bile or stones.

In case of large stones: mechanical lithotripsy, using strong forceps can be performed to facilitate removal of the gallbladder without enlarging/dilating incision, can take place. Subsequently after removal of the gallbladder the umbilical trocar is inserted and pneumoperitoneum restored. Under visual control the trocars are removed. Closure of the umbilical access incision as well as the other 10–12 mm trocar site fascia is mandatory to prevent a hernia. Use of local anaesthetics, injected at the access sides, should be considered if not done before placement of the trocars.

20.4 Intra-operative Complications

In presence of an acute cholecystitis or post-cholecystitis, fibrosis and shrinking of the gallbladder increase the chance of injury of the biliary tract and portal structures significantly. Meticulous operative technique and achieving CVS is critical in such cases. If clear identification of anatomy is impossible or IOC or IOS cannot be performed, conversion to open surgery should be considered. An alternative in high-risk patients is subtotal cholecystectomy. This procedure consists of resecting the fundus part of the gallbladder, removal of the stones and closing the remaining part of the gallbladder by suture while leaving a Foley-catheter in situ to drain any bile.

In case of bleeding from Calot's triangle, cystic plate or gallbladder bed, the first step is to tamponade the bleeding, using a swab or adequate instrument present in the operation area. In case of bleeding from the liver bed while the gallbladder has not yet been removed, the gallbladder can be used to tamponade the bleeding. Subsequently blood and cloths have to be removed, and the source of bleeding, if it is still ongoing, should be identified. Blind placement of clips or use of cautery in areas of Calot's triangle is not allowed. Use of clips or ligature should take place after visualization and identification of the bleeding structure. If the bleeding cannot get under control, conversion to open surgery should be considered. The use of cautery or use of haemostatic material to stop bleeding from the liver parenchyma or liver bed is recommended.

20.4.1 Bile Spillage and Stones Loss

To avoid infectious complications, fluid collections and abscess formation, all lost stones should be as far as possible removed without taking risks of causing complications. The operation field should be rinsed to remove debris and spilled bile. Use of Redon drain placed subhepatically should be considered to assure removal of fluids left.

20.4.2 Occurrence of Bile in Operative Field

If bile leaks from the gallbladder or from the liver bed a perforation or Luschka has to be excluded. An underlying lesion of the biliary tract has to be considered. One should try to identify the area of the bile leak. Ask for assistance of an experienced colleague, if possible. If bile appears in the area of triangle of Calot and the cystic duct can be cannulated, performing intraoperative cholangiography should be considered. Conversion only for assessment of the lesion is not recommendable. If a major lesion of the biliary tract or other portal structures is suspected or identified, repair procedure is only recommended if expertise is available (hepatobiliary surgery expert). Drainage and referring patient to a center of expertise is strongly recommended.

20.4.3 Conversion

Conversion to open surgery is not a complication but a step to safeguard best possible outcome for the patient. Main reasons for conversion are significant bleeding that cannot be controlled by laparoscopy, difficulty in visualisation, obscured/unclear anatomy, lack of progress during dissection for longer than 15–20 min. However, one should consider that in some situations conversion may not contribute to a better outcome. In such cases an alternative or a "bail-out" manoeuvre is performing a partial cholecystectomy.

References

1. Vettoretto N, Saronni C, Harbi A, Balestra L, Taglietti L, Giovanetti M. Critical view of safety during laparoscopic cholecystectomy. JSLS. 2011;15:322–5.
2. Soper NJ, Fernando Santos B. Laparoscopic cholecystectomy: complications and management. SAGES Manual Qual Outcomes Patient Saf. 2012;26:231–40.
3. Savader SJ, Lillemoe KD, Prescott CA, Winick AB, Venbrux QAC, Lund GB, et al. Laparoscopic cholecystectomy-related bile duct injuries: a health and financial disaster. Ann Surg. 1997;225:268–73.
4. Strasberg SM, Brunt LM. Rationale and use of the critical view of safety in laparoscopic cholecystectomy. J Am Coll Surg. 2010;211:132–8.
5. Gallstone disease. Dutch society of surgery. Available at: http://nvvh.artsennet.nl/richtlijnen/Bestaanderichtlijnen.htm [in Dutch]. Accessed July 2013. 2007.
6. Lee J, Miller P, Kermani R, Dao H, O'Donnell K. Gallblader damage control: comprised procedure for comprised patients. Surg Endosc. 2012;26:2779–83.
7. Jakimowicz J. Intraoperative ultrasonography in open and laparoscopic abdominal surgery: an overview. Surg Endosc. 2006;20:425–35.

Surgical Management of Ductal Calculi

21

Alessandro M. Paganini, Silvia Quaresima,
Andrea Balla, and Emanuele Lezoche

21.1 Introduction

Laparoscopic cholecystectomy (LC) is the standard treatment for patients with symptomatic gallstones and is one of the most commonly performed procedures in abdominal surgery. In patients undergoing laparoscopic cholecystectomy for symptomatic gallstones the prevalence of common bile duct (CBD) stones is between 8 and 15 % below age 60 and increases to 15–60 % in elderly patients [1]. Patients with symptomatic gallstones undergoing cholecystectomy should therefore be assessed for the presence of CBD stones and when these are confirmed they should be treated [1]. The methods for diagnosis and treatment of CBD stones are still debated.

Two-stage endo-laparoscopic management of gallstones and CBD stones (pre- or postoperative ERCP with endoscopic sphincterotomy (ES)), and laparoscopic cholecystectomy (LC), has long been standard practice for management of CBD stones, instead of traditional open choledocholithotomy and cholecystectomy. More recently, single-stage laparoscopic management of gallstones and CBD stones has been introduced. In a clinical trial set up by the EAES [2], the outcome of single-stage laparoscopic management of gallstones and CBD stones was equivalent to the two-stage approach, but with a shorter hospital stay. This finding was confirmed by a meta-analysis of randomized trials [3] comparing single-stage laparoscopic versus double-stage endolaparoscopic management, showing no advantage for pre- or post-operative ERCP/ES over laparoscopic surgery in elective patients but with a higher additional procedures' rate per patient in the endoscopic arm (Level of evidence 1a, Grade of recommendation A). The single stage laparoscopic approach was also associated with significantly less costs as compared with the two stage procedure, as demonstrated by reports from the U.S.A. [4] and from Europe [5].

21.2 Indications and Preoperative Work-Up

When evaluating a patient with symptomatic gallstones for LC, the possibility of an associated choledocholithiasis must be considered. The factors that should be evaluated include:

(a) patient factors, including the patient's eligibility criteria for LC and CBD exploration, and
(b) the predictors of bile duct stones.

21.2.1 Patient Factors

To plan the surgical procedure a series of data should be obtained. Useful information comes from the patient's history, from imaging studies and from laboratory tests.

21.2.1.1 History and Physical Examination

A good medical history provides valuable information concerning the ability of the patient to tolerate pneumoperitoneum and to rule out any bleeding disorder. A disease-specific history is also important to identify patients with previous episodes of acute cholecystitis, which may increase the risk of conversion to open surgery, as well as those at increased risk of choledocholithiasis (e.g., those who have had previous episodes of jaundice, pancreatitis, or cholangitis). Physical examination identifies patients whose body habitus, such as obesity, may make the operation more difficult and it reveals the presence of abdominal scars or incisional hernias from previous operations that may anticipate the presence of intraperitoneal adhesions.

A. M. Paganini, MD, PhD, FACS (✉) • E. Lezoche, MD, FACS
Chirurgia Generale, Specialita' Chirurgiche e Trapianti D'Organo "Paride Stefanini", Policlinico Umberto I, Rome, Italy
e-mail: alessandro.paganini@uniroma1.it

H.J. Bonjer (ed.), *Surgical Principles of Minimally Invasive Procedures*, DOI 10.1007/978-3-319-43196-3_21

21.2.1.2 Laboratory Tests

Preoperative blood tests should include liver function, renal function, electrolyte, and coagulation studies. Abnormal liver function test results, particularly alkaline phosphatase and gamma glutamyl transpeptidase levels, may be suggestive of biliary stasis from CBD stones.

21.2.1.3 Imaging Studies

Ultrasonography (US) is highly operator dependent, but in capable hands it can provide useful information. A shrunken gallbladder, a thickened gallbladder wall and peri-cholecystic fluid may be predictors of conversion to open cholecystectomy. The presence of a dilated CBD or CBD stones may predict choledocholithiasis that should be confirmed, however, either preoperatively (MRCP or EUS) or intraoperatively (fluoro-cholangiography or laparoscopic ultrasound), before their management is undertaken.

Other preoperative imaging studies of the CBD that are aimed at screening the patient for the presence of ductal stones include: (i) endoscopic retrograde cholangiopancreatography (ERCP), which should now be a purely therapeutic method, considering its morbidity; (ii) magnetic resonance cholangiopancreatography (MRCP), (iii) endoscopic ultrasonography (EUS), or CT cholangiography. MRCP and CT cholangiography have an advantage over ERCP and EUS in that they are less invasive. MRCP, however, cannot be employed in patients with metal prostheses, such as pacemakers, and in claustrophobic patients. CT cholangiography, on the other hand, cannot be employed in patients with previous known adverse reaction to iodinated contrast solutions. The frequency with which such imaging studies are obtained is usually inversely proportional to the technology and expertise for laparoscopic CBD exploration that are available in the individual center. When the technology and expertise for laparoscopic CBD exploration are lacking, a preoperative screening for ductal stones is usually performed in patients with positive predictors of choledocholithiasis (selective indication). Conversely, in centers where the technology and expertise for laparoscopic CBD exploration are present, the patient may skip preoperative screening of ductal stones altogether and proceed directly to LC with intraoperative cholangiography or laparoscopic ultrasound.

21.3 Technically Challenging Patients

The surgeon should be able to predict which patients are likely to be technically challenging. These include patients who have a particularly unsuitable body habitus from obesity, those who are likely to have multiple and dense peritoneal adhesions, and those with possible distorted anatomy in the region of the gallbladder from previous cholecystitis or pancreatitis. Morbidly obese patients present specific difficulties and necessitate higher inflation pressures to obtain adequate exposure. Patients with a history of multiple upper abdominal operations and those with a history of peritonitis may have multiple peritoneal adhesions which make access to the abdomen more risky and exposure of the gallbladder more difficult. Patients who have undergone gastroduodenal surgery, those with a history of acute cholecystitis, multiple recurrent biliary colics and severe pancreatitis may also be difficult candidates. These patients may present with dense adhesions in the region of the gallbladder, the anatomy may be distorted, the cystic duct may be foreshortened, and the CBD may be very closely and densely adherent to the gallbladder. Also the presence of a large gallbladder stone that is adherent to the walls of the infundibulum may make lateral retraction of the gallbladder difficult. These conditions are not absolute contraindications to a laparoscopic approach but the surgeon must be aware that in these cases conversion to open surgery, far from being a failure, should be considered at an early stage in the operation in the best interest of the patient. Failure to recognize this may lead to disastrous complications.

21.3.1 Predictors of Bile Duct Stones

The presence of stones in the CBD may be investigated preoperatively, intraoperatively, or postoperatively. Before elective LC, it is common practice to classify patients into one of three groups, based on the positive predictors of ductal stones:

(i) high risk group, includes patients with clinical jaundice or cholangitis and/or visible choledocholithiasis on US;
(ii) intermediate risk group, those who have hyperbilirubinemia, elevated alkaline phosphatase or gamma-GT levels, multiple small gallstones and a dilated CBD on US, and
(iii) low risk group, those with normal laboratory exams, no history of cholangitis or pancreatitis and normal sized CBD on US.

With the exception of cholangitis and/or visible ductal stones on US, which are the most reliable predictors of ductal stones, the positive predictive value of the indicators of ductal stones is low because the prevalence of choledocholithiasis, particularly in younger patients, is also low. If a policy of selective preoperative investigation of bile duct stones is followed in patients considered at high or intermediate risk of ductal stones, this may result in a 60–70 % rate of negative and therefore useless preoperative examinations, with increasing diagnostic burden for the patient, increasing duration of hospital stay and increasing costs. Moreover, both ERCP and ES carry their own risks and in patients who are candidates for LC these risks are additive with the risks of surgery.

ES is also associated with long-term morbidity. Late papillary stenosis is reported in 10–33 % of cases with recurrent stone formation and cholangitis. Increased incidence of bactibilia with chronic inflammation, of biliary hyperplasia or atypia and of bile duct cancer have been reported after ES. Therefore its use should be a matter of concern, particularly in younger patients.

Low risk patients usually do not undergo any preoperative diagnostic study and also intraoperative cholangiography is usually omitted in these patients, which results in a 2–4 % rate of unsuspected ductal stones which are left behind. In approximately two/thirds of these cases the ductal stones will not pass spontaneously through the papilla and will require ERCP/ES at a later date.

21.3.1.1 Intraoperative Screening of Common Bile Duct Stones

Intraoperative diagnosis of ductal stones with laparoscopic fluoro-cholangiography (IOC) is obtained during the same anesthesia and it does not increase the hospital stay. IOC during LC is associated with 98 % sensitivity, 94 % specificity and 100 % accuracy rates. It should be mandatory in academic centers where young surgeons are being trained and it is a useful technique for training in laparoscopic trans-cystic CBD exploration because the required cannulation maneuver is very similar. Shortly after cannulating the cystic duct, IOC provides excellent visualization of the entire biliary tree. It provides a road map of the biliary tree and the images remain for future reference. On the other hand, should an iatrogenic biliary injury have occurred, if correctly interpreted it allows the surgeon to identify it at an early stage, therefore avoiding ductal division and excision (Type III injury according to Way's classification), which continues to remain the most severe and most frequent type of biliary injury that is observed after LC.

Another interesting option for intraoperative screening of ductal stones is laparoscopic ultrasound (LUS), which is associated with 100 % PPV, 99.6 % NPV, 92.3 % sensitivity rate and 100 % specificity rate. LUS shares some of the advantages of IOC, being obtained during the same anesthesia and increasing the safety of LC, but it is strongly operator dependent. According to some authors, it is better than IOC as it is less invasive and takes less time to accomplish. The two imaging techniques are complementary one to the other, with IOC better indicated in case of uncertain biliary anatomy and when LUS is not available.

Most surgeons, however, advocate the use of selective intraoperative imaging of the biliary tree, mostly by IOC, during LC. One reason for this is to reduce the operating time. Another reason is that when ductal stones are discovered or confirmed at intraoperative imaging, most centers lack the technology, expertise and logistics that are required for intraoperative minimally invasive management of CBD stones, whether by laparoscopic or endo-laparoscopic rendez-vous techniques.

21.4 Patient Preparation

A peripheral central intravenous line is not required for laparoscopic CBD exploration. The same applies for the Foley catheter, unless a preoperative diagnosis of multiple and large CBD stones is present, and if the operation is expected to last more than 2 h. In this case a Foley catheter for the duration of the operation is indicated. A naso-gastric tube is positioned after general anesthesia is administered and it is removed before the end of the procedure.

21.4.1 Antibiotic Prophylaxis

Routine preoperative administration of antibiotics to all patients undergoing LC with ductal exploration is recommended to reduce peritoneal contamination from spillage of bile and stones into the peritoneal cavity.

21.4.2 Prophylaxis of DVT

The reverse Trendelemburg position and positive intra-abdominal pressure lead to venous pooling in the lower extremities. This may be minimized by using anti-embolic stockings and pneumatic compression devices in every patient, together with postoperative low-molecular weight heparin.

21.4.3 Patient Positioning

In the so called "North American" position, employed by the authors, the patient is supine on the operative table and the surgeon stands on the patient's left side (Fig. 21.1). The assistant holding the camera also stands on the patient's left side, to the left of the surgeon, while the second assistant stands on the patient's right side. The cart with video monitor, camera, light source, and carbon dioxide insufflator is positioned on the patient's right side at shoulder's level. A second light source and camera should be available on the same cart, together with a mixer connected to both cameras and video monitor, so as to display both the laparoscopic and the choledochoscopic images on the same screen. If a mixer is not available, then a second monitor should be positioned near the first one on the

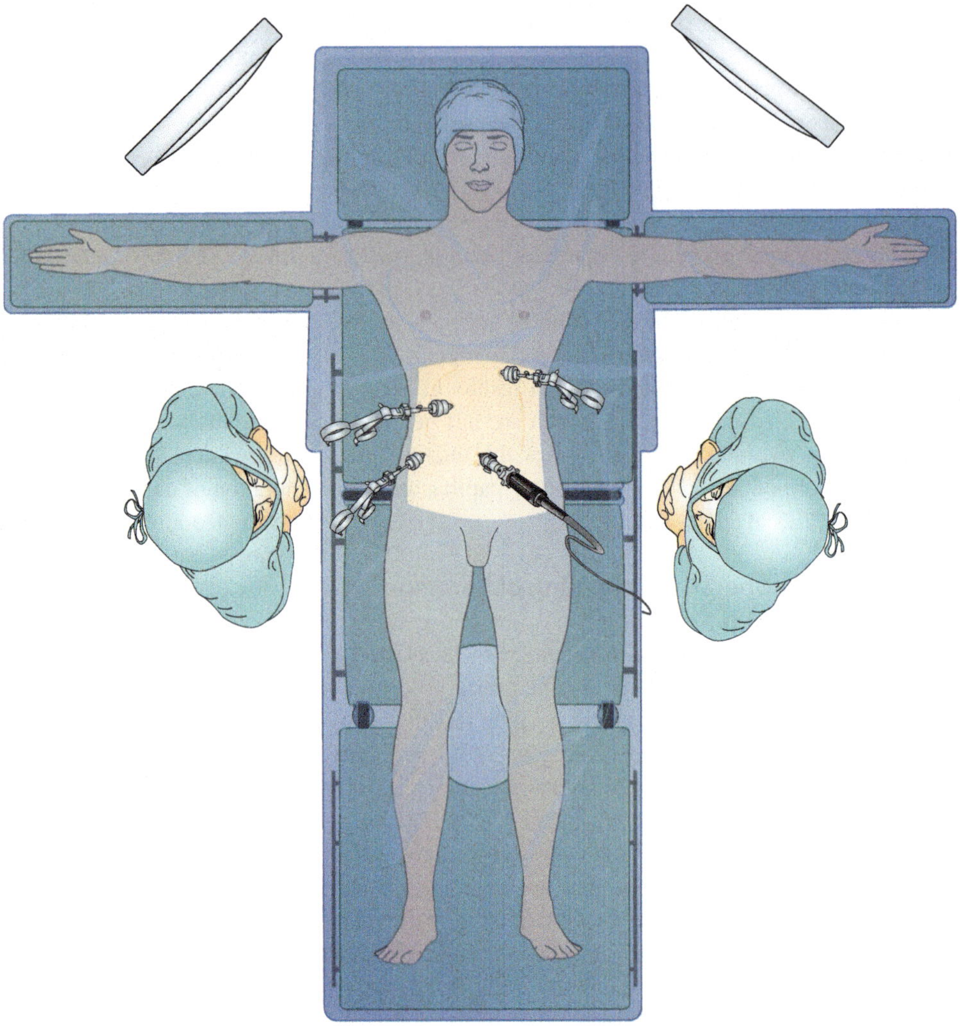

Fig. 21.1 Patient positioning for laparoscopic exploration of the common bile duct

patient's right side. It is necessary for the surgeon to have both the laparoscopic and choledochoscopic visions at the same time. If another video monitor for the second assistant is available, this should positioned on the left side of the patient's head.

Exposure is improved by tilting the operative table in reverse Trendelemburg position and rotating it with the patient's right side up. Gravity helps displacing the duodenum, colon, and omentum away from the gallbladder, increasing the working space.

21.5 Surgical Technique

After establishing supraumbilical pneumoperitoneum with open or closed technique, according to the surgeon's preference and to the presence of scars from previous abdominal operations, LC is initiated. Four trocars are usually employed (Fig. 21.2). Correct trocar position facilitates both IOC and laparoscopic CBD exploration.

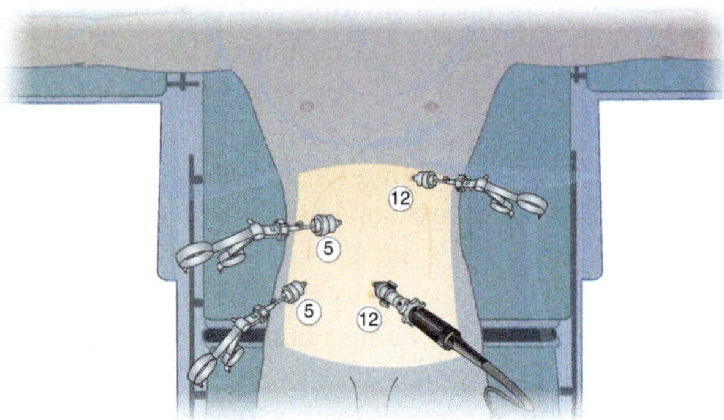

Fig. 21.2 Trocar positioning for laparoscopic exploration of the common bile duct

The first trocar (T1, 12 mm) is supra-umbilical, to accommodate an angled scope (30° or 45°) with camera. Three more trocars are then positioned under direct vision.

The second trocar (T2, 12 mm) is introduced two fingerbreadths left of the midline below the costal arch. Unlike

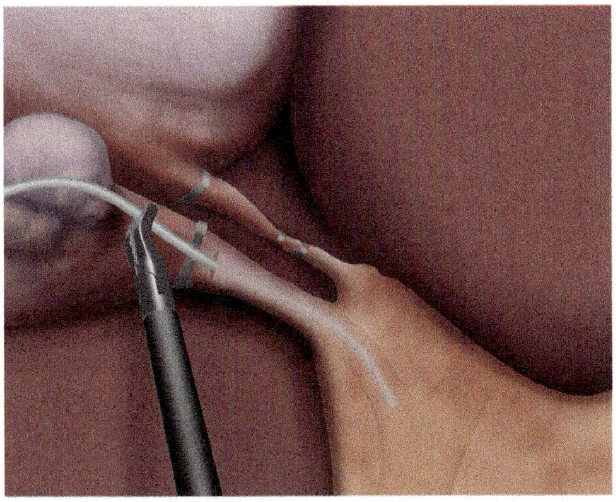

Fig. 21.3 Cholangiography catheter passed down the cystic duct into the common bile duct

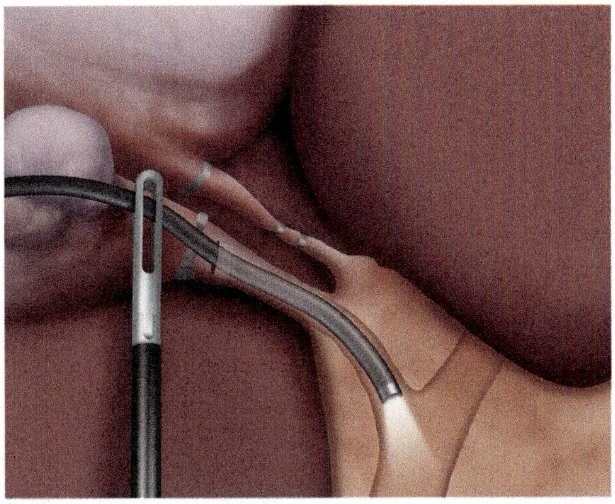

Fig. 21.4 Choledochoscope passed down the cystic duct for exploration of the common bile duct

other surgeons, who place this trocar along the midline or on the right of the midline, the authors believe the lateral shift of the epigastric trocar to the left of the midline to improve the coordination of the two operating instruments used by the surgeon, which end up to meet almost at right angles inside the peritoneal cavity. This facilitates suture of the choledochotomy, should this be required.

The third trocar (T3, 5 mm) is placed along the right anterior axillary line to provide firm cephalic traction to the fundus of the gallbladder with a grasper, so as to expose the inferior surface of the liver.

The fourth trocar (T4, 5 mm) is inserted just below the costal arch along the right midclavicular line in a position that corresponds to the cystic duct, after the grasper entering from T3 has exposed the inferior surface of the liver. This trocar position is important because after the infundibulum of the gallbladder and the cystic duct have been dissected free, the cystic duct can be aligned on the same axis of this trocar. By doing so, the cholangiography catheter may be safely pushed through the cystic ductotomy, taking advantage of the "vis-a-tergo" on the catheter itself and overcoming the resistance offered by continent Heister valves (Fig. 21.3).

As for any patient undergoing LC, the cystic duct is dissected free down to the lateral aspect of the common hepatic and common bile duct, to facilitate its cannulation with the cholangiogram catheter. The type of cholangiogram catheter that is commonly used is a 4 Fr. ureteral catheter, passed through a cholangiography clamp.

21.6 Trans-cystic or Choledochotomy?

The choice between a trans-cystic or a choledochotomy approach to explore the CBD is based on the individual patients' anatomy and ductal stones' characteristics, as shown at IOC. In general, the trans-cystic approach should be attempted first because it is less invasive as compared to a choledochotomy. A safe choledochotomy requires a CBD diameter of at least 8–10 mm and it is indicated when any of the following conditions are present: CBD stones considerably larger than the size of the cystic duct, multiple (more than 5) CBD stones; low and medial cystic duct – CBD junction; common hepatic duct stones (Fig. 21.4). In the absence of the above conditions, in the authors' opinion trans-cystic CBD exploration should be the treatment of choice.

21.6.1 Trans-cystic Approach

The grasper introduced from T3 is moved to grasp the infundibulum, to provide countertraction during the exploration maneuvers. All exploration maneuvers are performed through T4. If the size of the cystic duct is slightly smaller than the size of the CBD stone, it may be gently dilated up to a diameter of 6 mm with a balloon ureteral dilator catheter inflated with air. The CBD is first explored with a "blind basketing" technique. The cystic duct opening is entered with a flat wire stone extractor catheter which is advanced inside the CBD for 6–8 cm. When a resistance is encountered (sphincter tone), the outer sheath of the catheter is pulled backwards to open the basket. The basket is never opened by pushing it forward, to avoid trauma on the papilla or on the ductal wall. The catheter is then withdrawn from the CBD while it is being rotated along its axis, to facilitate capture of the stones by the basket. During the extraction manoeuvres, gentle external compression on the common hepatic duct is exerted with a grasper from the epigastric port to avoid stones inadvertently being swept proximal to the cystic duct into the common hepatic duct. This exploration manoeuvre is simple and it is repeated until all the stones identified at IOC have been removed. Next, a completion choledochoscopy is performed with a flexible choledochoscope or ureteroscope. When the cystic duct – CBD junction's anatomy is favourable, the choledochoscope may be directed to explore the common hepatic duct and the intrahepatic ducts. If control choledochoscopy is negative, the cystic duct may be closed with a clip as one would normally do during LC. If any stone is still present inside the CBD, it is removed under endoscopic control with a 3 Fr. flat wire basket passed through the working channel of the choledochoscope. Stones that are soft and friable may be fragmented during the exploration maneuvers with the basket. Harder stones that are impacted inside the CBD and that are difficult to mobilize with a basket, may be fragmented by electrohydraulic lithotripsy under endoscopic control. The lithotripsy fiber is passed through the working channel of the choledochoscope and its tip is placed against the stone under vision. The lithotripter is then activated, generating a spark that breaks the stone into fragments, which are subsequently removed with a basket under vision. It is important to avoid activating the lithotripter when the tip of its fibre is near the CBD wall because the spark that is generated may damage the ductal wall. Smaller stone fragments are flushed away with saline irrigation of the CBD through a trans-cystic catheter. To facilitate small fragments wash-out, the papilla itself may be gently dilated under fluoroscopic vision with a balloon ureteral dilator catheter inflated with air. Intravenous administration of 1 mg of glucagon may be associated at this time to relax the sphincter of Oddi. A completion trans-cystic fluorocholangiogram is routinely performed to check for the absence of retained CBD stones or fragments.

After completion of trans-cystic CBD exploration, the choice to position an external biliary drainage is taken according to the following indications:

1. if fibrin debris or bile sludge are still present inside the CBD at the end of the procedure;
2. if any instrumental maneuver on the papilla has been performed, such as papilla dilation or trans-papillary passage of the basket, which might be followed by papillary edema and possible cholangitis;
3. if a retained stone is demonstrated which cannot be removed laparoscopically for technical reasons.

The trans-cystic biliary drainage that is employed is derived from a 3 mm. latex T-tube after cutting away its transverse branches. One of the two ends is tapered off and a small extra hole is cut near this end. After introducing the biliary drainage completely inside the peritoneal cavity through the epigastric port, its tapered end is introduced through the cystic duct opening and is advanced by 2 cm. It is then fixed to the wall of the cystic duct with a 4/0 transfixing absorbable suture on straight needle. The suture is passed through both the cystic duct wall and the drainage wall, looping it on both sides around the cystic duct before knotting it. When a trans-cystic biliary drainage is not deemed necessary, the cystic duct is closed with clips. If the cystic duct wall is thickened by inflammation and the clip is not large enough to close it, the cystic duct may be closed with a 4/0 transfixing absorbable suture on straight needle.

21.6.2 Laparoscopic Choledochotomy

This technique was developed to treat large, multiple ductal stones. It is more challenging than the trans-cystic approach because it requires laparoscopic suturing expertise but the ductal exploration maneuver itself is easier since it is direct.

The authors prefer a transverse rather than a longitudinal choledochotomy [6]. The reason is that a transverse incision is less apt to be extended, should a larger stone be present. A short and transverse choledochotomy interrupts less ductal arterioles and its suture gives less ischemia (Fig. 21.5). If the stones are larger than the transverse choledochotomy, they are preferably fragmented with the lithotripter instead of extending the incision. On the other hand, there is a tendency to extend a longitudinal choledochotomy when large stones are present, and its suture may lead to an hourglass configuration of the CBD and subsequent risk of bile stasis. The maneuvers for direct CBD exploration follow the same steps as described for the trans-cystic duct approach. A choledochotomy approach allows one to easily explore the common hepatic duct as well, a manoeuvre that is usually more difficult to accomplish through the cystic duct.

After ductal exploration is completed as confirmed by completion choledochoscopy, the decision to place a biliary drainage is taken according to the previous indications. Biliary drainage is obtained either with a trans-cystic duct biliary drainage, according to the technique described above, or with a T-tube. Ideally, both choledochotomy and cystic duct are closed without biliary drainage.

The transverse choledochotomy is closed with one continuous suture on the left side of the T-Tube. Laparoscopic suturing with extracorporeal or intracorporeal knot-tying may be time-consuming, particularly at the beginning of the experience. A technique of continuous suture of the choledochotomy that avoids the use of knots and avoids placing metal clips in contact with the common bile duct was thus developed. The suture is an absorbable monofilament 4–0 on a straight needle. The thread carries an absorbable Poly-P-Dioxanone clip placed at 7 cm from the needle and arrested by a knot. After two or three stitches have been applied to

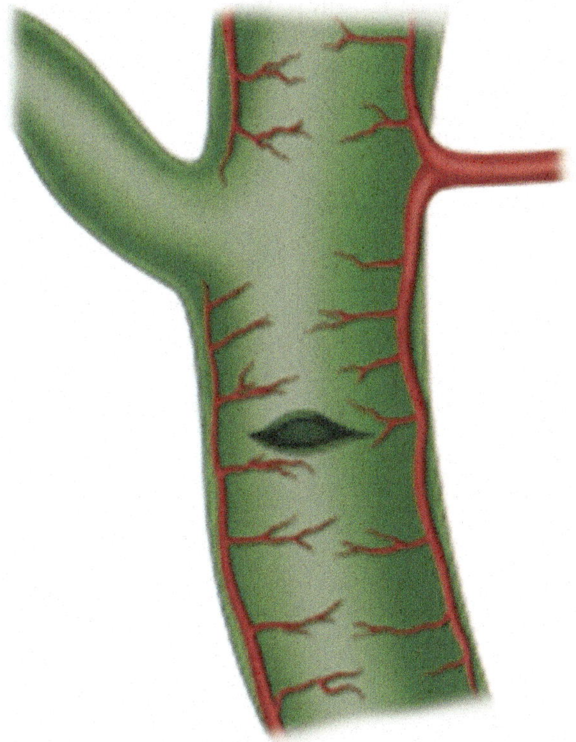

Fig. 21.5 Transverse choledochotomy for direct common bile duct exploration (*Source*: Lezoche E, Paganini AM, Guerrieri M. A new T-tube applier in laparoscopic surgery. Surgical Endoscopy 1996; 10:445–8)

approximate the edges of the choledochotomy, the suture is completed and it requires a second knot. At this point, a second absorbable clip is placed on the suture, which is kept under tension by the needle-holder.

After the suture is completed, the suture line is tested by injecting saline through the T-tube. Should leakage occur, the continuous suture may be tightened by pulling at one end and applying one more absorbable clip on the suture. A completion cholangiogram through the T-tube is taken for documentation.

If T-tube drainage is not used, the incision is closed by a continuous suture with the same technique and the completion cholangiogram is done through the cystic duct. Laparoscopic cholecystectomy is completed in the usual manner, and a drain is placed in the subhepatic space near the T-tube.

21.7 Postoperative Care

When a biliary drainage has been positioned intraoperatively, the patient undergoes a direct cholangiography on the first postoperative day. If the cholangiogram is negative and there is free flow of contrast material through the papilla, the drainage is closed, it is placed under a medication and the patient is discharged. If a residual CBD stone or stone fragment is demonstrated at postoperative cholangiography, the biliary drainage is used to flush the CBD with saline to aid in clearance of the residual stone fragment. The patient is then discharged with the biliary drainage closed and placed under a medication. The biliary drainage is removed 30 days after the operation, as a day-hospital procedure, with a direct cholangiogram prior to its removal to check again for the absence of residual stones. This time interval is required for the development of a mature sinus tract around the biliary drainage.

If a residual stone is identified prior to biliary drainage removal, the mature sinus tract allows to explore the CBD percutaneously with the 7.5 Fr. choledochoscope in the radiology suite under fluoroscopic vision and local anaesthesia. First, a soft-tip guide-wire is introduced under fluoroscopic control through the biliary drainage into the CBD and through the papilla into the duodenum. The biliary drainage is then removed leaving the guide-wire in place. Next, the guide-wire is introduced inside the working channel of the choledochoscope, which is then advanced through the sinus tract until it enters the CBD. After guide-wire removal, the residual stone is extracted with a 3 Fr. basket under choledochoscopic vision. The electrohydraulic lithotripter should be available at this time to deal with any residual stone that may be difficult to remove with a basket. When the percutaneous approach fails, or in patients with suspected residual stones in the absence of a biliary drainage, ERCP and endoscopic sphincterotomy are employed. In the occasional patient with an impacted CBD stone, extracorporeal shockwave lithotripsy (ESWL) may be employed, with ERCP and endoscopic sphincterotomy.

21.8 Follow Up

After completing the treatment plan, all patients enter a prospective follow-up protocol, which includes: interview by the same investigators, aimed at revealing the recurrence of biliary symptoms, laboratory exams and ultrasound at 6 and 12 months for the first year. If any laboratory sign of bile stasis appears, MRCP is obtained.

References

1. Scientific Committee of the European Association for Endoscopic Surgery (E.A.E.S.). Diagnosis and treatment of common bile duct stones (CBDS). Results of a consensus development conference. Surg Endosc. 1998;12(6):856–64.
2. Cuschieri A, Croce E, Faggioni A, Jakimowicz J, Lacy A, Lezoche E, Morino M, Ribeiro VM, Toouli J, Visa J, Wayand W. EAES ductal stone study. Preliminary findings of multi-center prospective randomized trial comparing two-stage vs single-stage management. Surg Endosc. 1996;10(12):1130–5.

3. Martin DJ, Vernon DR, Toouli J. Surgical versus endoscopic treatment of bile duct stones. Cochrane Database Syst Rev. 2006;(2):CD003327.
4. Urbach DR, Khajanchee YS, Jobe BA, Standage BA, Hansen PD, Swanstrom LL. Cost-effective management of common bile duct stones: a decision analysis of the use endoscopic retrograde cholangiopancreatography (ERCP), intraoperative cholangiography, and laparoscopic bile duct exploration. Surg Endosc. 2001;15(1):4–13.
5. Topal B, Vromman K, Aerts R, Verslype C, Van Steenbergen W, Penninckx F. Hospital cost categories of one-stage versus two-stage management of common bile duct stones. Surg Endosc. 2010;24(2):413–6.
6. Lezoche E, Paganini AM, Guerrieri M. A new T-tube applier in laparoscopic surgery. Surg Endosc 1996;10:445–8.

Part VIII

Pancreas

22 Laparoscopic Surgery of Pancreatic Body and Tail

Laureano Fernández-Cruz

22.1 Introduction

Distal pancreatic resection is commonly performed in patients with inflammatory pancreatic disorders for chronic pancreatitis and tumours localized in the body and tail of the pancreas. The technique, however, varies from surgeon to surgeon.

In general, distal pancreatectomy is performed en-bloc along with resection of the spleen. Most of the time, the en-bloc pancreatic-spleen resection is performed for technical reasons; it makes the operation short and easy but does not offer any special advantage for the patient. Overwhelming sepsis in patient after distal pancreatectomy and splenectomy has been reported. Kimura et al. [1] have described the technique of preserving both the splenic artery and vein. In addition, Warshaw [2] has described a technique of distal pancreatectomy in which splenic vessels are ligated both at the level of transection of the pancreas and again at the splenic hilum, leaving the spleen to survive on blood flow through the short gastric vessels. Others have described techniques whereby the pancreas is dissected off the splenic vessels completely.

In recent years, the laparoscopic approach bas been introduced with all the advantages of a minimally invasive procedure [3–5]. The primary differences between the open and laparoscopic approaches are the method of access, the method of exposure, and the extent of operative trauma. The clinical advantages of the laparoscopic approach are the reduced length of hospitalization, the reduction in postoperative pain, absence of wound related complications and faster recovery.

L. Fernández-Cruz, MD, FRCS Ed (Hon) FCRSI (Hon)
Professor of Surgery, University of Barcelona, Department of Surgery, Hospital Clinic i Provincial de Barcelona, Villarroel 170, escalera 6, 4ª planta, 08036 Barcelona, Spain
e-mail: lfcruz@clinic.ub.es; laurefcruz@gmail.com

22.2 Laparoscopic Surgery

For suspected benign lesions in the tail of the pancreas the patient is placed in the half-lateral position with the left side up (Fig. 22.1). The surgeon and assistant stand on the left side of the patient and the camera person and scrub nurse on the opposite side. However, when suspected malignant lesions or big tumors the Lloyd-Davis position of the patient is preferable and the surgeon is placed between the patient's legs.

Four 10–5 mm trocars are inserted in the abdominal wall 3–4 cm above the umbilicus, on the xiphoid area, subcostal on the midaxilary line and subcostal to the midclavicular line (Fig. 22.2.).

Pneumoperitoneum is established with CO_2. Abdominal pressure is monitored and maintained at less than 14 mmHg. A 30° scope is used. The liver is explored visually and by laparoscopic ultrasonography (7.5 MHz probe, 10 mm diameter; B-K Medical, Gentolfe, Denmark), (LapUS).

22.3 Spleen-Preserving Distal Pancreatectomy with Splenic Vessels Preservation

Step 1 The first step is to start with sectioning the splenorenal ligament and dissecting the subjacent fascia lateral to the spleen. The splenocolic ligament is divided using harmonic scalpel or the Ligasure™ device. The splenic flexure of the colon is mobilized downward. The gastrocolic omentum is widely opened up to the level of the mesenteric vessels, and the body-tail of the pancreas is then visualized. The anterior aspect of the pancreas is exposed by dividing the adhesions between the posterior surface of the stomach and the pancreas. Care must be taken to preserve the short gastric and the left gastroepiploic vessels. Careful placement of a liver retractor creates a substantial working space. A complete dissection of the superior border of the pancreas in front of the common hepatic artery allows identification of the anterior surface of the portal vein. The dissection is continued along the coeliac trunk to identify the left gastric artery and the splenic artery.

H.J. Bonjer (ed.), *Surgical Principles of Minimally Invasive Procedures*, DOI 10.1007/978-3-319-43196-3_22

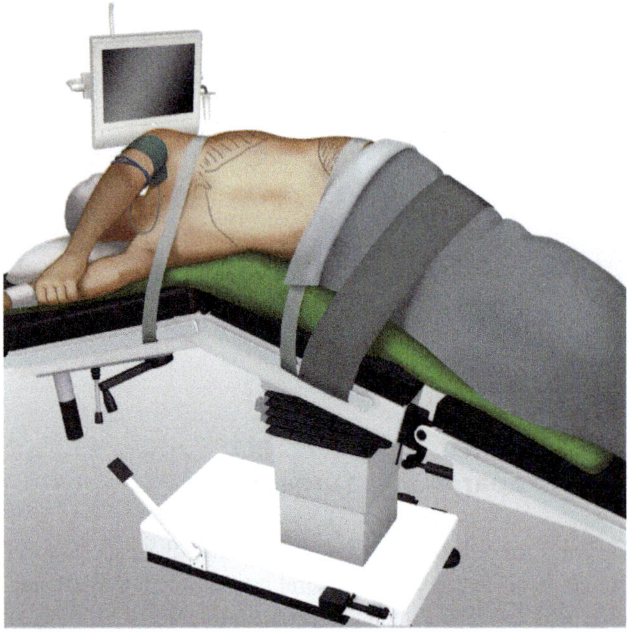

Fig. 22.1 Patient positioning for laparoscopic surgery of the body and tail of the pancreas

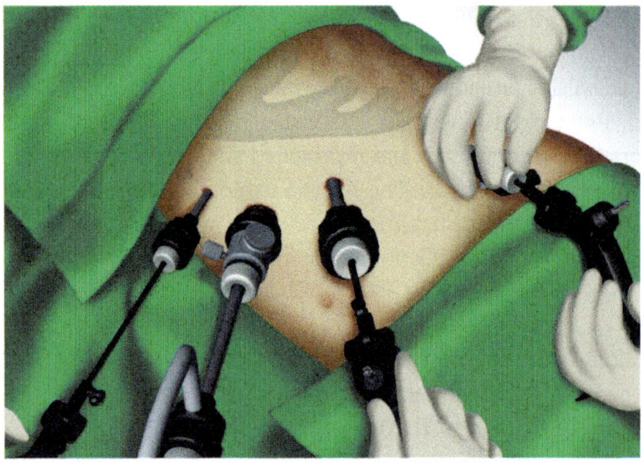

Fig. 22.2 Trocar positioning for laparoscopic surgery of the body and tail of the pancreas

Step 2 The inferior border of the pancreas is dissected and the body and tail of the pancreas are completely detached from the retroperitoneum (Fig. 22.3).

This mobilization of the left pancreas allows visualization of the posterior wall of the gland, were the splenic vein is easily identified (Fig. 22.4).

The splenic vein is pushed away from the posterior pancreatic wall with gentle blunt dissection. Visual magnification through the laparoscope permits excellent control of the small pancreatic veins, which are coagulated using the Ligasure™ device, the harmonic scalpel, or clipped with titanium clips. A tunnel is created between the splenic vein and the pancreas. The splenic artery is identified again through this space using blunt careful dissection with a curve dissector (Fig. 22.5).

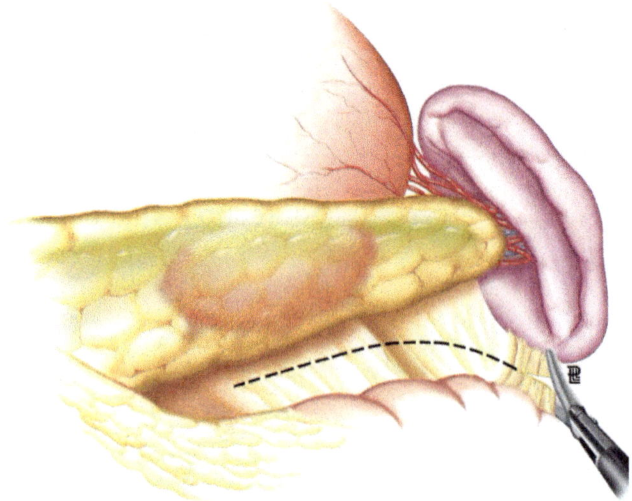

Fig. 22.3 Transecting the splenocolic ligament and opening the retroperitoneum (Reproduced with permission of Prof. Laureano Fernandez Cruz)

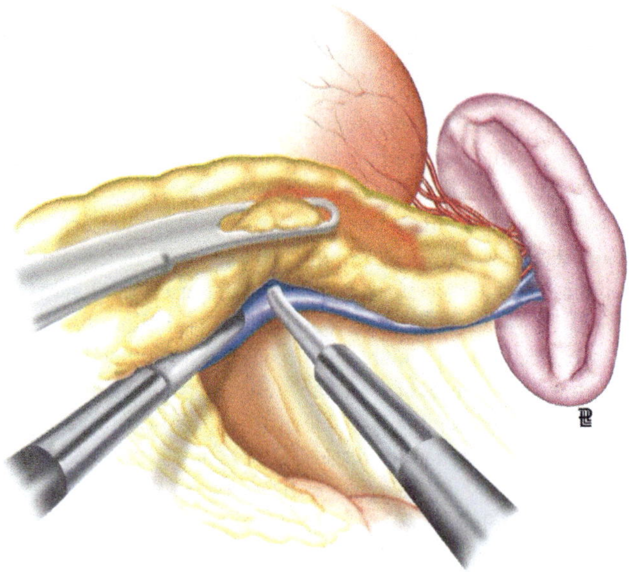

Fig. 22.4 Visualization of the posterior surface of the pancreatic body and tail (Reproduced with permission of Prof. Laureano Fernandez Cruz)

Step 3 The pancreas is then transected with a 60 mm endoscopic linear stapler (Fig. 22.6).

Step 4 The tail of the pancreas is then grasped and retracted anteriorly with a 5 mm forceps, and traction is applied to expose the small branches of the splenic artery and vein, which are coagulated using the Ligasure™ device (Fig. 22.6).

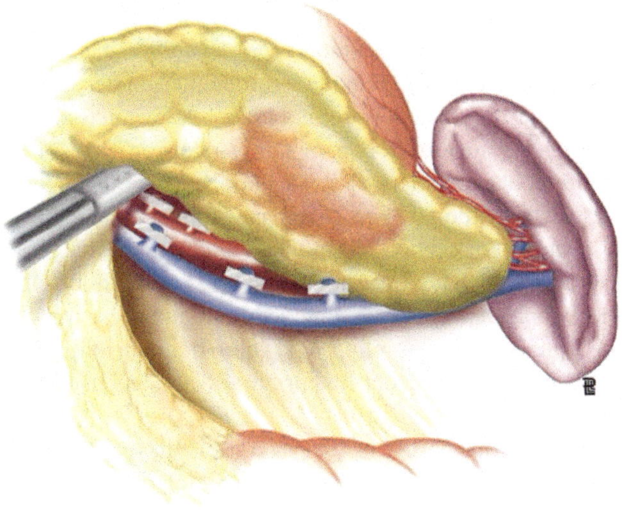

Fig. 22.5 Ligation of branches of the splenic vein and artery (Reproduced with permission of Prof. Laureano Fernandez Cruz)

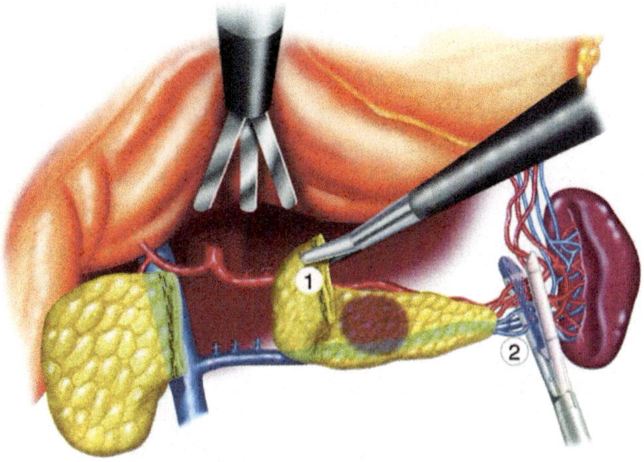

Fig. 22.6 Staple transection of the pancreas (Reproduced with permission of Prof. Laureano Fernandez Cruz) the splenic vein and exposure of the splenic artery (Reproduced with permission of Prof. Laureano Fernandez Cruz)

The dissection is continued laterally until the splenic hilum. The vascular area connecting the end of the tail of the pancreas and the spleen is transected with a 30 mm endoscopic linear stapler (EndoGIA). Another option is to expose the vessels connecting the tail of the pancreas with the splenic vessel, which are coagulated.

22.4 Spleen-Preserving Distal Pancreatectomy Without Splenic Vessels Preservation

The technique of spleen-preserving distal pancreatectomy *without splenic vessels preservation* follows the same surgical step 1 as described above (Fig. 22.7).

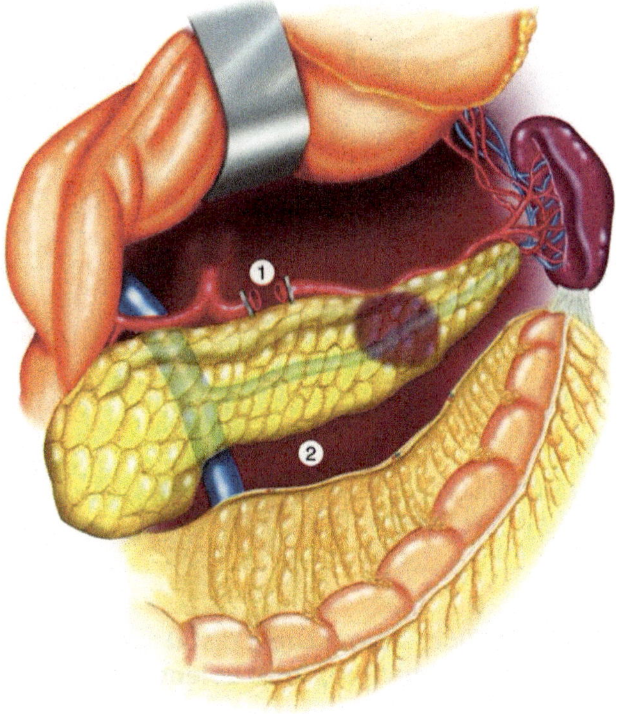

Fig. 22.7 Central transection of the splenic artery (Reproduced with permission of Prof. Laureano Fernandez Cruz)

Step 2 Lymphadenectomy in the area of common hepatic artery, celiac artery and left gastric artery. The splenic artery is clipped (7 mm titanium clips) and divided 1–2 mm from its origin of the coeliac trunk (Fig. 22.7).

Step 3 The inferior border of the pancreas is dissected and the body-tail of the pancreas is completely detached from the retroperitoneum. The mobilization of the left pancreas allows visualization of the posterior wall of the gland, where the splenic vein is easily identified. At this point, the splenic vein is divided between 7 mm clips (Fig. 22.8).

Step 4 The pancreas is then transected with a 60 mm endoscopic linear stapler (Fig. 22.8).

Step 5 The left pancreas is then lifted up and mobilized posteriorly with the splenic artery and vein. The latter are clipped and divided or transected with endoGIA as they emerge from the pancreatic tail to enter the hilum of the spleen.

Step 6 The spleen is kept vascularized solely from the short gastric vessels and the left gastroepiploic vessels (Fig. 22.8).

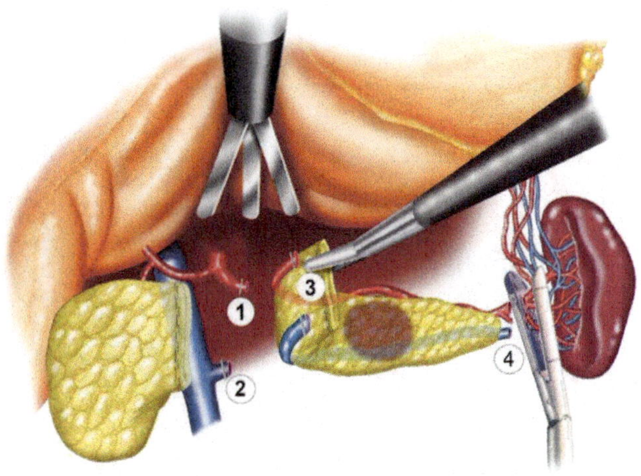

Fig. 22.8 Transection of the splenic vein (Reproduced with permission of Prof. Laureano Fernandez Cruz)

22.5 En-Bloc Laparoscopic Distal Pancreatectomy with Splenectomy

En-bloc laparoscopic distal pancreatectomy with splenectomy (Lap SxDP) is performed in patients with suspected pancreatic malignancy and in patients with ductal adenocarcinoma of the body–tail of the pancreas. The principles of this operation follow the technique described by Strasberg et al. in 2003, called radical antegrade modular pancreatosplenectomy (RAMPS) [6]. The technical details of this operation performed laparoscopically are as follows: The patient is placed in the Lloyd-Davis position with the table tilted head up. The operating surgeon stands between the patient's legs, and two assistants stand on each side of the patient. Four ports are placed: a 10 mm port in the midline above the umbilicus for the laparoscope, a 10 mm port in the left midclavicular line, 1–3 cm below the costal margin; an 11 mm port in the left mid-axillary line below the costal margin; and 11 mm port in the right midclavicular line. The first step is to divide the lienorenal ligament and dissect the adjacent fascia lateral to the spleen. The splenocolic ligament is divided using the harmonic scalpel. The splenic flexure of the colon is mobilized downward. The gastrocolic omentum is widely opened up to the level of the mesenteric vessels, and the body–tail of the pancreas is then visualized. The anterior aspect of the pancreas is exposed by dividing the adhesions between the posterior surface of the stomach and the pancreas. The omentum is opened to facilitate identification of the coeliac trunk and its branches to perform regional lymphadenectomy. Careful placement of a liver retractor creates a substantial working space. A grasping forceps is then passed behind the stomach from left to right to facilitate anterior and lateral retraction of the stomach. A large lymph node is usually present in the hepatoduodenal ligament and the hepatic artery can usually be found just cephalic to this. The common hepatic artery is then identified proximal and distal to the gastroduodenal artery; at this point, the lymph nodes are mobilized. A complete dissection of the superior border of the pancreas in front of the common hepatic artery allows identification of the anterior surface of the portal vein. This manoeuvre is usually bloodless and the dissection is continued along the coeliac trunk to identify the left gastric artery and the splenic artery. Once the lymphadenectomy is completed around these vessels, the splenic artery is clipped (7 mm titanium clips) and divided 1–2 mm from its origin of the coeliac trunk (Fig. 22.9).

The inferior border of the pancreas is dissected and the body and tail of the pancreas are completely detached from the retroperitoneum. This mobilization of the left pancreas allows visualization of the posterior wall of the gland, where the splenic vein is easily identified. At this point, the splenic vein is divided between 7 mm clips. The pancreas is then transected with a 60 mm endoscopic linear stapler. The left pancreas is then lifted up and mobilized posteriorly with the splenic artery and vein. The lymph nodes along the superior border of the body and tail are mobilized. The dissection then proceeds to expose the anterior surface of the superior mesenteric artery; in this area, the lymph nodes, fat, and fibrous tissue are taken. The dissection is continued posteriorly and the inferior attachments of

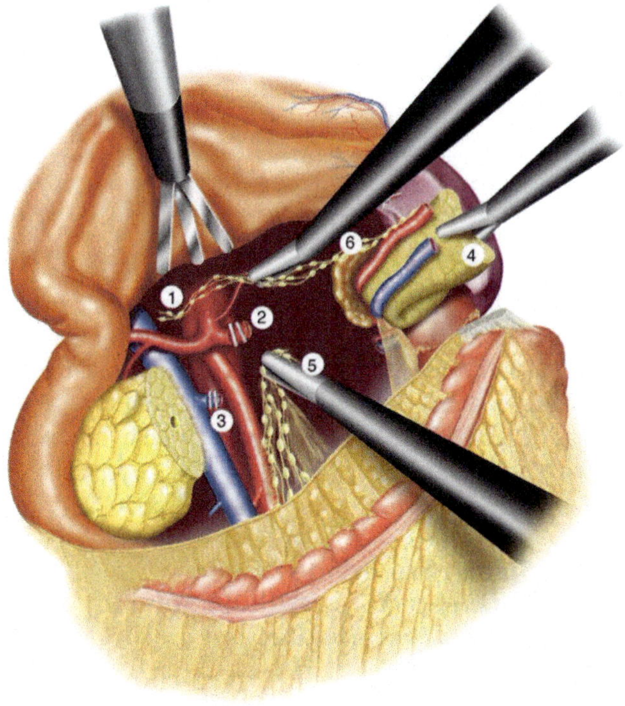

Fig. 22.9 En-bloc distal pancreatectomy with splenectomy (Reproduced with permission of Prof. Laureano Fernandez Cruz)

Table 22.1 Laparoscopic pancreatic resection: technical options

	Presumed benign lesions	Suspected or malignant lesions
Position of the patient	Half-lateral with the left side up	Lloyd Davis
Surgeon	On the left side of the patient	Between the patient's legs
Surgical Steps		
1	Division of splenocolic ligament Splenic flexure of the colon is mobilized downward Gastrocolic omentum is widely opened	
2	Inferior border of the pancreas dissected Body and tail of the pancreas completely detached from the retroperitoneum	
3	The splenic vein is visualized and clipped	Identification of celiac trunk and its branches
4	The pancreas is transected. The left pancreas is retracted anteriorly and traction is applied to expose the splenic artery	Lymphadenectomy in the areas of common hepatic artery, celiac artery and left gastric artery
5	The splenic artery is clipped at its origin	The splenic artery is clipped at its origin
6	Preservation of the short gastric vessels	The neck of the pancreas is transected
7	Transection in the area between the tail of the pancreas and the hilum of the spleen	The splenic vein is clipped at its junction with the mesenteric vein
8	Preservation of the spleen	Lymphadenectomy on the superior border of the pancreas
9		Lymphadenectomy along the superior mesenteric artery
10		Fatty tissue, lymph nodes and nerves are removed between the posterior wall of the pancreas and the adrenal gland and left kidney. Adrenalectomy when there is adrenal invasion
11		The Gerota's fascia attached to the lateral border of the pancreas is removed
12		The short gastric vessels are coagulated and divided
13		Pancreatosplenectomy

the pancreas are divided. The inferior border of the pancreas is dissected including Gerota's fascia on the superior surface of the kidney. This dissection is continued anterior to the adrenal gland which is resected if invaded by tumor. When pancreatosplenectomy is indicated, division of the lienorenal ligament and division of the short gastric vessels are the last step in the procedure. Table 22.1 describes the surgical steps using the laparoscopic approach for presumed benign lesions and for suspected or overt malignant lesions.

22.6 Enucleation

Laparoscopic enucleation of pancreatic lesions is usually performed for neuroendocrine tumors or benign cystic tumors assuming do not communicate with the pancreatic duct. Bleeding tends to be minimal, there is no reconstruction required and enucleation is associated with low morbidity and mortality.

The use of intraoperative laparoscopic ultrasonography is an integral part of the laparoscopic procedure. After the pancreatic tissue is opened at the appropriate site the tumor is enucleated taking care not to damage the pancreatic duct (Fig. 22.10).

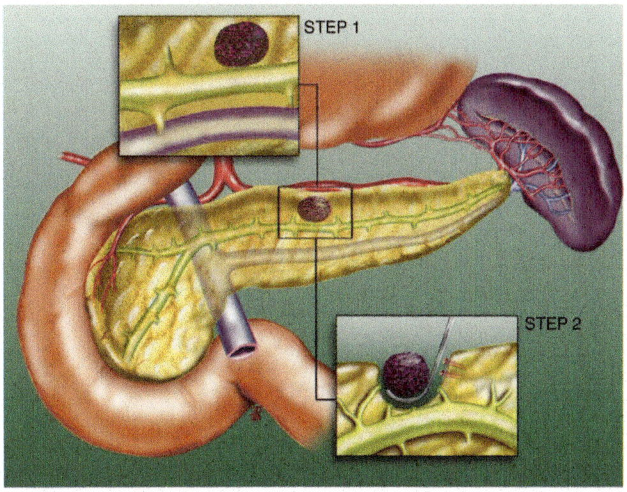

Fig. 22.10 Enucleation of neuro-endocrine pancreatic tumours (Reproduced with permission of Prof. Laureano Fernandez Cruz)

References

1. Kimura W, Inone T, Futawake N, Shiukai H, Han I, Muto T. Spleen preserving distal pancreatectomy with conservation of the splenic artery and vein. Surgery. 1996;120:885–90.
2. Warshaw AL. Conservation of the spleen with distal pancreatectomy. Arch Surg. 1988;123:550–3.

3. Fernández-Cruz L, Martínez I, Gilabert R, Cesar-Borges G, Astudillo E, Navarro S. Laparoscopic distal pancreatectomy combined with preservation of the spleen for cystic neoplasms of the páncreas. J Gastrointest Surg. 2004;8:493–501.
4. Mabrut JY, Fernández-Cruz L, Azagra JS, Bassi C, Delvaux G, Weerts J, Fabre JM, Boulez J, BaulieuxPeix JL, Gigot JF. Laparoscopic pancreatic resection: results of a multicenter European study of 127 patients. Surgery. 2005;137:597–605.
5. Fernández-Cruz L, Cosa R, Blanco L, Levi S, López-Boado MA, Navarro S. Curative laparoscopic resection for pancreatic neoplasms: a critical analysis from a single institution. J Gastrointest Surg. 2007;11:1607–22.
6. Strasberg SM, Drebin JA, Linehan D. Radical antegrade modular pancreatosplenectomy. Surgery. 2003;133:521–7.

23 Laparoscopic Pancreaticoduodenectomy

Igor E. Khatkov, Victor V. Tsvirkun, Roman E. Izrailov, and Pavel S. Tyutyunnik

23.1 Introduction

Laparoscopic pancreaticoduodenectomy has been recently adopted as a minimally invasive procedure in pancreatic surgery. The first laparoscopic pancreaticoduodenectomy was performed by Gagner and Pomp in 1992 [1]. According to current data laparoscopic pancreaticoduodenectomy is still technically challenging but it seems to be effective for patients with pancreatic head and periampullary cancer with all the benefits of minimally invasive surgery [2–6]. Probably because of its technical difficulties laparoscopic pancreaticoduodenectomy is routinely performed by few surgical centers in the world. The technique of laparoscopic pancreaticoduodenectomy is not standardized and as a result the initial learning curve may be difficult.

23.2 Patient Selection

Laparoscopic pancreaticoduodenectomy is performed for a variety of malignant and benign diseases of the pancreas. Still today, surgery is the most effective treatment for the pancreatic head cancer, cancer of lower common bile duct and peri-ampullary cancer.

Criteria for performing laparoscopic pancreaticoduodenectomy are well established and are the same as for open pancreaticoduodenectomy.

Patients with meromorphic type of constitution with a lower common bile duct tumor with a size between 2 and 3 cm are the most appropriate candidates for the first laparoscopic pancreaticoduodenectomy. Increasing surgical experience will lead to widening of the indications. Laparoscopic resection of portal or mesenteric vein is now technically feasible and safe in experienced centers.

If a surgeon has experience in performing major laparoscopic procedures in general and pancreatic surgery, it is possible to start any case by laparoscopic approach. Intraoperatively, after laparoscopic assessment of the tumor by inspection and mobilization, the surgical team needs to decide whether to continue laparoscopically or to convert to open surgery.

General cancer principles in surgery should not be compromised while using the laparoscopic approach to performing laparoscopic pancreaticoduodenectomy. Extended lymphadenectomy does not have any influence on long-term survival but is valuable for more accurate staging and prognosis.

23.3 Operating Room Set Up

The patients is placed with both legs in stirrups to allow the primary surgeon to stand between the legs and the first and second assistant to the left and right side of the patient. The positioning of the patient is shown in Fig. 23.1.

Usually the first trocar is placed right under the umbilicus. If the distance between xiphoid process (XP) and umbilicus is short (less than half the length of the laparoscopic instrument), the first trocar should be placed 2–3 cm lower than the umbilicus. After diagnostic laparoscopy, additional trocars are inserted as shown in Fig. 23.2.

The following instruments are used: three fenestrated bowel graspers, Maryland dissector, short right angle dissec-

I.E. Khatkov, MD, PhD
Director, Moscow Clinical Scientific Center,
Shosse Entuziastov, 86, 111123, Moscow, Russia

Head of Surgical Department, Moscow State University of Medicine and Dentistry, Ulitsa Delegatskaya, 20-1,127473 Moscow, Russia

V.V. Tsvirkun, MD, PhD
Moscow Clinical Scientific Center,
Shosse Entuziastov, 86, 111123 Moscow, Russia

R.E. Izrailov, MD, PhD • P.S. Tyutyunnik, MD (✉)
Moscow Clinical Scientific Center,
Shosse Entuziastov, 86, 111123 Moscow, Russia

Moscow State University of Medicine and Dentistry,
Ulitsa Delegatskaya, 20-1, 127473 Moscow, Russia
e-mail: tiutiunnikk@gmail.com

H.J. Bonjer (ed.), *Surgical Principles of Minimally Invasive Procedures*, DOI 10.1007/978-3-319-43196-3_23

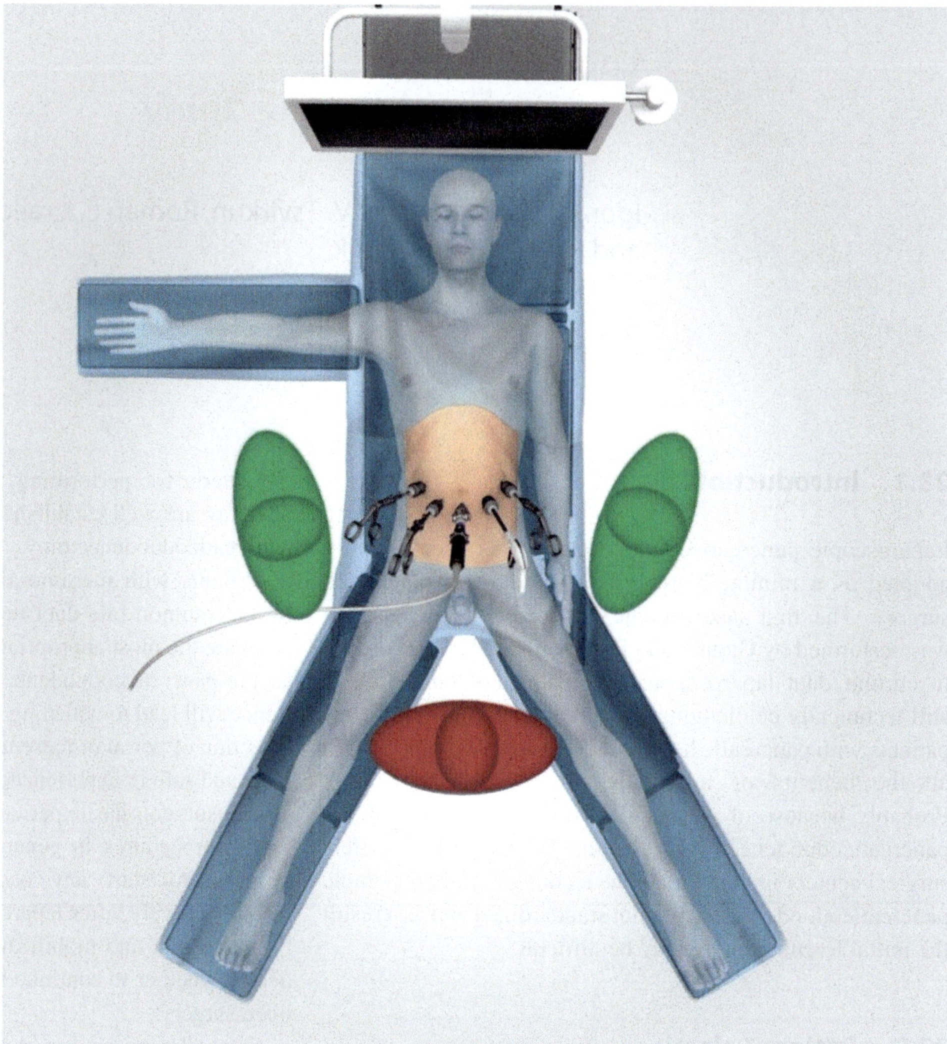

Fig. 23.1 Positioning of the patient

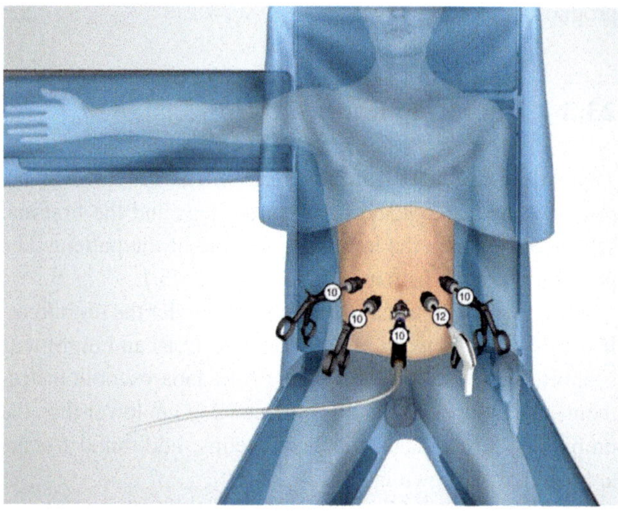

Fig. 23.2 Trocar positioning for laparoscopic pancreaticoduodenectomy

tor, firm grasper, curved needle driver, ultrasonic dissector (Harmonic Scalpel®), pair of scissors, Goldfinger (Ethicon EndoSurgery®), straight needle for liver fixation, suction and irrigation device, clip applier and endobag. A 30° optics is employed.

A straight needle is inserted just next to the xyphoid. The liver is lifted and secured in an up right position to the abdominal wall by 1–0 suture by means of a straight needle.

The *first* surgical step is dividing the gastrocolic ligament. The gastrocolic ligament is kept stretched with fenestrated graspers and divided in a cranio-caudal fashion from the short gastric vessels down to the pylorus using an harmonic scalpel. In this way the right gastroepiploic artery and vein are divided separately using the harmonic scalpel after double clipping. Lymphadenectomy of group number 4 and 6 lymph nodes according to the Japanese Gastric Cancer (JGCC) is consequently performed.

The *second* step involves dissection along the lower edge of the pancreas and identification of the superior mesenteric vein (SMV). The second assistant tilts the stomach and the

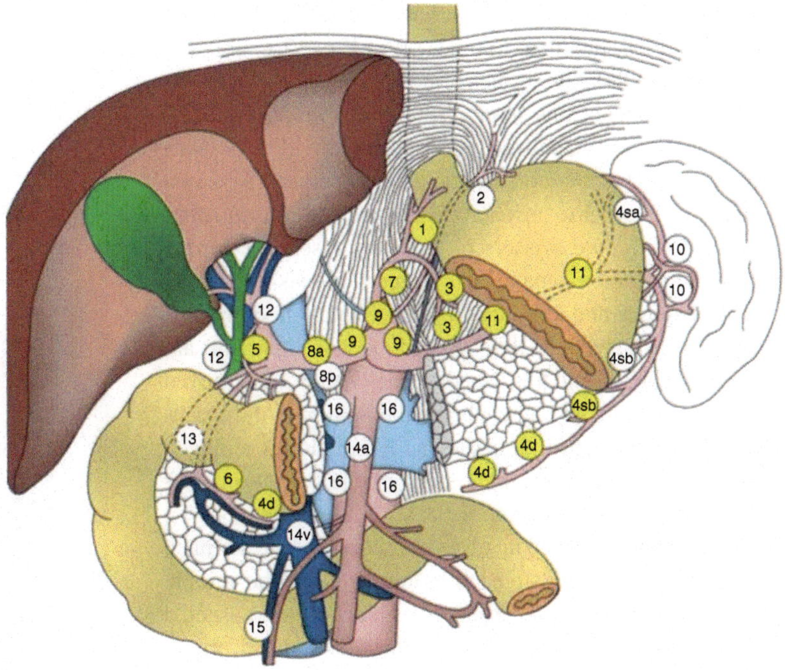

Fig. 23.3 Regional lymph nodes pancreas (*Source*: Perspectives in the treatment of gastric cancer Dimitrios H Roukos and Angelos M Kappas *Nature Clinical Practice Oncology* (2005) 2, 98–107)

peritoneum is opened along the lower edge of the pancreas. The incision begins at the proximal part of the pancreatic tail up to the head of the pancreas. After dissection at the level of the middle colic vein, the Superior Mesenteric Vein (SMV) is identified. Lymphadenectomy of number 14 lymph nodes is performed (Fig. 23.3).

If possible (no adhesion or tumor infiltration) the initial steps of tunneling the neck of the pancreas from the SMV and PV are performed. If any difficulties are encountered, it will be better to first perform the Kocher maneuver.

The *third* surgical step is the Kocher maneuver which is performed as deeply as possible. This maneuver starts with division of the peritoneum 1 cm lateral to the descending part of the duodenum. The first assistant pulls the duodenum to the right by a fenestrated grasper whereas the second assistant pushes the right colon with fat tissue in the opposite direction. Lymphadenectomy of lymph nodes number 13a and 13b is then performed. The dissection is performed by the surgeon with an harmonic scalpel. An incision on the upper part of duodenum's peritoneum is carried out on the right side of the hepatoduodenal ligament up to the liver. Lymphadenectomy of lymph nodes number 12c and 12 b1 is performed. When the mobilization of the pancreaticoduodenal complex reaches the lower horizontal part of the duodenum, the second assistant pushes the duodenum to the left whereas the first assistant pushes the transverse mesocolon down. The dissection of the lower part of the duodenum is carried out when the most distal part of the duodenum is mobilized during the transection of the ligament of Treitz. Lymphadenectomy of lymph nodes 13a and 13 b is then performed at this stage of the operation.

Mobilization of the uncinate process becomes possible after the last two steps of Kocher maneuver. The mobilization is started from the deepest part of the lower horizontal part of the duodenum toward the end of the incision of the peritoneum of the lower edge of the pancreas. The surgeon has to be very gentle and precise. He has to clip carefully and transect the short veins of the uncinate process. Uncontrolled dissection at this point may cause bleeding that is quite difficult to stop.

The *fourth* surgical step is inter-aorto-caval lymphadenectomy. The anterior wall of the inferior vena cava (IVC), the left renal vein and the anterior wall of the aorta are clearly visible after Kocher maneuver. Fat tissue with lymphatic nodes in the aorto-caval space is dissected at the level of the uncinate process up to the left renal vein. (lymph nodes no.16$b_{1)}$. The anterior and left lateral wall of the aorta are clearly visible. The prevertebral fascia is a posterior edge of the lymphadenectomy in this region.

Inter-aorto-caval lymphadenectomy is still one of the controversial points of discussion in the treatment of pancreatic and periampullary cancer. Nevertheless, the inter-aorto-caval lymphadenectomy is reasonable because it is safe and provides better staging.

Dissection of the hepatoduodenal ligament and cholecystectomy is the *fifth* surgical step of pancreaticoduodenectomy. The operation proceeds to the hepatoduodenal ligament. It starts with dividing the lesser omentum (from the left to the right) along the lower margin of the left lobe of the liver and initial mobilization of the gallbladder. It is easier to find the left hepatic artery and dissect it in the proximal direction up to the proper hepatic artery. Then, using the harmonic scalpel, all the fat tissue with lymph nodes of the hepatoduodenal ligament (no.$12a_1$,$12a_2$,$12b_2$,$12p_2$ are dissected). The gallbladder is then removed (pulled down by the second assistant) at this stage of the operation. The gastroduodenal artery is visualized, dissected and divided between double clips. The common hepatic duct is occluded by a vascular clamp in order to prevent bile leakage and consequently transected with cold scissors in order to preserve a normal wall of the common hepatic duct for anastomosis.

The posterior and left fatty tissue and lymph node groups no $12p_1$,12h 12p1f of the hepatoduodenal ligament are removed to the left and transected. Partially, they are removed separately from the specimen, being the right part of the hepatoduodenal ligament's fat tissue and lymph nodes removed with the specimen at the final stage of the operation after portal vein (PV) mobilization.

The *sixth* surgical step involves transection of the stomach or the duodenum. The stomach is transected in the middle third using a linear stapler. Sometimes it could be transected during lymphadenectomy along the hepatoduodenal artery. It allows lymphadenectomy performed more easily.

During the laparoscopic pylorus preserving PD, the transection of the duodenum is performed not less than 2 cm below the pylorus in order to preserve its function. It is important to do that in the direction from the greater to the lesser curvature of the stomach, because it provides the most appropriate situation for the duodenojejunostomy (DJA).

Transection of the jejunum is the *seventh* surgical step. The deep Kocher maneuver in the lower part of the duodenum is finished by mobilization of the horizontal part of the duodenum. At that moment the surgeon pulls the duodenum forward and up with the left hand. The first assistant pushes the superior mesenteric vein with the surrounding fat tissue back, down and left. The surgeon, using an harmonic scalpel with the right hand, dissects the distal part of the duodenum free. Dissection under the transverse mesocolon is completed with transection of ligament of Treitz. With the help of the second assistant the jejunum is pulled into the upper part of the abdominal cavity. The mesentery of the jejunum is transected near the wall of the jejunum using the harmonic scalpel 10–15 cm distally of Treitz and the jejunum is transected by the linear stapler (45 mm). The transection of the mesentery of the jejunum is continued proximally up to the uncinate process and the superior mesenteric vein. At this stage, if possible, it is useful to see the superior mesenteric artery right below the superior mesenteric vein by pulling the complex strongly forward and to the left (Fig. 23.4). But, if it is difficult for some reason, it could be done later.

The *eighth* surgical step is transection of the pancreas. The final tunneling is performed by blind and sharp dissection using the harmonic scalpel. The pancreas is transected by means of harmonic scalpel. It is important to transect pancreatic duct by cold scissors in order to provide an adequate passage of the pancreatic juice later. The distal part of the pancreas is mobilized 3 cm and covered by cotton wool in

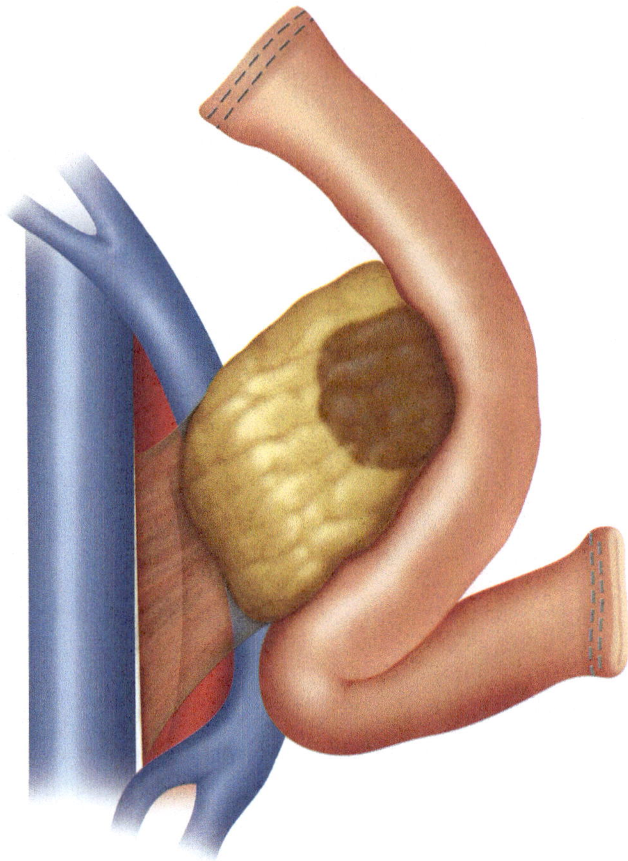

Fig. 23.4 Exposure of the uncinated process and the superior mesenteric vein

order to prevent the pancreatic juice leaking into the abdominal cavity.

Final mobilization is the *ninth* step pancreaticoduodenectomy. The specimen is pulled to the right. At this moment the dissection continues towards to the superior mesenteric vein and portal vein, dissecting and clipping all short vessels to the uncinate process. Pulling the specimen forward, up and right (by the surgeon and the second assistant) and pushing the superior mesenteric vein to the left (by the first assistant). In the majority of cases, it is possible to visualize the superior mesenteric artery just below the superior mesenteric vein (Fig. 23.4). Sometimes it is necessary to push the whole specimen to the left side of the patient and pull it to the left together with the superior mesenteric vein in order to perform the dissection along the superior mesenteric artery.

Sometimes the wall of the aorta has to be visualized and fat tissue along the wall of the superior mesenteric artery has to be dissected. To perform safe dissection without any bleeding requires dissection close to the wall of the artery using the harmonic scalpel. With the dissection along the superior mesenteric vein and the superior mesenteric artery, the mobilization part of the procedure is finished.

The *tenth* surgical step is resection of the superior mesenteric vein. If the tumor infiltrates the portal vein, it is possible to mobilize the specimen complex without damaging the vein. If portal vein invasion has taken place, it would be possible to perform resection of the portal vein. The resection might be a wedge or circular. In such cases, the whole specimen is mobilized as usual, and after this the portal vein, superior mesenteric vein and splenic vein are mobilized and controlled by vascular clamps. If the invasion is localized, a partial wedge resection might be carried out and the opening of the vein will be sutured using 4.0 Prolene®. When it is necessary to perform a circular resection of the infiltrated part of the vein, this will be done using cold scissors. If there is no tension, an end-to-end anastomosis by 4.0 Prolene can be performed. A vascular graft may be used for a patient with extended resection of the vein. The choice of the graft depends on the diameter of the portal vein or superior mesenteric vein. The saphenous vein or an artificial graft are both appropriate for such a case. The circular vascular anastomosis could be carried out with running suture by 4.0 Prolene®.

Reconstruction follows the ten surgical steps to dissect and resect the pancreatic head. Obviously, dissection and resection are the most difficult and challenging part of pancreaticoduodenectomy particularly when a large tumor invading the superior mesenteric vein is present. Reconstruction is a more straightforward and standardized stage of laparoscopic pancreaticoduodenecomy but the quality of reconstruction will influence the postoperative morbidity and mortality.

All anastomosis are performed on one jejunum loop using intracorporeal suturing. For this reconstruction, the surgeon works through the trocars on either side of the optics.

For the *pancreatojejunostomy,* we use in all cases a single layer end-to-side dunking anastomosis with interrupted sutures. About 20–30 cm of the jejunum loop is carried up through the supramesocolic compartment and duodenal bed to the upper part of abdominal cavity. It is necessary to control the jejunum mesentery's position in order avoid any torsion. The pancreaticojejunostomy is done with 2.0 or 3.0 nonabsorbable multifilament material. The pancreatic stump is stitched from the anterior to the posterior surface 2–2.5 cm from the cut edge and 0.7–1 cm from the inferior part. The jejunum loop is stitched 4–6 cm distal from the stump in the middle of the posterior semicircle. The double knot is tied with the help of both assistants. The first assistant holds the pancreatic stump and carries out light traction of the stump to the front. The second assistant pushes the jejunum loop as close as possible to the pancreas. At the same, time the surgeon ties the knot onto the jejunum wall rather than on the pancreas. All the other posterior sutures are performed by stitching the pancreatic stump along its surface 2 cm distal to the cut edge. All the sutures should be quite superficial in order not to damage the main pancreatic duct. The distance between sutures is about 1 cm. The last suture of the posterior wall is performed the same way as the very first one. Using an harmonic scalpel the incision of the jejunum is performed along the pancreatic edge, 1 cm from the row of sutures. The length of the incision should be 1 cm less than the diameter of the pancreatic stump (Fig. 23.5).

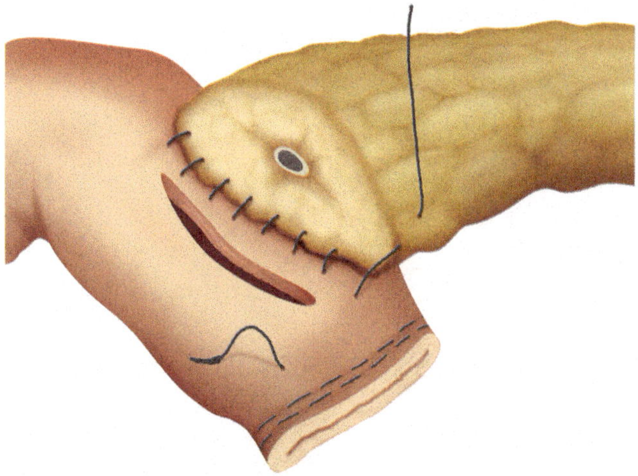

Fig. 23.5 Pancreaticojejunostomy

The anterior row is performed in the same manner as the posterior one (parallel to the posterior row of the pancreas). It is better to make the upper and the lower sutures one after another (an upper at first, after that lower one and finally 2–3 stitches between). While the surgeon is inserting the stitch, the first assistant pushes the pancreatic stump inside the jejunum.

The *hepaticojejunostomy* is performed by two running semicircular sutures with 4.0 monofilament. If the common bile duct is narrow (less than 5 mm), it should be performed by interrupted sutures. The incision of the jejunum wall is performed 10–15 cm distal from the pancreaticojejunostomy using the harmonic scalpel. The length of the incision should be equal to the diameter of the common bile duct. The first stitch is performed at 9 o'clock. The free end of the filament (without a needle) should be about 3 cm long to enable the second assistant to hold it and push towards the patient's right shoulder and elevate the liver at the same time (Fig. 23.6).

The first assistant pulls the jejunum in the opposite direction so the line of anastomosis becomes parallel to the axis of the needle driver. The surgeon stitches the back layer of anastomosis with a running suture 2 mm apart. A knot is tied at 3 o'clock in order to prevent the stricture of the hepaticojejunostomy. The front row of the hepaticojejunostomy is performed by the same filament and is finished at 9 o'clock by tying a knot with the free end of the first stitch.

The *gastrojejunostomy or duodenojejunostomy* is the next reconstructive step. In both options the jejunum loop is pulled up in antecolic position and an anastomosis is performed 30–40 cm below the hepaticojejunostomy.

For a *gastrojejunostomy,* the jejunum loop is fixed to the lowest part of the gastric stump on the greater curvature by

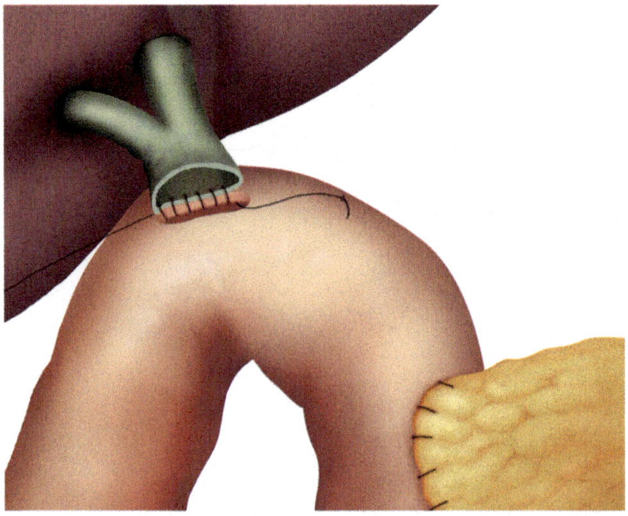

Fig. 23.6 Hepaticojejunostomy

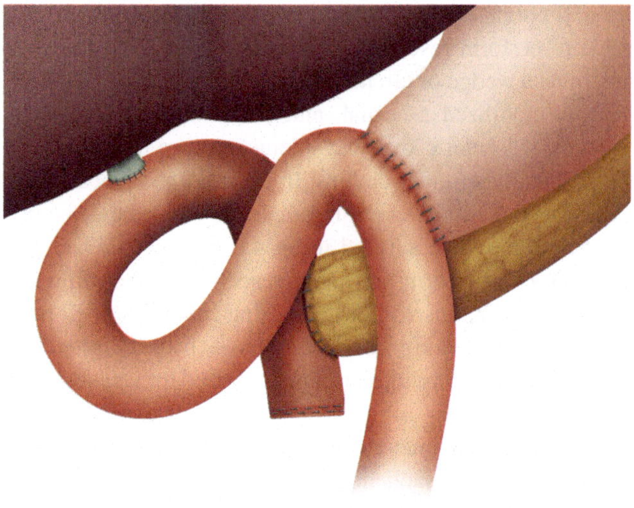

Fig. 23.7 Completed reconstruction after pancreaticoduodenectomy

one stitch. The incisions in the stomach and jejunum are performed by monopolar cautery hook, the stapler is inserted: one branch in the stomach next to the greater curve and another in the jejunal loop. The 45 mm blue cartridge is used. The fixation knot is cut off after that and the common incision aperture is sutured from the lower part in the upper direction by one row running absorbable filament material.

For a *duodenojejunostomy,* an end-to-side anastomosis is performed by hand made two row suture. It is not possible to use stapler suture in order to preserve the pylorus. The first row is performed through the stapled layer of the duodenum and jejunum wall parallel to its mesentery by running suture. The duodenum and jejunum walls are opened in a longitudinal direction by monopolar cautery hook. Accordingly, the internal row of the anastomosis is performed by the same running suture and the external row is finished by seromucosal running sutures. The final situation after reconstruction is depicted in Fig. 23.7.

At the end of the operation, the abdominal cavity is examined for any damage or bleeding and any fluid is evacuated. Two drains (in the pancreaticojejunostomy and hepaticojejunostomy areas) are inserted through ports 4 and 5. The greater omentum is pulled up to cover the pancreaticojejunostomy so that the gastrojejunostomy or duodenojejunostomy are not in direct contact with the pancreaticojejunostomy.

The greater omentum is fixed in this position by 2–3 clips. It can be done to prevent delayed gastric emptying postoperatively. The endobag with specimen complex is removed through the widened (3–5 cm) umbilical incision. The wounds are closed.

Conclusion

Laparoscopic pancreaticoduodenectomy is a difficult but feasible and safe procedure. Laparoscopic approach provides good exposure of the operative field to all members of the surgical team and permits a more precise and safer operation. It allows the surgeon to perform lymphadenectomy following all the principles of cancer surgery. The essential criteria for success are to have a motivated team of professionals with experience in pancreatic surgery and major laparoscopic procedures.

References

1. Gagner M, Pomp A. Laparoscopic pylorus-preserving pancreatoduodenectomy. Surg Endosc. 1994;8:408–10.
2. Kendrick ML, Cusati D. Total laparoscopic pancreaticoduodenectomy: feasibility and outcome in an early experience. Arch Surg. 2010;145:19–23.
3. Palanivelu C, Rajan PS, Rangarajan M, Vaithiswaran V, Senthilnathan P, Parthasarathi R, et al. Evolution in techniques of laparoscopic pancreaticoduodenectomy: a decade long experience from a tertiary center. J Hepatobiliary Pancreat Surg. 2009;16:731–40.
4. Zureikat AH, Breaux JA, Steel JL, Steven J. Hughes can laparoscopic pancreaticoduodenectomy be safely implemented? J Gastrointest Surg. 2011;15:1151–7.
5. Kim SC, Song KB, Jung YS, Kim YH, Park DH, Lee SS, Seo DW, Lee SK, Kim MH, Park KM, Lee YJ. Short-term clinical outcomes for 100 consecutive cases of laparoscopic pylorus-preserving pancreatoduodenectomy: improvement with surgical experience. Surg Endosc. 2013;27:95–103.
6. Boggi U, Amorese G, Vistoli F, Caniglia F, De Lio N, Perrone V, Barbarello L, Belluomini M, Signori S, Mosca F. Laparoscopic pancreaticoduodenectomy: a systematic literature review. Surg Endosc. 2014;15.

24 Treatment of Severe Complicated Pancreatitis

Alfred Cuschieri

24.1 Introduction and Pathogenesis

Whilst in the majority of patients, acute pancreatitis is a self-limiting disease, in 15–20 % of patients a severe necrotising pancreatic/peri-pancreatic process develops accompanied by a systemic inflammatory response characterised by an activated cytokine cascade and including a destructive exaggerated leukocyte tissue response, resulting in a life-threatening disorder with a reported mortality exceeding 20 % [1]. There are two subtypes of the necrotizing severe disease: (i) early severe acute pancreatitis (ESAP) defined as presence of organ failure on admission or soon after and accounts for 30 % of patients and (ii) late or delayed severe acute pancreatitis. The main factor predisposing to ESAP is extensive pancreatic necrosis (odds ratio, 3.8) and in practice, ESAP more frequently requires necrosectomy and carries an overall higher mortality than the delayed onset severe disease [2]. There are different serum markers used as indices of severe pancreatitis: interleukin-1β, interleukin-6, interleukin-18, s-ICAM, C-reactive protein, anti-proteases, trypsinogen activation peptide (TAP), carboxypeptidase B activation peptide (CAPAP), PMN-elastase and activated complement factors.

Bacterial infection of pancreatic necrosis is the most frequent local complication and is associated with the development of systemic complications which are responsible for the majority of deaths [3, 4]. Organ failure is more frequent in patients with infected necrosis and in those with extensive pancreatic necrosis. The aetiology of the pancreatitis influences the microbiology of infected pancreatic necrosis and cultures are more often positive in biliary than alcoholic disease (74 % vs. 32 %). Gram-positive bacteria predominate in alcoholic pancreatitis whereas Gram-negative bacteria account for the majority of infections in severe biliary pancreatitis. Candida infection of the pancreatic necrosis is a major problem and is associated with a poor prognosis [5]. Recent clinical studies have confirmed that gut permeability is increased in patients with severe acute pancreatitis (impaired gut barrier function) with increased risk of bacterial/endotoxin translocation from the gut to the systemic circulation [6]. The early use of antibiotics and continuous regional arterial infusion of protease inhibitor has been proposed in order to reduce the mortality [7–13]. The best available guidelines for the management of severe acute pancreatitis are those proposed by the Japanese in 2009 (see Table 24.1 – reference [14]).

24.1.1 Treatment Options

Although necrosectomy is traditionally performed by laparotomy [15–18], in the last 5–10 years minimal access and radiologically-guided approaches [19–23] are increasingly used and the growing number of published reports indicates that they reduce morbidity (bleeding and intestinal injuries) and improve survival significantly. The retroperitoneal approach (RPA) allows direct and complete removal of necrotic infected tissues and is currently popular [17, 24], but the author's experience is with the operation of infracolic pancreatic necrosectomy [25, 26] with continuous irrigation and drainage of the lesser sac with the Beger's technique (reference [16]). This procedure is described fully in this chapter. It is also used to drain infected pseudocysts via a cysto-jenunostomy.

24.2 Indications for Surgical Treatment and Treatment Options

Treatment of sterile necrosis should be conservative in the first instance and should include systemic high dose antibiotic (elaborate). However, persistent organ failure that does not respond to therapy in the presence of extensive pancreatic

A. Cuschieri, MD, ChM, FMed Sci, FRCS, FACS, FIBiol
Department of Surgery and Molecular Oncology, Ninewells Hospital and Medical School, Dundee, Scotland, UK
e-mail: a.cuschieri@dundee.ac.uk

H.J. Bonjer (ed.), *Surgical Principles of Minimally Invasive Procedures*, DOI 10.1007/978-3-319-43196-3_24

Table 24.1 Evidence-based Japanese (JPN) guidelines for the surgical management of acute pancreatitis, excluding gallstone pancreatitis

1. Computed tomography-guided or ultrasound-guided fine-needle aspiration for bacteriology should be performed in patients suspected of having infected pancreatic necrosis;
2. Infected pancreatic necrosis accompanied by signs of sepsis is an indication for surgical intervention;
3. Patients with sterile pancreatic necrosis should be managed conservatively, and surgical intervention should be performed only in selected cases, such as those with persistent organ complications or severe clinical deterioration despite maximum intensive care;
4. Early surgical intervention is not recommended for necrotizing pancreatitis;
5. Necrosectomy is recommended as the surgical procedure for infected pancreatic necrosis;
6. Simple drainage should be avoided after necrosectomy, and either continuous closed lavage or open drainage should be performed;
7. Surgical or percutaneous drainage should be performed for pancreatic abscess;
8. Pancreatic abscesses for which clinical findings are not improved by percutaneous drainage should be subjected to surgical drainage immediately;
9. Pancreatic pseudocysts that produce symptoms and complications or the diameter of which increases should be drained percutaneously or endoscopically; and
10. Pancreatic pseudocysts that do not tend to improve in response to percutaneous drainage or endoscopic drainage should be managed surgically.
11. Computed tomography-guided or ultrasound-guided fine-needle aspiration for bacteriology should be performed in patients suspected of having infected pancreatic necrosis;
12. Infected pancreatic necrosis accompanied by signs of sepsis is an indication for surgical intervention;
13. Patients with sterile pancreatic necrosis should be managed conservatively, and surgical intervention should be performed only in selected cases, such as those with persistent organ complications or severe clinical deterioration despite maximum intensive care;
14. Early surgical intervention is not recommended for necrotizing pancreatitis;
15. Necrosectomy is recommended as the surgical procedure for infected pancreatic necrosis;
16. Simple drainage should be avoided after necrosectomy, and either continuous closed lavage or open drainage should be performed;
17. Surgical or percutaneous drainage should be performed for pancreatic abscess;
18. Pancreatic abscesses for which clinical findings are not improved by percutaneous drainage should be subjected to surgical drainage immediately;
19. Pancreatic pseudocysts that produce symptoms and complications or the diameter of which increases should be drained percutaneously or endoscopically; and
20. Pancreatic pseudocysts that do not tend to improve in response to percutaneous drainage or endoscopic drainage should be managed surgically.

necrosis (>50%) even if this is not infected is an indication for necrosectomy. Infected pancreatic necrosis diagnosed by radiologically fine needle aspiration of the necrotic area for bacteriology (FNAB) constitutes an absolute indication for necrosectomy.

24.3 Preoperative Work-Up

Patients with established pancreatic necrosis require serial contrast enhanced computed tomography or preferably MRI and if infection is suspected, FNAB is essential. In some centres ultrasound is used for procurement of FNAB. MRI is increasingly preferred to contrast-enhanced CT as serial imaging is usually needed in the individual patient and this creates radiation risks with CT. There are still unresolved issues in the management of severe pancreatic necrosis, including antibiotic prophylaxis, indications for and frequency of repeat imaging and FNAB, and the role of enteral feeding. However a recent Cochrane review reported that early antibiotic prophylaxis reduces the risk of infection of pancreatic necrosis.

24.4 Laparoscoic Infracolic Necrosectomy

The technique of laparoscopic necrosectomy was first undertaken in Dundee in 1998. It reproduces the classical open necrosectomy to date has been accompanied by reduced morbidity and a significant increase in survival rate (90%). It may be carried out totally laparoscopically, or through the hand-assisted laparoscopic approach.

Special Instruments The procedure is greatly facilitated by 30° forward oblique laparoscope, curved co-axial instruments and flexible ports, prehensile grasper for atraumatic gasping of the transverse colon and good pulsed irrigation system.

Position of Patient and Ports The patient is placed in the supine position with the surgeon and camera person on the right side of the patient and the assistant and scrub nurse on the opposite side (Fig. 24.1).

Following induction of capnoperitoneum, the 11.0 mm optical port is inserted through the umbilicus and a 10 mm 30° forward oblique laparoscope is introduced. Two flexible instruments ports (for use with curved coaxial instrument)

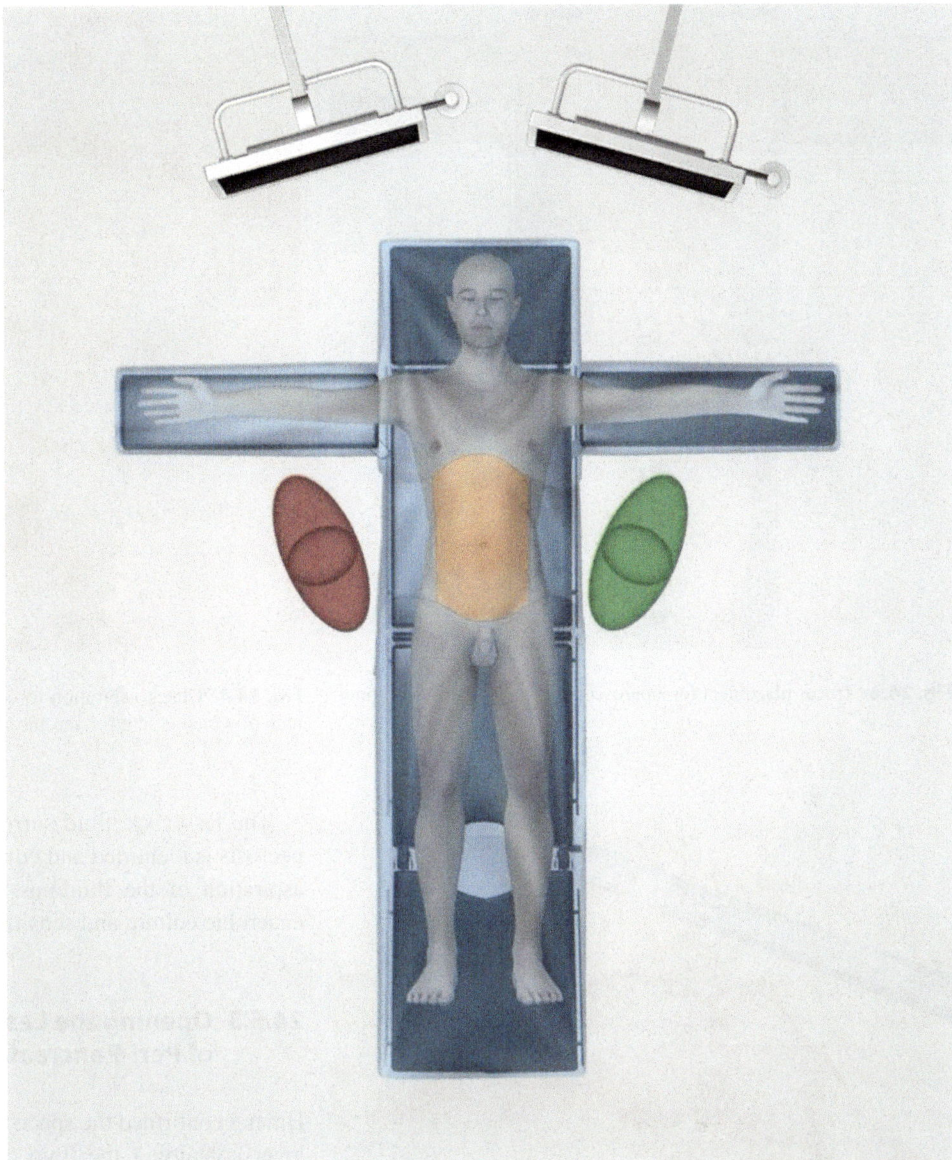

Fig. 24.1 Patient positioning for laparoscopic infracolic necrosectomy

are then placed on each side of the laparoscope. These serve as the instrument ports for the surgeon (Fig. 24.2).

The curved coaxial instruments (Storz, Tuttlingen, Germany) greatly facilitate the manipulations particularly when the lesser sac is entered, but the procedure can be carried out with straight laparoscopic instruments.

24.5 Steps of the Laparoscopic Infracolic Necrosectomy

24.5.1 Elevation of Transverse Colon

This initial step provides the necessary infracolic exposure of the lesser sac. The greater omentum is lifted upwards by two atraumatic graspers of intestinal clamps until the transverse colon is exposed behind it. This may require initial division of adhesions binding the greater omentum to loops of the small intestine.

The exposed transverse colon is then grasped by a prehensile articulating grasper (Storz, Tuttlingen, Germany) or large atraumatic intestinal clamp and elevated upwards to expose the inferior surface of the transverse mesocolon and hold it stretched over the bulging lesser lessee sac and contents behind it. At this stage the patient is tilted slightly head-down to improve the exposure. The advantage of the prehensile grasper is that it allows 'ring holding' of the transverse colon and hence reduces the risk of damage to the bowel.

The transverse mesocolon is the rolled over to enhance the tense bulge in the lesser sac containing the pancreatic necrosis and peri-pancreatic fluid which becomes clearly visible at its lower margin as a 'blue line' stretching horizontally up to the duodeno-jejunal junction/ligament of Treitz (Fig. 24.3).

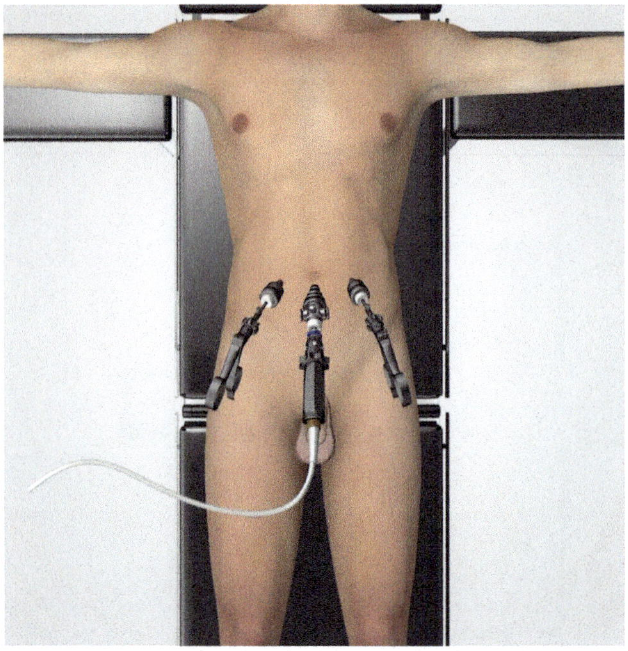

Fig. 24.2 Trocar placement for laparoscopic infracolic necrosectomy

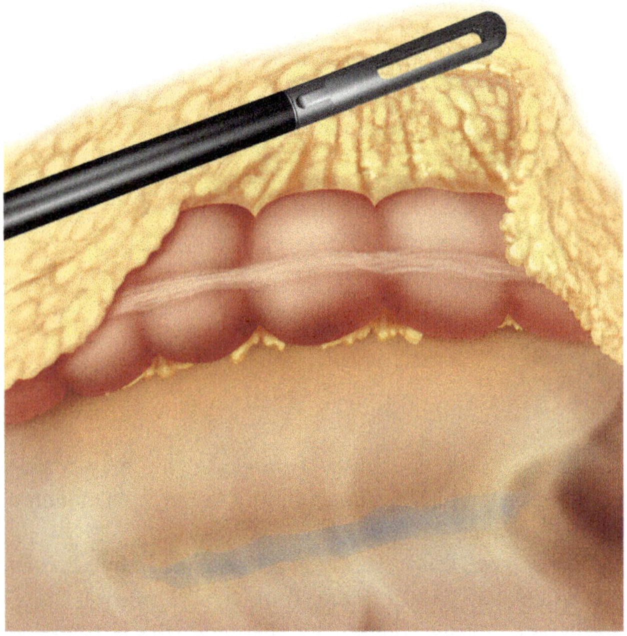

Fig. 24.3 The blue line on the inferior aspect of the root of the transverse mesocolon is an indicator of dark peri-pancreatic fluid in the lesser sac and confirms pancreatic necrosis

24.5.2 Division of the Peritoneum of the Inferior Leaf of the Transverse Colon

The peritoneum at the base of the inferior leaf of the transverse mesocolon to the left of the middle colic vessels and over the bulging lesser sac is coagulated and divided along the blue line by curved scissors to expose the bulging 'fascia' encasing the pancreatic sequestrum and peri-pancreatic fluid.

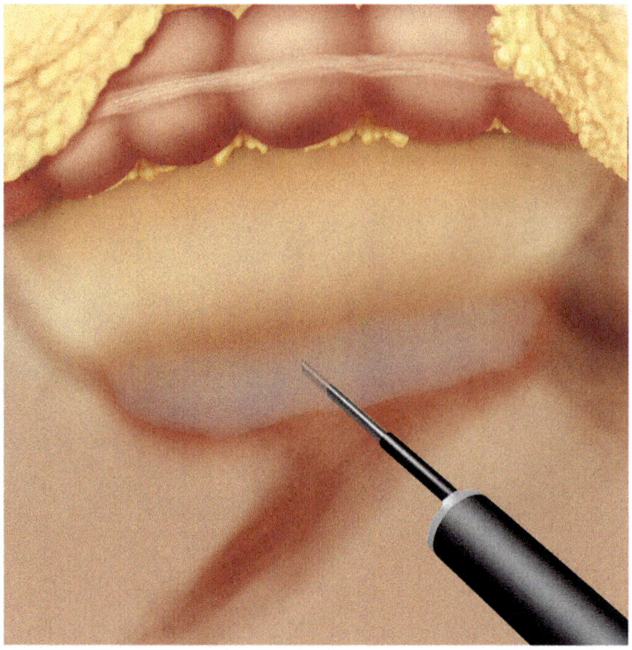

Fig. 24.4 Check aspiration to confirm peri-pancreatic fluid, a specimen of which is sent for aerobic and anaerobic culture

The lesser sac fluid surrounding the pancreatic infected necrosis is identified and confirmed by needle puncture with aspiration of the fluid/pus which is sent for aerobic and anaerobic culture and sensitivity (Fig. 24.4).

24.5.3 Opening the Lesser Sac and Aspiration of Peri-Pancreatic Space

Having confirmed the space by needle aspiration, the fibrous layer containing the fluid and the necrosed pancreas and peripancreatic fat is divided by scissors just enough to enable the insertion of the sucker into the lesser sac. This is used to aspirate and wash the closed lesser sac before it is opened further for the necrosectomy. This repeated aspiration and irrigation by at least 1.0 l of saline of the closed lesser sac is very important for reducing the risk of significant bacterial contamination of the peritoneal cavity.

Thereafter, the opening in the lesser sac is sac is extended (Fig. 24.5) to provide sufficient access for the necrosectomy, taking care to avoid damage to the middle colic vessels.

24.5.4 Necrosectomy

The visually-guided necrosectomy is carried by a combination of 'pulsed pressure' irrigation, suction and piecemeal removal of the necrotic segments using non-crushing/non-tooth graspers or intestinal clamp. The co-axial curved Babcocks and intestinal claps instruments are ideally suited for insertion into the lesser sac and grasping the pancreatic slough.

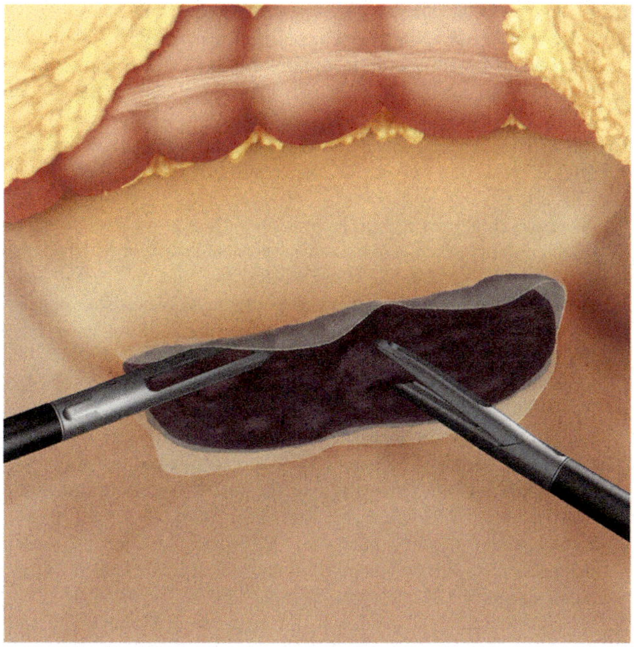

Fig. 24.5 Widening the opening in the mesocolon providing access to the lesser sac

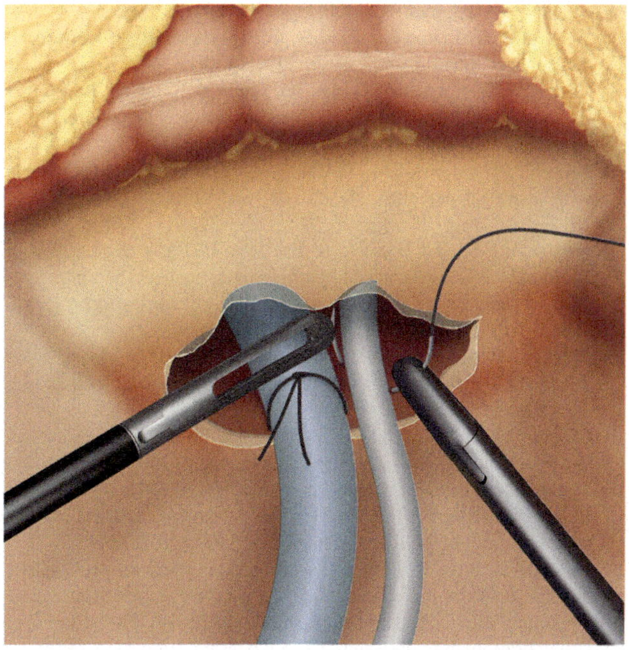

Fig. 24.6 Suture fixation of the drains to prevent dislodgement after the operation

The irrigation is used both to clean the cavity and to dislodge the necrotic pancreatic tissue. Only the loose or loosened necrotic pancreatic slough is grasped and removed. The necrosectomy entails piecemeal removal of all the loose sequestrum provided there is no bleeding when the necrosectomy is stopped. Adherent slough must not be removed forcibly, i.e., only picking and gentle detachment is allowed. Once the necrosectomy is completed, the cavity is given a final saline wash and inspected by the laparoscope.

24.5.5 Evacuation of the Pancreatic Slough

The necrotic segments may be removed piecemeal each time a fragment is picked up. However, to reduce instrument traffic it is better to place them all in a water and rip-proof bag, which is exteriorised at the end of the operation through the wound made to introduce the large port in the left flank. Apart from anything else, this saves on operating time, and probably reduces contamination.

24.5.6 Insertion of Drains for Closed Irrigation of the Lesser Sac

This is a crucial step. Large silicon (10 mm) inflow and outflow drains are inserted through separate stab wounds and their internal ends guided inside the lesser sac. Both drains are secured to the edges of the opening in the fibrous capsule by absorbable sutures to prevent dislodgement from the lesser sac into the peritoneal cavity (Fig. 24.6). They are also fixed to the exit site by skin sutures.

These drains should lie side by side or on top of each other. They are used for postoperative hypertonic crystalloid irrigation of the lesser sac. For this reason, the irrigation system should be checked by injecting saline through the inflow drain. Once the necrosectomy cavity has filled fluid, the turbid effluent should return via the outflow drain.

The transverse colon and greater omentum are then released and placed gently on top of the drains and the root of the small bowel mesentery.

All the port wounds are irrigated with antibiotic solution (gentamycin) prior to closure.

24.5.7 Postoperative Management

The patients are nursed in HDU or ICU (depending on need for respiratory support) after surgery. The irrigation of the lesser sac (2 l per 24 h) with hyperosmolar dialysate solution is continued until the returning fluid is clear of necrotic bits, usually 7–10 days. Antibiotic therapy (imipenem) is maintained for 7 days.

References

1. Isenmann R, Rau B, Beger HG. Early severe acute pancreatitis: characteristics of a new subgroup. Pancreas. 2001;22(3):274–8.
2. Gloor B, Muller CA, Worni M, Martignoni ME, Uhl W, Buchler MW. Late mortality in patients with severe acute pancreatitis. Br J Surg. 2001;88(7):975–9.
3. Raty S, Sand J, Nordback I. Difference in microbes contaminating pancreatic necrosis in biliary and alcoholic pancreatitis. Int J Pancreatol. 1998;24(3):187–91.

4. Buchler MW, Gloor B, Muller CA, Friess H, Seiler CA, Uhl W. Acute necrotizing pancreatitis: treatment strategy according to the status of infection. Ann Surg. 2000;232(5):627–9.
5. Gotzinger P, Wamser P, Barlan M, Sautner T, Jakesz R, Fugger R. Candida infection of local necrosis in severe acute pancreatitis is associated with increased mortality. Shock. 2000;14(3):320–3.
6. Juvonen PO, Alhava EM, Takala JA. Gut permeability in patients with acute pancreatitis. Scand J Gastroenterol. 2000;35(12): 1314–8.
7. Nordback I, Sand J, Saaristo R, Paajanen H. Early treatment with antibiotics reduces the need for surgery in acute necrotizing pancreatitis--a single-center randomized study. J Gastrointest Surg. 2001;5(2):113–8.
8. Slavin J, Neoptolemos JP. Antibiotic prophylaxis in severe acute pancreatitis--what are the facts? Langenbecks Arch Surg. 2001;386(2):155–9.
9. Gloor B, Schmidt O, Uhl W, Buchler MW. Prophylactic antibiotics and pancreatic necrosis. Curr Gastroenterol Rep. 2001;3(2):109–14.
10. Shrikhande S, Friess H, Issenegger C, Martignoni ME, Yong H, Gloor B, Yeates R, Kleeff J, Buchler MW. Fluconazole penetration into the pancreas. Antimicrob Agents Chemother. 2000;44(9):2569–71.
11. Villatoro E, Bassi C, Larvin M. Antibiotic therapy for prophylaxis against infection of pancreatic necrosis in acute pancreatitis. Cochrane Rev. Prepared and maintained by The Cochrane Collaboration and published in The Cochrane Library. 2009; Issue 1. http://www.thecochranelibrary.com.
12. Matsukawa H, Hara A, Ito T, Fukui K, Sato K, Ichikawa M, Yoshioka M, Seki H, Takeda K, Sunamura M, Shibuya K, Kobari M, Matsuno S. Role of early continuous regional arterial infusion of protease inhibitor and antibiotic in nonsurgical treatment of acute necrotizing pancreatitis. Digestion. 1999;60 Suppl 1:9–13.
13. Takeda K, Matsuno S, Ogawa M, Watanabe S, Atomi Y. Continuous regional arterial infusion (CRAI) therapy reduces the mortality rate of acute necrotizing pancreatitis: results of a cooperative survey in Japan. J Hepatobiliary Pancreat Surg. 2001;8(3):216–20.
14. Isaji S, Takada T, Kawarada Y, et al. JPN Guidelines for the management of acute pancreatitis: surgical management. J Hepatobiliary Pancreat Surg. 2006;13(1):48–55. doi:10.1007/s00534-005-1051-7. PMCID: PMC2779397.
15. Lankisch PG, Struckmann K, Assmus C, Lehnick D, Maisonneuve P, Lowenfels AB. Do we need a computed tomography examination in all patients with acute pancreatitis within 72 h after admission to hospital for the detection of pancreatic necrosis? Scand J Gastroenterol. 2001;36(4):432–6.
16. Beger HG, Rau B, Isenmann R. Necrosectomy or anatomically guided resection in acute pancreatitis. Chirurg. 2000;71(3): 274–80.
17. Nakasaki H, Tajima T, Fujii K, Makuuchi H. A surgical treatment of infected pancreatic necrosis: retroperitoneal laparotomy. Dig Surg. 1999;16:506–11. doi:10.1159/000018777.
18. Wyncoll DL. The management of severe acute necrotising pancreatitis: an evidence-based on review of the literature. Intensive Care Med. 1999;25(2):146–56.
19. Gouzi JL, Bloom E, Julio C, Labbe F, Sans N, el Rassi Z, Carrere N, Pradere B. Percutaneous drainage of infected pancreatic necrosis: an alternative to Surgery. Chirurgie. 1999;124(1):31–7.
20. Carter CR, McKay CJ, Imrie CW. Percutaneous necrosectomy and sinus tract endoscopy in the management of infected pancreatic necrosis: an initial experience. Ann Surg. 2000;232(2):175–80.
21. Kam A, Young N, Markson G, Wong KP, Brancatisano R. Case report: inappropriate use of percutaneous drainage in the management of pancreatic necrosis. Gastroenterol Hepatol. 1999;14(7):699–704.
22. Oria A, Ocampo C, Zandalazini H, Chiappetta L, Moran C. Internal drainage of giant acute pseudocysts: the role of video-assisted pancreatic necrosectomy. Arch Surg. 2000;135(2):136–40.
23. Horvath KD, Kao LS, Wherry KL, Pellegrini CA, Sinanan MN. A technique for laparoscopic-assisted percutaneous drainage of infected pancreatic necrosis and pancreatic abscess. Surg Endosc. 2001;15(10):1221–5.
24. Castellanos G, Serrano A, Pinero A, Bru M, Parraga M, Marin P, Parrilla P. Retroperitoneoscopy in the management of drained infected pancreatic necrosis. Gastrointest Endosc. 2001;53(4): 514–5.
25. Cuschieri SA, Jakimowicz JJ, Stultiens G. Laparoscopic infracolic approach for complications of acute pancreatitis. Semin Laparosc Surg. 1998;5(3):189–94.
26. Hamad GG, Broderick TJ. Laparoscopic pancreatic necrosectomy. J Laparoendosc Adv Surg Tech A. 2000;10(2):115–8.

Part IX

Spleen

25 Laparoscopic Surgery of the Spleen

Eduardo M. Targarona Soler

25.1 Introduction

Splenectomy may be indicated in the treatment of a number of diseases including benign and malignant hematological conditions, cysts, trauma or splenic aneurysms. An organ situated deep in the left hypochondrium and difficult to access, the spleen remains poorly understood with regard to its physiology and function. Delaitre (Paris), Carroll (Los Angeles) and Poulin (Montreal) were the first to report successful laparoscopic splenectomy in humans [1–6].

The spleen is a fragile and highly vascularized organ, receiving as much as 20 % of the cardiac output. Many hematological diseases for which splenectomy may be indicated are associated with a reduced platelet count, which increases the risk of bleeding and spleen enlargement. As well as being deeply recessed, the spleen is directly attached to several organs. These factors all contribute to the level of difficulty in the performance of laparoscopic splenectomy and advanced training on the part of the surgeon is required.

25.2 Indications and Contraindications

Laparoscopic splenectomy has been applied across the spectrum of splenic diseases. Its best indication is the treatment of benign hematologic conditions with a normal or slightly enlarged spleen, as is seen in ITP (idiopathic thrombocytopenic purpura), AIDS-related ITP, hemolytic anemia, or spherocytosis. Laparoscopic splenectomy for malignancy is more controversial because it may require additional resection of lymph nodes or even the removal of an intact specimen.

Although splenomegaly is a relative contraindication for laparoscopic splenectomy, it is feasible in cases of moderate splenomegaly, with a spleen weighing up to 1500 g or a maximal dimension of 25 cm. Massive splenomegaly is not an absolute contraindication. Experience with devices for 'hand-assisted' laparoscopic splenectomy indicates that massive splenomegaly could be a good indication for this technical alternative. Portal hypertension, on the other hand, does not appear to be a good indication, but experience is as yet scarce.

25.3 Set-Up and Patient Positioning

Patients undergoing elective laparoscopic splenectomy do not require any special preparation. A preoperative CT or ultrasonography is recommended to evaluate the size of the spleen or to rule out the existence of accessory spleens (AS) whose intraoperative identification may be difficult.

Many indications for laparoscopic splenectomy are related to low platelet counts where the risk for intraoperative hemorrhage is increased. Several preoperative measures have been proposed to increase the number of platelets and/or diminish the risk of hemorrhage. These include an intravenous bolus of corticosteroids or incremental doses of immune gamma globulins, mainly in patients with autoimmune thrombocytopenic purpura. Poulin et al. proposed preoperative splenic artery embolization to occlude terminal vascular branches and diminish the risk of bleeding as well as to reduce spleen size. Patients who underwent splenic artery embolization showed significantly less intraoperative blood loss and consequently a lower rate of emergency blood transfusion (up to 10 % less). Splenic artery embolization is an invasive procedure and is associated with pain, hemorrhage and hepatic or splenic abscesses. Although preoperative splenic artery embolization is not recommended routinely for laparoscopic splenectomy, it may play a role in massive spleens measuring more than 25 cm in their maximum dimension. An additional intraoperative method to achieve normal platelet count could be fresh platelet transfusion. This method is, however, usually restricted to patients with ITP related to HIV infection, due to the theoretically increased risk of other viral infections through pooled platelet transfusion.

E.M.T. Soler, MD, PhD
Department of Surgery, Hospital de Sant Pau, Barcelona, Spain
e-mail: etargarona@santpau.cat

H.J. Bonjer (ed.), *Surgical Principles of Minimally Invasive Procedures*, DOI 10.1007/978-3-319-43196-3_25

Polyvalent pneumococcal, meningococcal and H. influenzae vaccines are administered prior to surgery. Antibiotic prophylaxis is initiated immediately preoperatively. Laparoscopic splenectomy is performed under general endotracheal anaesthesia. Decompression of the stomach with an oral gastric tube is recommended. It is removed upon completion of the surgery.

Preoperative anti-aggregant therapy is warranted, especially in patients with additional risk factors such as myelofibrosis.

25.4 Instrument Checklist

Laparoscopic splenectomy can be performed in any operating room suitable for conventional laparoscopy and does not require any special equipment. When available, mobile booms and shelves can serve to support video monitors and other laparoscopic equipment, reducing operating room clutter. The use of *two video monitors* improves the surgeon's comfort and efficiency. Laparoscopic splenectomy is usually performed using *three or four trocars*. The laparoscope is often moved between the trocars to enhance visualization. If a 10 mm scope is used, at least two of the ports must be **10–12** mm in size whereas if a 5 mm (or smaller) scope is used, only one port needs to be **10–12** mm. An *angled (30° or 45°)* laparoscope is most commonly used for LS, although some surgeons prefer to use the 0° optic. Most grasping, dissecting and cutting instruments used in this procedure are 5 mm in diameter. It should also be mentioned that mini laparoscopic (2–3 mm) instrumentation is being used more widely, especially for pediatric patients.

Different methods for hemostasis should be readily available in the operating room such as: endoloops, clip appliers, endovascular stapling devices, electrocautery (mono or bipolar), and computed controlled bipolar cautery (Ligasure™). The ultrasonic dissector (Ultracision™) is also a very useful tool for spleen dissection. Clips should be used with care to avoid their placement in sites where an endostapler may also be applied as they can block the functioning of the stapler. Endovascular staplers are very useful, mainly for control of splenic hilar structures. A durable nylon sack should be considered key equipment for laparoscopic splenectomy. Such a sack must be able to withstand the rigors of the final morcellation process once the spleen is in the bag and prior to specimen extraction.

25.5 Surgical Anatomy

The important anatomical aspects of the spleen are its vascularization and its great number of relationships with adjacent organs. The spleen has in essence a double blood supply: short gastric vessels and a main hilar vascular trunk. Although highly variable, splenic anatomy has been classified into two main patterns: the distributed and the magistral types. The more common distributed type (70 %) consists of a short splenic trunk with numerous long branches entering the splenic hilum. In the magistral type, a long main splenic artery divides into short terminal branches in the hilum. There are also accessory polar vessels and anastomoses with gastroepiploic vessels. These anatomic details require that the surgeon be completely familiar with the variable and anomalous extrasplenic vascular anatomy.

The spleen is fixed by several ligaments and peritoneal folds to the colon (splenocolic ligament), the stomach (gastrosplenic ligament), the diaphragm (phrenosplenic ligament), the kidney, adrenal gland and tail of pancreas (lienorenal ligament). These attachments are avascular and can be safely sectioned under the direct vision and magnified image of the laparoscope with the help of the ultrasonic dissector.

Despite the fragility of the splenic parenchyma, its capsule is solid and can be manipulated without rupture if handled with care. Prior to extraction of the spleen, the morcellation process (within a durable bag) is facilitated by the frail structure of the spleen.

25.6 Lateral Approach

The patient is placed in the right lateral decubitus position with the flank at the level of the articulating point of the operating table. The table is broken 20–30° below level in both cephalad and caudad portions and the patient is placed in moderate reverse Trendelenburg position (Fig. 25.1). This serves to maximize the window of access between the patient's left iliac crest and costal margin.

Three trocars are then inserted in the patient's left upper quadrant. An 11 mm port is inserted in the anterior axillary line superior to the patient's anterior superior iliac spine. This trocar is used for the endovascular stapler and ultimately for the removal of the spleen. The trocar that is most frequently used for the camera is placed in the rim of the umbilicus in pediatric and slender patients. For larger patients it is often necessary to move this site into the left upper quadrant. A left subcostal or subxiphoid trocar is also inserted for a retracting or grasping instrument. Finally, a dorsal trocar (2 or 5 mm) is placed under direct vision below the twelfth rib in the mid to post axillary line. A retracting forceps to elevate the lower pole of the spleen is passed through this trocar (Fig. 25.2).

Dissection begins with mobilization of the splenic flexure of the colon (Fig. 25.3). This is done with a combination of sharp dissection and the ultrasonic dissector. The lateral peritoneal attachments of the spleen are then incised. A cuff of peritoneum is left along the spleen. The retracting forceps can be used either to grasp the peritoneal cuff and mobilize the spleen medially or placed under the inferior pole to elevate it. In this way the spleen is never grasped directly.

Dissection of the splenic hilum is begun from the lower pole and continued in a cephalad progression. A lower pole splenic vessel is often present and should be divided between clips or with the ultrasonic dissector.

Once the lower pole of the spleen has been mobilized and the polar vessels have been divided, entry into the lesser sac is facilitated. With the spleen elevated, the short gastric vessels and main vascular pedicle are tented. The short gastric vessels can be divided with the ultrasonic dissector, clips or the endovascular stapler. The tail of the pancreas is often visible at this point of the dissection. The splenic pedicle is well exposed and can easily be accessed. The main artery and vein, once dissected free, are divided by separate applications of the endovascular stapler (Fig. 25.4).

If a concomitant procedure such as cholecystectomy is to be performed, the patient will need to be rolled supine and a further (2 or 5 mm) port introduced into the patient's right upper quadrant.

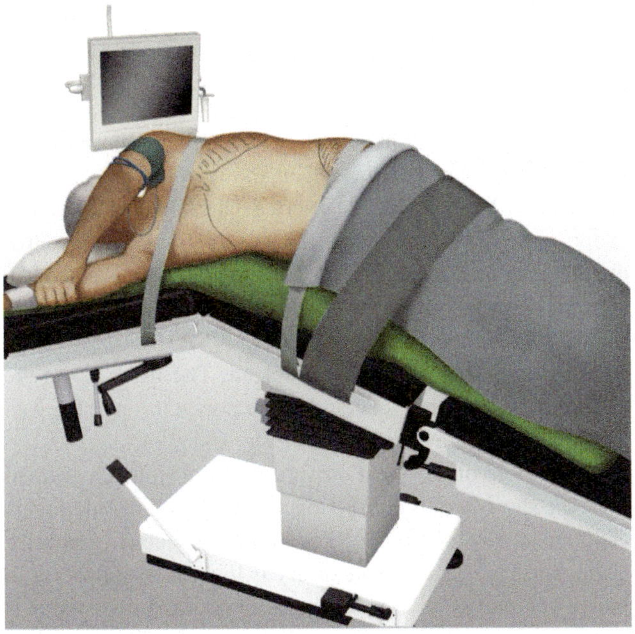

Fig. 25.1 Patient positioning for laparoscopic splenectomy in lateral position

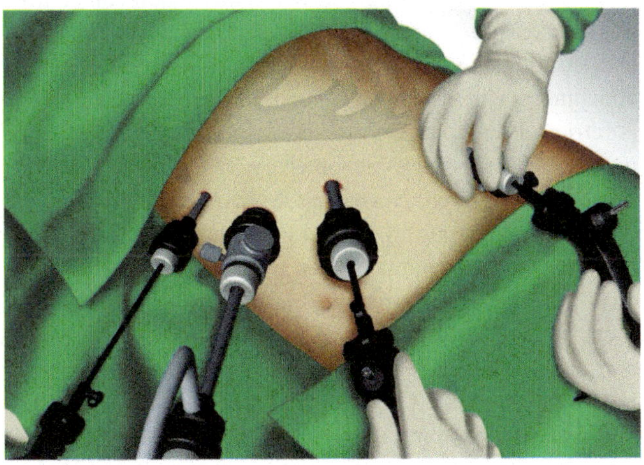

Fig. 25.2 Trocar placement for laparoscopic splenectomy

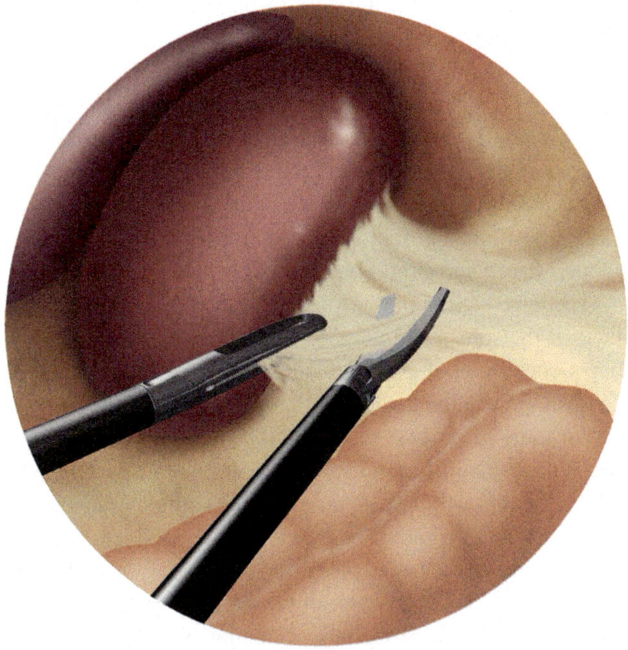

Fig. 25.3 Dissection of the splenocolic ligament

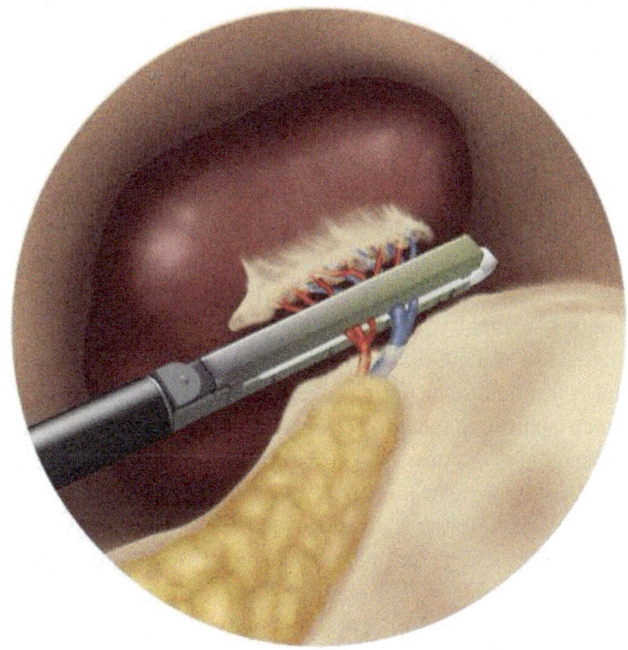

Fig. 25.4 Stapling of splenic artery and vein

25.7 Extraction of the Specimen

Once the remaining splenic hilar and short gastric vessels have been divided, a small cuff of avascular splenophrenic ligament is temporarily left in situ. This serves to hold the spleen in its normal anatomic position and will greatly facilitate placing it into a sack for extraction. The sack is introduced and unfurled. It is then maneuvered over the relatively immobile spleen. The final spleno-phrenic attachments are then divided and the drawstring on the sack is closed. The neck of the sack is withdrawn through the 11 mm trocar. Within the sack the spleen is morcellated with blunt clamps or by finger fracure and extracted piecemeal. As intra-abdominal contamination from splenic material and subsequent splenosis are to be avoided, great care must be taken to insure that the bag is not ruptured. Furthermore, a change of gloves after extracting the spleen is recommended. Once the entire specimen and sack have been removed, a final laparoscopic survey and irrigation are performed.

The introduction of the spleen into the bag may prove difficult if the spleen is enlarged and can be made easier if the bag's opening is of a large diameter with an aperture device controlled from the exterior.

On some occasions, such as in the case of rare primary or secondary splenic tumours, the spleen should be retrieved intact, though pathologists usually have sufficient diagnostic material with the morcellated specimen. In the event that it is necessary to extract the spleen intact, an accessory incision must be used. This incision can be made in various locations on the abdomen or through the widening of a trocar incision, or a Pfannestiel or umbilical incision can be made. A posterior culpotomy has also been suggested for extraction of the specimen.

25.8 Hand-Assisted Laparoscopic Splenectomy

In the hand-assisted laparoscopy splenectomy procedure, the patient is placed in right lateral decubitus position. With massive splenomegaly, the lateral position is reduced to 30–45° to prevent the spleen from falling. A pneumoperitoneum is created with a Veres needle inserted into the right iliac fossa at a good distance from the spleen. A 12 mm trocar is inserted in the periumbilical area to perform an exploratory laparoscopy and to select the best site for an accessory incision (7–7.5 cm) to insert the hand. It is usually made in the right hypogastrium, but in cases of massive splenomegaly it is made in the right subcostal area or in the right iliac fossa (Fig. 25.5). Once the incision is made, the device (Lapdisc, Ethicon, Somerville, NJ, USA; Omniport, Advanced Surgical Concepts Ltd, Dublin, Ireland; Handport, Smith Nephew, Andover, MA, USA) is introduced. Usually,

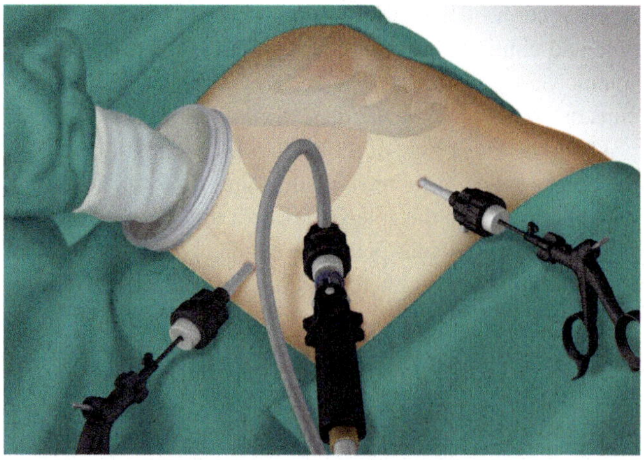

Fig. 25.5 Placement of hand port and trocars for hand port assisted laparoscopic splenectomy

the non-dominant left hand is then inserted into the abdomen to examine the shape of the spleen and surrounding anatomy. A second 12 mm trocar is inserted laterally to the laparoscope under manual control. All the instruments are introduced using this trocar. When additional retraction is needed, a 5 mm trocar is placed in the left flank and an endoretractor (Endoflex, Genzyme, Tucker, GA, USA) is inserted to expose the anterior face of the spleen. The first step in the procedure is to access the retrogastric pouch through the gastrosplenic omentum.

The whole of the great curvature of the stomach is freed until the short vessels are sectioned with the ultrasonic shears (Ultracision™, Ethicon, US) or bipolar device (Ligasure™, Valleylab, US). The splenic artery is located by palpation in the upper border of the pancreas and a ligature or clip is placed to interrupt the inflow of blood into the spleen. The hand then mobilizes the spleen medially to expose its posterior surface and the retroperitoneal adhesions are dissected. The splenic hilum and pancreatic tail are bluntly dissected with the hand. Using this dissection, the endostapler can be placed in the splenic hilum in such a way that it can be fired without tension, sparing the pancreatic tail. Once the hilum is controlled, the upper pole is dissected from the posterior attachments and the spleen is freed. In most cases, the spleen is retrieved intact through the accessory incision. However, in cases of massive splenomegaly, a sterile plastic bag (Endocatch II, Tyco, Norwalk, CN USA) or a bag used for liver harvesting during liver transplantation is introduced into the abdomen and the spleen is placed inside it and then morcellated. It is then removed in large pieces through the 7 cm incision. Although most authors prefer the surgeon's non-dominant hand for intra-abdominal insertion, some favor the assistant's.

Partial splenectomy may be indicated in selected cases. Anatomical requirements for partial splenectomy include a distributed vascular irrigation of the spleen, with segmental branches originating out of the spleen. The segmental anatomy of the spleen facilitates partial splenectomy, because a clear transection line is easily observed after the ligature of the branches that irrigate the area to be excised. Partial splenecomy is particularly indicated in children and with localized splenic diseases such as masses or cysts located in either pole of the spleen.

25.9 Specific Complications of the Technique(s), How to Avoid Them, and Management of Complications

Independently of any complications inherent to laparoscopic surgery in general (e.g. related to pneumoperitoneum, injuries from trocars), laparoscopic splenectomy is associated with several potential perioperative complications that the surgeon should be aware of and be able to treat. The greatest potential problem is hemorrhage, which can be of three types: from a small calibre vessel (short gastric or polar vessels), a larger vessel of the hilum, or the splenic parenchyma. The first type of hemorrhage, though not life threatening, can become quite a hindrance to the operation as rapidly accumulating blood may impede vision, but it can also be easily stopped with clips, electrocoagulation or the ultrasonic dissector. Hemorrhage from a larger vessel may be an indication for immediate conversion to laparotomy. It is best prevented by delicate dissection of the artery and vein to prevent rupture of smaller splenic and pancreatic blood vessels. The dissected artery and vein should then be clipped prior to any movement of the spleen. The rigidity of the clamping instruments alone can suffice to injure these vessels. Hemorrhage originating in the parenchyma is less dangerous and can be managed either by clamping the artery or applying slight pressure with gauze, or electrocoagulation.

Another potential complication of laparoscopic splenectomy is injury to the tail of the pancreas. Proper dissection and placement of the endostapler can avoid this problem. The use of the lateral approach to laparoscopic splenectomy allows the splenic hilum to lengthen and this permits the endostapler to be used without risk of damaging the pancreatic tail. A further possible complication of laparoscopic splenectomy is perforation of the diaphragm during dissection of the superior pole of the spleen. A small puncture may be quickly amplified by the presence of pneumoperitoneum, causing a pneumothorax. This can be controlled laparoscopically and with a pleural drain.

Other complications reported with laparoscopic splenectomy include deep vein thrombosis, portal vein thrombosis, pulmonary embolus and wound infection. Recent reports have suggested a higher incidence of portal thrombosis with laparoscopic splenectomy. No clear relation to pneumoperitoneum has been found, but close monitoring of postoperative thrombocytosis and preoperative antiaggregant therapy is warranted, especially in patients with additional risk factors such as myelofibrosis. It is interesting to note that particularly in the largest series of laparoscopic splenectomy, there is a remarkably low incidence of deep surgical infection or subphrenic abcess.

25.10 Limitations, Caveats and Controversies Related to the Technique(s)

While performing LS the surgeon must always be mindful of the possibility of the existence of accessory spleens, particularly in the treatment of ITP or spherocytosis. Accessory spleens are present in 10–30 % of patients and can be found in the splenic fossa next to the colon or the stomach as well as in the omentum or below the mesocolon. They should be excised at the beginning of the procedure, otherwise they may be mistaken for hematomas as the operation progresses. Laparoscopic ultrasonography or a radioisotope detection probe for intraoperative identification of accessory spleens has been suggested but their efficiency has not been established. Accessory spleens may cause therapeutic failures of splenectomy and can require repeat intervention. Some cases of laparoscopic treatment of accessory spleen left in situ have been published.

Moderate splenomegaly (spleens of less than 20 cm in length or approximately 1000 g) does not constitute a clear contraindication to LS yet may be associated with greater technical difficulty in performing the procedure. This is especially true during the steps of mobilization of the spleen and its introduction into the sack. It should be noted that dissection of the splenic hilum is not rendered more difficult in cases of splenomegaly because the vascular structures remain in their normal anatomic position and may even become somewhat elongated and therefore easier to ligate and divide. The advantages of laparoscopic splenectomy for massive splenomegaly are not yet well established. Liberation of the posterolateral ligaments of the superior pole of an enlarged spleen can be particularly difficult. When the spleen is elevated with endoseparators, access to the posterior aspect of the superior pole is blocked. When the organ size is such that it crosses the midline and reaches all the way to the iliac crest, it is extremely difficult to introduce the spleen into a sack intracorporeally and it is preferable to extract the specimen through an accessory incision. It has been proposed that the spleen be fragmented into five or six pieces within the abdomen and then be extracted through a Pfannestiel incision, but this method is not generally endorsed due to the risk of subsequent splenosis.

25.11 Laparoscopic Treatment for Other Splenic Disorders

An interesting indication for laparoscopic surgery of the spleen is in the treatment of primary *cysts* or (secondary) cysts following splenic trauma. The most accepted treatment approach is the observation of lesions of less than 5 cm, but larger cysts require excision due to the risk of rupture, hemorrhage, or infection. Splenectomy has been considered the treatment of choice for benign cystic lesions of the spleen. Other less invasive alternatives such as percutaneous aspiration often lead to recurrence of the cysts. In the last few years, organ conserving techniques have been developed and reported with good results, including partial splenectomy and partial excision of the cysts. In 1985, Salky et al. performed the first laparoscopic treatment of a splenic cyst, aiding in the wider application of laparoscopic surgery. Extirpation of the cyst is safe, effective and less aggressive than splenectomy. If the cyst is located in a difficult area for a conservative approach (hilum or superior pole), total splenectomy is recommended.

The laparoscopic approach has also been suggested for the treatment of splenic aneurysms. Hashizume et al. successfully treated an aneurysm of the splenic artery, ligating both ends of the aneurysm while preserving the spleen.

The use of laparoscopy for the diagnosis of intra-abdominal injuries has been recommended for years but was not widely used until laparoscopic cholecystectomy became common and videolaparoscopy caught the interest of abdominal surgeons. Many studies throughout the 1970s and 1980s proved the usefulness of laparoscopy in the detection of intra-abdominal injuries. Two prospective randomized studies comparing exploratory laparoscopy with peritoneal lavage have demonstrated similar sensitivities (100%), although laparoscopy showed superior specificity. These studies suggest that laparoscopy may serve a role in the exploration of cases where peritoneal lavage has not produced a definitive diagnosis.

Therapeutic laparoscopy has also been described for splenic injuries. The techniques most commonly used are aspiration of clots, application of a hemostatic agent for capsular splenic tears, and placement of an absorbable mesh in the case of a highly mobile spleen.

Specific "Tips and Tricks"

1. Carefully evaluate the anatomy of the spleen (CT scan) and the patient's biological status (coagulation parameters).
2. Select the table position (full lateral, semilateral or supine) depending on the volume and shape of the spleen.
3. Consider using the Hasson technique and avoid tearing the spleen when inserting a trocar.
4. After laparoscopic examination, consider conversion to HALS if the size of the spleen hampers its mobilization.
5. If HALS is used, consider making the port incision below the sternum or costal margin as it permits conversion through a subcostal incision.
6. Control the artery first. It is easily located and simple clipping or ligature permits a reduction in spleen volume.
7. A large upper or lower pole located near the midline implies increased technical difficulty.
8. Locate the tail of the pancreas. Enlarged nodes may hamper localization.
9. Assure hemostasis, as it may be more difficult than after open surgery.
10. Drainage is advised in the presence of clotting anomalies or oozing surgical field.

References

1. Park A, Gagner M, Pomp A. The lateral approach to laparoscopic splenectomy. Am J Surg. 1997;173:126–30.
2. Poulin EC, Mamazza J, Schlachta CM. Splenic artery embolization before laparoscopic splenectomy. An update. Surg Endosc. 1998;12:870–5.
3. Poulin EC, Thibault C. The anatomic basis for laparoscopic splenectomy. Can J Surg. 1993;36:484–8.
4. Targarona EM, Gracia E, Rodriguez M, et al. Hand-assisted laparoscopic surgery. Arch Surg. 2003;138:133–41.
5. Targarona EM, Espert JJ, Balagué C, Piulachs J, Artigas V, Trias M. Splenomegaly should not be considered a contraindication for laparoscopic splenomegaly. Ann Surg. 1998;228:35–9.
6. Uranues S, Alimoglu O. Laparoscopic surgery of the spleen. Surg Clin North Am. 2005;85:75–90.

Part X

Small Intestine

Adhesiolysis for Bowel Obstruction

26

Wilhelmus J.H.J. Meijerink

26.1 Introduction

Laparoscopic treatment of bowel obstruction is one of the most challenging procedures in laparoscopic surgery. Adhesions can be wide spread through the abdomen, both omentum and bowels can be adhered to the anterior and lateral abdominal wall (Fig. 26.1). The presence of dilatation of bowel loops make the procedure even more complex. Almost in all cases small bowel is involved (Fig. 26.2). The ascending and descending colon are less involved in adhesions as they are already attached to the lateral bowel wall. The transverse colon and flexures are frequently involved in adhesions with omentum but are less frequently involved in complete obstruction because of a relative wide lumen and strong muscles. Sigmoid can be obstructed in the pelvis due to severe adhesions and cause functional outlet obstruction.

Two distinct clinical situations have to be considered: surgical therapy with adhesiolysis in the acute situation with a clear obstructive moment and the presence of an ileus, or a more chronic obstruction in which intermitted (partial) obstruction and chronic abdominal pain are the major complaints.

In obstruction it is important to consider the cause of functio laesa. Advanced malignant processes may cause both obstruction of loops with metastases, but also cause obstruction with ingrowth in abdominal and intestinal nervous system. Especially gynecological malignancies are known for this fenomenen. Adhesiolysis in widespread ovarian or colorectal cancer very rarely resolves obstruction due to bowel paralysis by nerve injury. Also in prior untreated inflammatory bowel disease, treatment is generally conservative with high-dose steroids and biologicals. Surgical treatment is necessary when conservative treatment fails. Intra-abdominal abbesses are primarily treated with CT scan guided drainage. In case of multiple (interloop) abscesses (laparoscopic) surgical treatment might be necessary.

26.2 Acute Bowel Obstruction

Acute bowel obstruction is a medical emergency. Morbidity and mortality are dependent of early recognition and treatment. Evaluation, diagnosis and treatment must be started immediately as the patient arrives in the hospital. Bowel obstruction can vary from a single fibrotic string somewhere distal from the duodenum to multiple incarcerated loops in complex obstructions. Symptoms however are similar with (severe) abdominal pain, abdominal distention, vomiting and constipation. Depending from the level of obstruction, vomiting, distention or lack of stools can be the most prominent signal. After resuscitation and diagnostic tests, a decision for further treatment can be made. Diagnostic tools include monitoring of vital signs, laboratory results, X-ray, CT scan or ultrasound. Present radiological imaging techniques can reliably distinguish between simple obstructions and more complex situations with volvulus, closed loops, incarcerated (internal) hernia's or inflammatory masses (e.g. Crohn). Level and severity of the obstruction has to be estimated en depending from results, treatment can be conservatively or in many cases surgical. Postoperative adhesions are the most common cause of bowel obstruction (60 %) and chronic abdominal complaints. Adhesions are more seen after appendectomy, colorectal surgery and gynecological procedures. Previous surgery in the pelvis and lower abdomen, are more prone to adhesions and obstruction the upper GI surgery. Other causes of adhesions (even in the absence of previous surgery) include inflammatory processes, (subclinical) appendicitis, Diverticular disease, and especially after fecal peritonitis. Diffuse obstruction such as in Crohn's disease, peritoneal carcinomatosis or radiation enteritis are commonly treated conservatively, whereas acute obstruction in a "virgin" abdomen, incarceration, bowel ischaemia or volvulus need emergency surgical treatment.

W.J.H.J. Meijerink, MD, PhD
Department of Gastro-Intestinal and Advanced Laparoscopy, VU University Medical Center, Amsterdam, The Netherlands
e-mail: j.meijerink@vumc.nl

H.J. Bonjer (ed.), *Surgical Principles of Minimally Invasive Procedures*, DOI 10.1007/978-3-319-43196-3_26

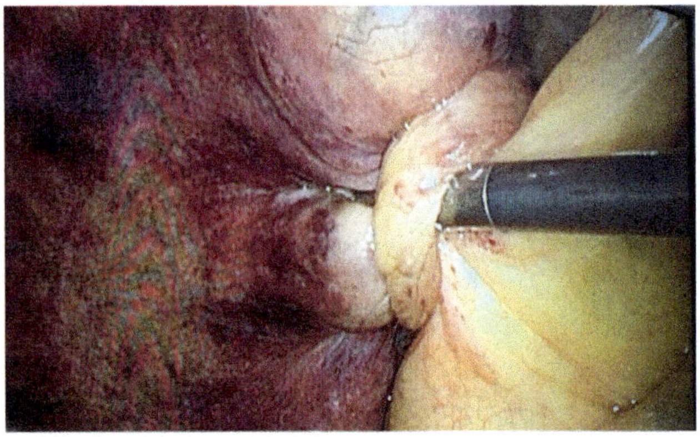

Fig. 26.1 Adhesive band causing ischemia of small bowel

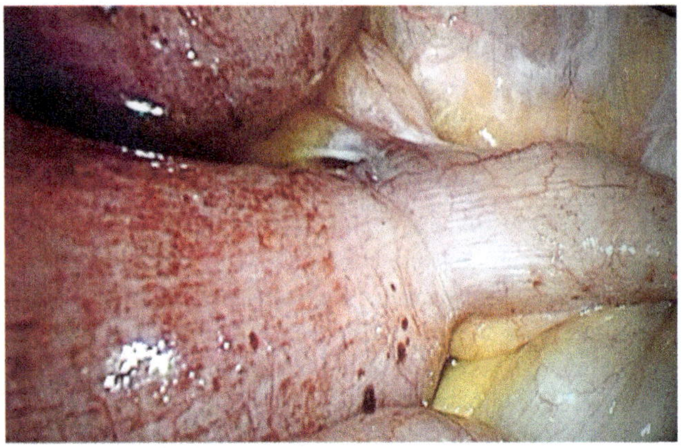

Fig. 26.2 Small bowel after lysis of adhesive band

In acute bowel obstruction the role of laparoscopy is limited and timing is extremely important. Delaying surgery increasingly complicates the laparoscopic treatment because of the ongoing dilatation of bowel loops and a progressive loss of working space in the abdomen. Also bowel loops become more and more vulnerable to surgical trauma and lack of adequate visualization hampers adequate laparoscopic treatment. The advantage in case of conversion could be the proper place of incision.

26.3 Chronic Bowel Obstruction

Chronic and intermittend bowel obstruction are difficult situations both for the patient and the surgeon. Chronic abdominal pain and obstruction as seen for example in severe postoperative adhesions, radiation enteritis, multiple intraperitoneal metastases or sclerosing peritonitis are not easily resolved with surgery. (Extensive) Resection of bowel segments or cutting adhesions usually only relieves symptoms for a very short period of time. Preoperative surgical counseling is crucial to limit patients' expectations towards the final result of surgical treatment.

26.4 Procedural Considerations in Acute Bowel Obstruction

An adequate and extensive anamnesis is crucial. Previous (surgical) history and underlying disease are of utmost importance to understand the cause and possible localization of adhesions and obstruction. An anamnestic distinction between a high or low bowel obstruction often can be made based on patients information and symptoms (nausea, vomiting, constipation). The severity, duration and associated complaints are important.

Physical examination starts with observation. Is abdominal distension present? Umbilicus can be flattened as symptom of an extension of the abdomen. One should look for possible herniae either in previous scars as in the groin. On auscultation peristalsis can vary from clear and present bowel movements in case of a mechanical obstruction, to absent in case of a paralytic ileus. Percussion is high tympanic in case of extended bowels. On palpation the abdomen is tender and painful over the abdomen.

26.5 Diagnosis

Laboratory results do not reveal information about localization and cause of obstruction. In case of bowel obstruction serum chemistry including urea and creatinine and complete blood count are indicative for severity and duration of obstruction. C-reactive protein and white blood cell count indicate accompanying inflammation and duration of obstruction. Elevated lactate dehydrogenase tests are indicative for acute mesenterial ischemia or bowel necrosis.

Plain abdominal x-rays in 2 views are in over 60 % accurate in simple obstructions. Sonographie has a high negative productive value in small bowel obstruction, but in case of extended bowel loops filled with air, the added value of sonography is limited. CT scanning is in majority of cases study of choice. Intravenous contrast combined with oral contrast enhance the diagnostic quality of the CT-scan. Distention of bowel loops, free abdominal air, inflammatory masses, free fluids, abscesses, affected parts of the bowel and absence of air in the distal bowel parts can easily be identified. Stenotic traject can be visualized in most cases and are indicative for the cause of obstruction. Except for clear obstructing fibrotic strings, adhesions can not be visualized. (MRI-) Enteroclysis has limited value in the acute situation. In partial, chronic or intermittent small bowel obstruction, enteroclysis may add valuable information about stenotic bowel loops and localization.

26.6 Treatment

Initial emergency treatment is directed to resuscitation of the patient. Aggressive fluid administration combined with gastrointestinal decompression by nasogastric tube, analgesia and anti-emetic drugs and stabilization of blood pressure and respiratory function is dependent of the initial presentation of the patient. After initial stabilization of the patient, early surgical treatment in strangulated and complete bowel obstruction is warranted. In simple complete bowel obstruction initial conservative treatment may be followed by surgical treatment within 24–48 h when conservative therapy fails.

26.7 Set-Up

- Requirements for laparoscopic adhesiolysis
- Basic laparoscopic instruments and atraumatic bowel graspers
- Sealing devices are needed sporadicly in case of resection
- 0 or preferably 30° scope. A 5 mm HD scope facilitates different port positions
- Screens on both sides of the patients

26.8 Required Skills

Excellent dexterity and intracorporal suturing capabilities.

26.9 Port Placement

An open introduction of the first port is mandatory in all cases with expected adhesions and/or dilated bowel loops caused by obstruction. In case of previous midline scars, other possible entry points should be considered, preferably outside the area with expected adhesions and adhered bowel loops. A balloon port (Hassontrocart) can be very useful to prevent loss of pneumoperitoneum during the procedure. After entry of the abdomen laparoscopic inspection is done to judge if laparoscopic treatment is possible. Next ports are placed under direct vision at appropriate places, depending from the adhesions and expected working area.

26.10 Procedure

After open introduction, inspection and port placement, a sharp dissection of adhesions can be done. One should refrain from electrocoagulation as much as possible to prevent thermal injuries to adhered bowel loops. Serosal tears should be oversewn by intracorporal sutures with braided or monofilament threads. One should look for the transition of dilated bowel loops to collapsed loops. This is suggestive for the presence of a fibrotic string. In case of a string, one can cut the string with scissors. The involved bowel segment should be inspected carefully to exclude focal necrosis and subsequent perforation. In many cases, adhesions are multiple, without one specific obstruction. The complete small bowel should be inspected to exclude other obstructive moments. Non-obstructive adhesions can be left. Preventive (total) adhesiolysis is considered to be ineffective.

If a malignant process or intraperitoneal metastases are present, one or more segment resections can be necessary. A small laparotomy can facilitate the resection. In case of gross metastases and involved radix of the mesentery with multiple enlarged loops, surgical therapy is less successful as bowel nerve involvement is likely. Bowel strangulation rarely occurs when carcinomatosis is present. A long postoperative recovery can be expected in these cases and in some cases patients are dependent on parenteral nutrition for a prolonged period.

Incarceration and adhesions of bowel loops after surgery in the small pelvis can be very challenging. Adhesions to the pelvic wall and especially the promontory and sacrum after excision of the mesorectum can be very dense and fibrotic. The presence of ureters, iliac vessels and sacral venous vessels, make this procedure even more challenging. Laparoscopic management of these adhesions is extremely difficult. A small pfannenstiel incision and open adhesiolysis is recommended.

Adhesiolysis in incarcerated hernia can be easier than they look at first sight. Careful retraction of entrapped bowel loops reveal adhesions to the anterior abdominal peritoneum and hernia sac. Sharp dissection without cautery is advised. Concomitant exterior manipulation of the hernia (by preference by using one hand of the operating surgeon) can facilitate reduction of bowel loops and expose adhesions which would otherwise be difficult to expose. The incarcerated bowel has to be inspected closely for possible serial tears and (partial) necrosis. When no necrosis is present and segment resections are not necessary, a laparoscopic hernia repair can be considered in the same procedure.

Bibliography

1. Di Saverio S, Cocclini F, Galati M, et al. Bologna guidelines for diagnosis and management of adhesive small bowel obstruction (ASBO): 2013 update of the evidence-based guidelines from the world society of emergency surgery ASBO working group. World J Emerg Surg. 2013;8(1):42.
2. Diaz JJ, Bokhari F, Sohn MJ, et al. Guidelines for management of small bowel obstruction. J Trauma. 2008;64:1651–64.
3. Cirocchi R, Abraha I, Farinella E, et al. Laparoscopic versus open surgery in small bowel obstruction. Cochrane Database Syst Rev. 2010;(2):CD007511.
4. Zerey M, Sechrist CW, Kercher KW, et al. The laparoscopic management of small bowel obstruction. Am J Surg. 2007;194:882–7.
5. Khaikin M, Schneidereit N, Cera S, et al. Laparoscopic vs. open surgery for acute adhesive small-bowel obstruction: patients' outcome and costt-effectiveness. Surg Endosc. 2007;21:742–6.
6. Williams SB, Greenspon J, Young HA, et al. Small bowel obstruction: conservative vs surgical management. Dis Colon Rectum. 2005;48:1140–6.
7. Maglinte DD, Kelvin FM, Sandrasegaran K, et al. Radiology of small bowel obstruction: contempory approach and controversies. Abdom Imaging. 2005;30:160–78.

Part XI

Colon and Appendix

27 Diagnostic Laparoscopy in Suspected Appendicitis and Laparoscopic Appendectomy

Agneta Montgomery

27.1 Introduction

Acute appendicitis is the most common inflammatory disease of the abdominal cavity. Open appendectomy has been the gold standard for treatment. After the introduction of the laparoscopic appendectomy by Semm in 1983 it has spread world-wide and is now a routine operation in many hospitals [1]. Numerous studies have been performed comparing laparoscopic appendectomy to open appendectomy and a summary of some meta-analyses is given below.

In a meta-analysis of 39 randomized control trials (RCT) comparing laparoscopic appendectomy to open appendectomy included almost 6000 patients. Laparoscopic appendectomy was associated with; earlier resumption of liquid and solid intake, shorter duration of hospital stay, reduced analgesic consumption, earlier return to work and normal life, less wound infections, better cosmesis, similar hospital costs but a longer operative time [2].

Laparoscopic appendectomy compared to open appendectomy in children demonstrated only reduced hospital stay in uncomplicated appendicitis after laparoscopy. In complicated appendicitis laparoscopic appendectomy was associated with fewer complications over all, lower rate of wound infections, shorter hospital stay, fewer bowel obstruction episodes but an increased incidence of intra-abdominal abscesses and a longer operation time [3]. A total of 100,000 patients were included in these analyses.

In another meta-analysis, 15,000 patients older than 60 years of age were included [4]. Laparoscopic appendectomy was associated with lower mortality, fewer complications and shorter hospital stay. No differences were seen in operative time, wound infections or intra-abdominal collections compared to open appendectomy.

A. Montgomery, MD, PhD
Department of Surgery, Skåne University Hospital, Malmö, Malmö, Sweden
e-mail: agneta.montgomery@skane.se

When comparing laparoscopic appendectomy to open appendectomy in obese patients the laparoscopic technique showed fewer wound infections, shorter hospital stay, no difference in intra-abdominal abscess rate but a longer operation time resulting in a 50 % reduction in morbidity and a 66 % reduction in wound infections [5].

In conclusion, laparoscopic appendectomy seems favourable in most situations and no major disadvantage has been demonstrated compared to open appendectomy. When adding the possibility to perform a diagnostic laparoscopy as introduction of the operation the advantages seem even more tempting for the patient.

27.2 Indications

Almost all patients would gain from a diagnostic laparoscopy that will confirm a diagnosis. The laparoscopic approach shows most benefits in fertile women because gynaecological disorders can mimic appendicitis. A benefit is also seen in obese patients due to fewer postoperative infectious complications [6].

Contraindications for laparoscopy in the acute abdomen are few. After former abdominal surgery one should avoid the area of scars while placing the first trocar. The sub-costal areas are recommended, in scarless areas, where adhesions usually are minimal. From this position one could decide, due to the competence of the surgeon, whether to proceed laparoscopically or to convert. Most elderly patients with co-morbidities can tolerate a laparoscopic procedure when using low intra-abdominal pressure and careful tilting. These patients are the once to gain the most from minimally invasive surgery after the operation. There is no contraindication for laparoscopy when general peritonitis is present confirmed by the SAGES guidelines [6]. Laparoscopic appendectomy is not recommended in ongoing pregnancy. A meta-analyse suggests with available low-grade evidence that laparoscopic

H.J. Bonjer (ed.), *Surgical Principles of Minimally Invasive Procedures*, DOI 10.1007/978-3-319-43196-3_27

appendectomy in pregnant women might be associated with a greater risk of fetal loss than in open appendectomy [7].

27.3 Preoperative Work-Up

Acute appendicitis is mainly a clinical diagnosis and the indication for operation is based on medical history and clinical findings of local peritonitis in the right lower quadrant. Ultrasound (US) is non-invasive and might be a useful complement for differential diagnosis particularly in children. Computed tomography (CT) is a second choice that could be considered to exclude other disorders particularly in elderly and obese patients.

Blood chemistry including electrolytes, haemoglobin, white leukocyte count and CRP is standard in former healthy patients. A validated appendicitis inflammatory response score, developed by Andersson et al, is a useful tool for the diagnosis of acute appendicitis [8]. This is shown to outperform the well-known Alvarado score.

27.4 Operating Room

A single dose of prophylactic antibiotics is given immediately before surgery and thrombo-embolic prophylaxis in risk patients according to local routines. A peripheral i.v. line is usually sufficient in low risk patients. A naso-gastric tube and a Foley catheter are recommended in all patients. An empty bladder is important in order to minimize the risk of harming the bladder at the supra-pubic trocar placement. This is especially important in children were also an empty bladder could reach above the symphysis pubis and care should be taken at trocar insertion.

The patient is positioned flat on the operating table with the left arm along the side. No anaesthetic arc is used in order to have the camera assistant comfortable positioned at the left shoulder according to Fig. 27.1. The patient is tilted slightly head down and rolled towards the left for maximal comfort of the working team and for good surgical access.

27.5 Surgical Technique

27.5.1 Accessing the Abdominal Cavity

The operation is always initiated by a systematically planned diagnostic laparoscopy. An open access to the abdominal cavity is recommended using a small skin incision transversally hidden in the umbilical fold for maximal aesthetics. A trocare placement above the umbilicus could be recommended to get a somewhat larger distance to the right fossa. This is especially valuable in children and people with a short torso. The Verres needle technique has been shown to be the only associated factor for complications when accessing the peritoneal cavity [9]. To use the safest possible technique for access is especially important in emergency laparoscopies. The technique is to be used around-the-clock,

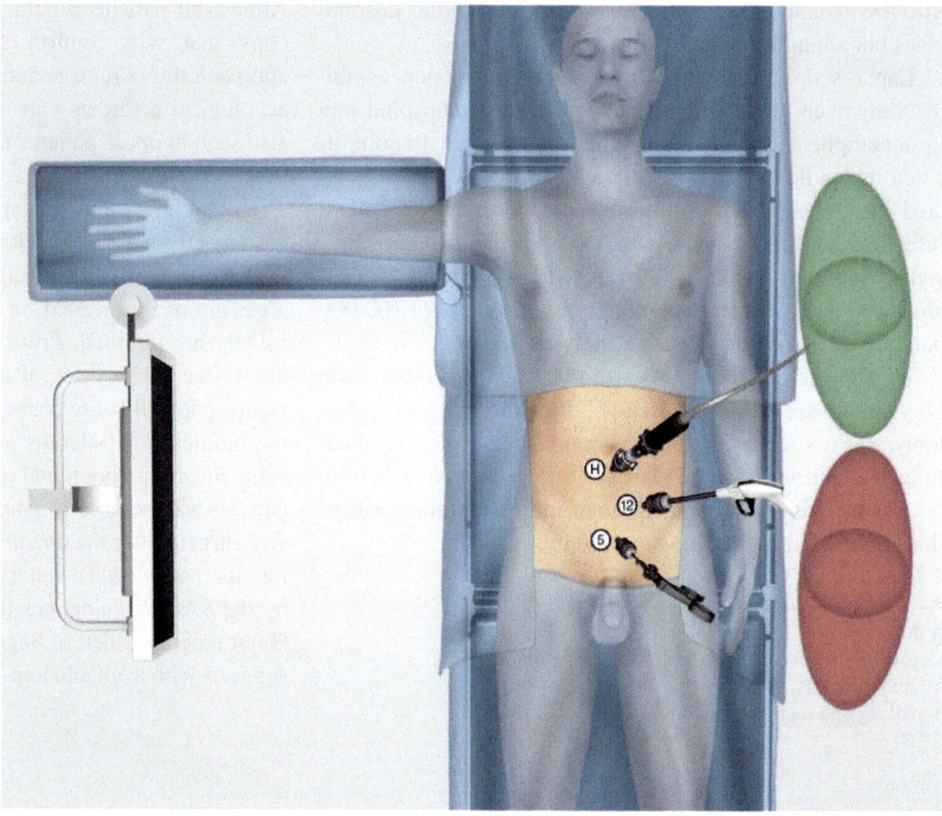

Fig. 27.1 Patient positioning for laparoscopic appendectomy

by residents and surgeons that might have less experience in laparoscopic surgery in their ordinary day practice. Patients might have paralysis and distended bowels or peritonitis. Patients with suspected appendicitis are usually young and many are children. A special precaution is needed in young patients since the peritoneum contains more collagen than in elderly and is very resistant to penetration by a trocar. These patients are also often slim and the large vessels are close to the abdominal wall. The open access technique has been proved to be easy to use and safe [10, 11].

The intra- abdominal trocar position is checked by the camera and the insufflation is initiated. It is recommended to keep a low pressure level since several emergency patients with peritonitis and associated diseases could be sensitive to high pressure levels, but also to extreme tilting. An intra-abdominal pressure above 10 mmHg is nearly never needed and 7 mmHg is almost always enough. To roll the patient to either side can often be enough for accessing the abdominal cavity instead of extreme tilting. The latter can induce cardiac arrhythmia. It is wise as a surgeon to be able to follow the Electrocardiography (ECG) monitor in order to predict the anaesthesiologist complaining. The abdominal cavity is roughly checked for pathology, peritonitis and fluid collections.

Two more trocars are used. The second, a 5 mm trocar, is placed under vision of the camera in the left lower quadrant lateral to the epigastric vessels and in case of unclear diagnose another 5 mm trocar is placed, to later be covered in the hair line, above the symphysis pubis. It is wise to use a grasper on the inside as an anvil, especially in children, at the third trocar placement. In case of a clear appendicitis judged as accessible for laparoscopic appendectomy a 12 mm trocar can be placed directly (Fig. 27.2). It is recommended to make an incision in the fascia longitudinally including the peritoneum to facilitate the 12 mm trocar placement, which could be very hazardous especially in children.

27.6 Diagnostic Laparoscopy

The operation is always initiated by a systematically planned diagnostic laparoscopy. The right lower quadrant is initially viewed to localise and judge the status of appendix if possible. In case of a normal appendix a thorough systematically diagnostic laparoscopy is eligible for diagnosis.

Start to examine the peritoneum for local or generalised peritonitis and omental reactions (oedematous and/or adherent to organs or to the abdominal wall). Proceed to examine the pelvic area and to look for fluid collections of different kinds (serous, bloody, bile, pus, intestinal content). Fluid collections are also commonly seen lateral to the right liver lobe in the Morrison´s pouch and provide a clue of the pathology at hand.

The gynaecologic organs are thoroughly examined in females and rectum and sigmoid colon are checked for pathology. In case of gynaecological pathology a second

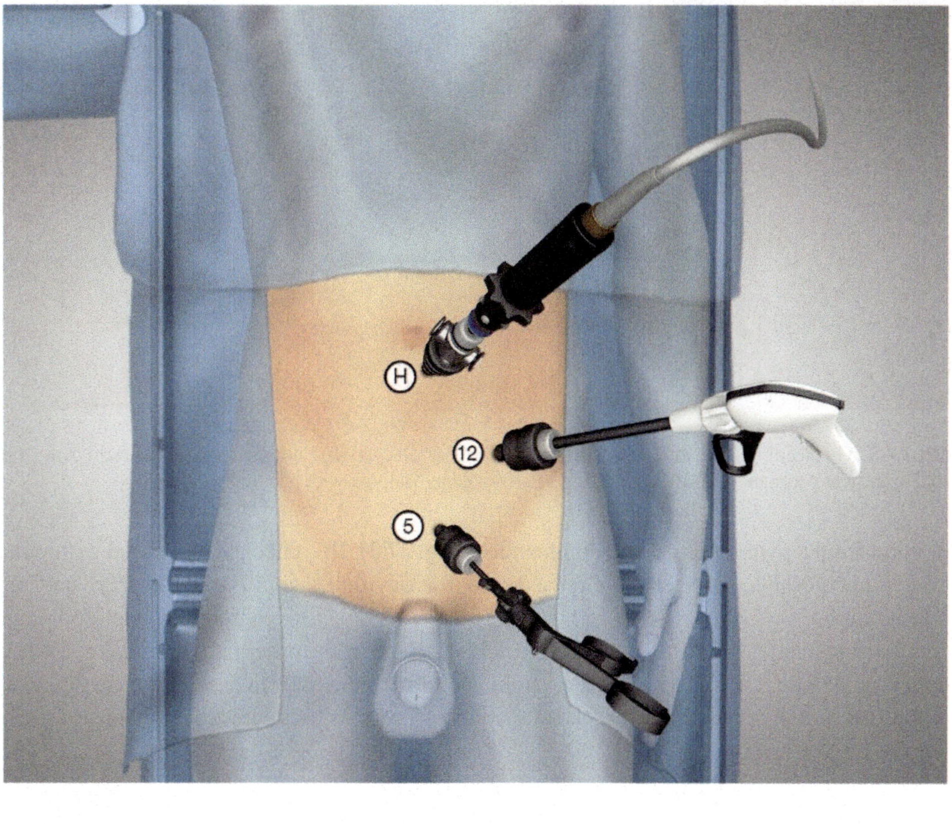

Fig. 27.2 Trocar placement for laparoscopic appendectomy

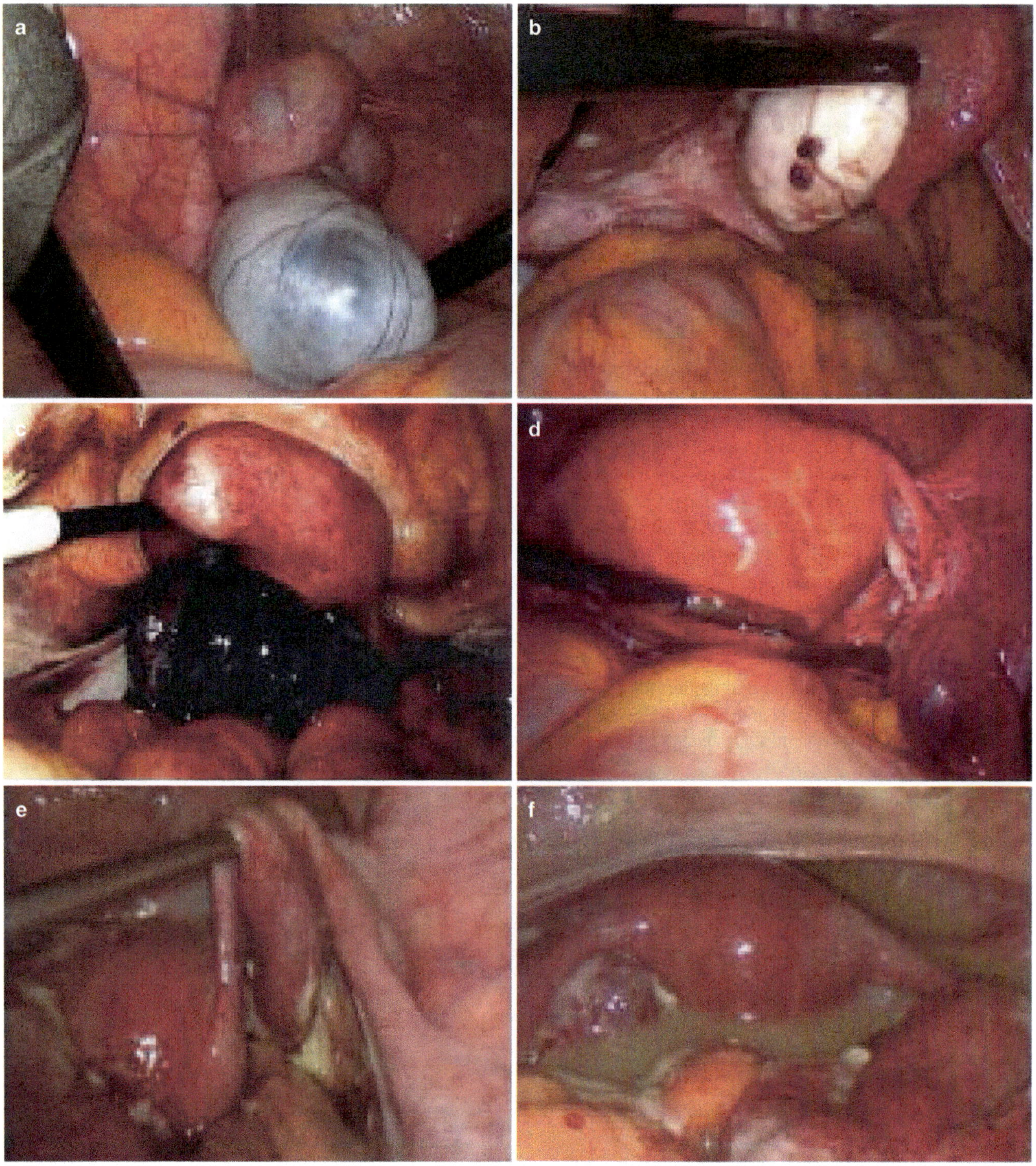

Fig. 27.3 Gynaecological disorders at laparoscopy. (**a**) ovarian cyst. (**b**) Endometriosis of the right ovary. (**c**) Torsion of the adnexa with gangrene. (**d**) Intra-tuber pregnancy. (**e**) Pyosalphinx. (**f**) Perforated pyosalpinx with pus in the pelvis

opinion from a gynaecologist is recommended (Fig. 27.3). If this is not possible, images should be saved for daytime consultation.

The diagnostic laparoscopy goes clockwise; the right colon, gallbladder, liver, duodenum, stomach, transverse colon, left colon is checked. At last the small intestine is checked by careful manipulation, using non-traumatic graspers in a gentle way, starting from the ilio-caecal angel in a retrograde manner looking for a Meckels diverticulum or other pathology (Fig. 27.4).

In case of a clear diagnosis of appendicitis a reduced procedure for diagnostic laparoscopy can be performed taking

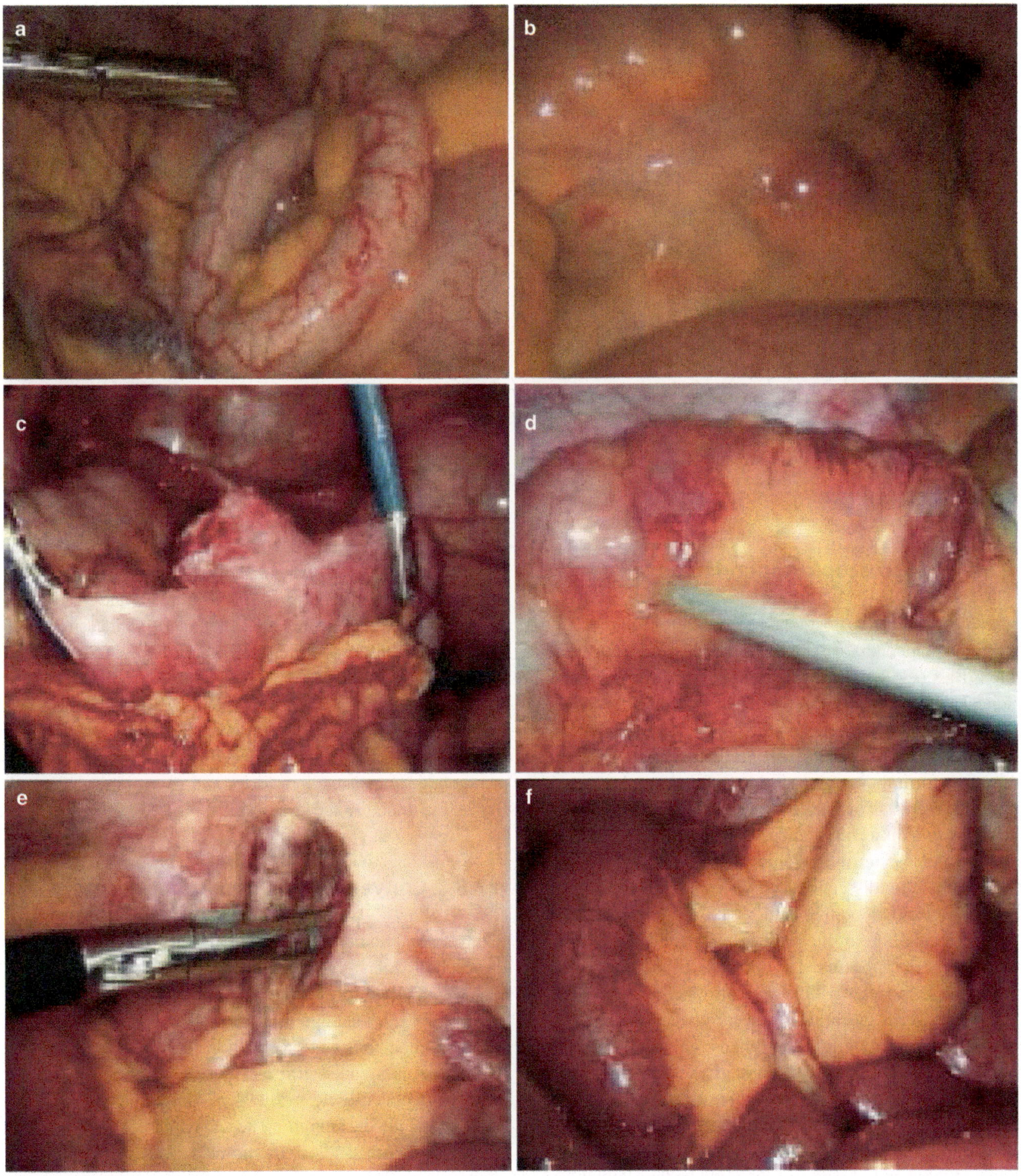

Fig. 27.4 Other differential diagnosis at laparoscopy. (**a**) Normal appendix. (**b**) Lymfadenitis in the mesentery of the small bowel in the ileo-caecal angel. (**c**) Perforated Meckels diverticulum. (**d**) Sigmoid diverticulitis. (**e**) Torsion of appendicis epiploica. (**f**) Mesenteric band causing small intestinal obstruction

the clinical situation into account. A gynaecological examination in females is though mandatory.

In case of no identified pathology a macroscopically normal looking appendix should be left in place. A diagnostic laparoscopy can safely be performed with a very low complication rate [12]. The complication rate after removing a healthy appendix equals that of removal of a gangrenous appendix [13].

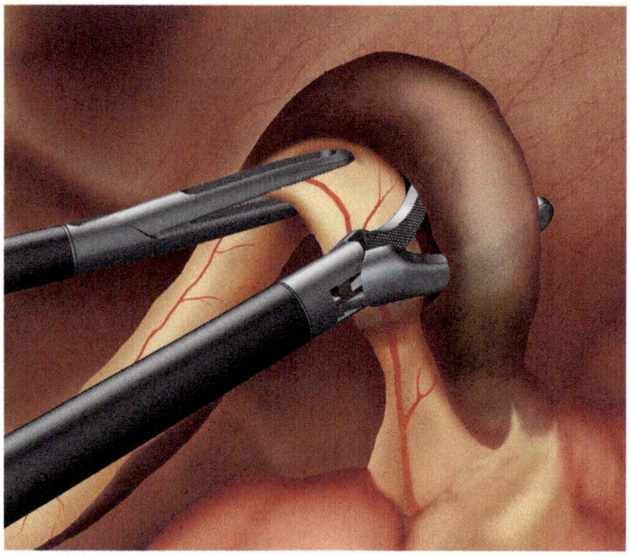

Fig. 27.5 Creating a 'window' between the base of the appendix and the meso-appendix

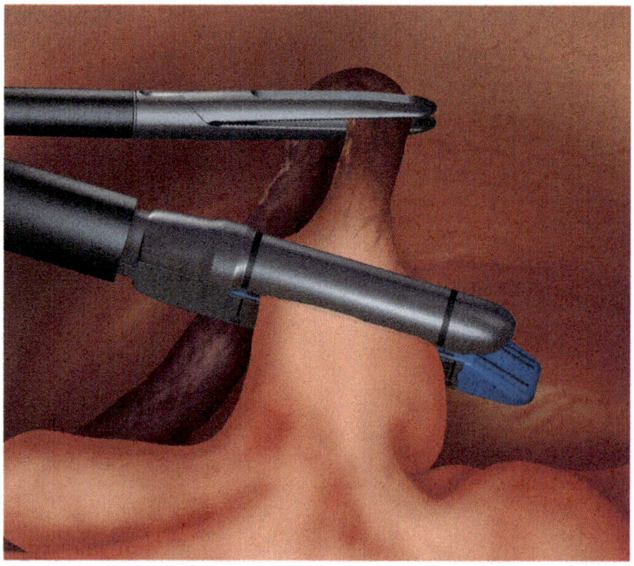

Fig. 27.6 Stapler transection of the base of the appendix

27.7 Laparoscopic Appendectomy

The meso-appendix is grabbed in order not to harm an unperforated appendix using an atraumatic grasper or preferable a Babcock that can host some volume of tissue without squeezing it. The dissection follows the appendix leaving a "lump" of the meso-appendix distally on appendix for grabbing. This way the artery will be divided distally avoiding bleeding form the mesoappendix and making the specimen easier to extract. The dissection can be done with a monopolar hook or a dissecting forceps (Fig. 27.5). In heavy inflammation and/or a retro-caecal position an ultrasonic shears is of great help for dissection also for security reasons in keeping a clean and blood free field.

The taenia libre of the right colon is followed to identify the base of the appendix. The appendix is preferable divided using a linear stapler with a blue cartridge, Fig. 27.6. This is definitely worth the price for security reasons. This is an emergency operation involving many surgeons on call. The stapling technique is easy to learn, gives a secure staple line, easy to inspect, and is fast. The simplest 30 mm device can be used. When using these as a routine, the prize can be negotiated with the company and the prize will hopefully equal the prize of three endo-loops, which would be the alternative.

The appendix is grasped including the linear stapler line for retrieval, retracted and covered within the 12 mm port before extraction of the port. A retrieval bag should be used when the appendix does not fit within the port. For larger specimens the fascial insicion can be elongated (skin usually not needed) by cutting along port in the midline if needed. The appendix is sent untouched (in order not to destroy for diagnosis) for pathological examination.

The abdominal cavity is cleaned. In contaminated situations a culture is recommended. Meticulous cleaning is recommended of the pelvic area, the right fossa and Morrison's pouch using suction only. Installation of saline should be avoided, or only used very locally, in order not to spread the contamination.

Ports are retrieved under camera vision. The fascia is sutured for port-sites >5 mm, except in children, were all port-sites are closed. Intra-cutaneous wound closure is recommended for cosmetic reasons and to avoid an extra call for staple or suture retrieval.

27.8 Conversion to Open Appendectomy

Conversion should be performed when operation does not proceed or when a complication occurs. A second opinion is always good before converting if available. One should always consider using a midline incision since better exposure could be achieved especially when a resection is forthcoming. An extended grid incision usually ends by cutting into the rectal muscle medially and dividing muscles and inter-costal nerves laterally. The end result of this is often an incisional hernia and/or chronic pain. This can be avoided using the midline were a hernia is fare easier to repair and leaves the patient with less sequels.

27.9 Learning Curve

There are no studies to indicate the number of operations needed to become a skilled surgeon for LA. A total of 20 LA is attained in a few works of resident training in the Guidelines on LA from Italy [14]. Initial experience of laparoscopic surgery in an elective setting is of course of main importance to become skilled also in an emergency setting. The learning curve is always individual, but a thorough mentorship is mandatory around the lock in order to keep up the quality of LA. One suggestion is to have an official license at the department in two steps, first for DL followed by a second for LA. This is a successful tool used in our department for years. This licence system increases confidence for the competence of the operating surgeon for staff members at OR, for the resident and for the surgeon on call.

27.10 New Techniques

Single Incision Laparoscopic Surgery (SILS) using a special multiport umbilical trocar is an increasing trend with the aim to reduce trauma to the abdominal wall by having just one trocar site. The technique is basically the same as ordinary LA to the price of loss of triangulation, need of special instruments and higher costs. There is no difference in outcome demonstrated in a meta-analysis by Pisanu et al. [15]. Caution on interpreting the results should be taken since the results are based mainly on observational studies.

Natural Orifice Transluminal Endoscopic Surgery (NOTES) must be regarded as experimental surgery so far. In a European register, “EURO-NOTES”, 33 appendectomies were reported to be performed either trans-gastric or trans-vaginal [16].

27.11 Postoperative Care

Naso-gastric tube and Foley catheter could usually be removed after finishing the operation. Antibiotics and trombo-embolic treatment postoperative should follow local routines. Patients are normally put back on oral diet the day after operation if no contraindication has been identified. Patients with a phlegmonous or non perforated appendix can usually leave the hospital within 24 h after operation. Information on the operation and on the risk of complications should be carefully explained. Follow up is performed following the routines of the department.

Patients in need of intravenous antibiotics or having had a serious infection would need hospital care until recovery. Postoperative ileus is often seen in these patients. In prolonged fever, deep infection should be suspected, and an US should be performed and a drainage be inserted if appropriate. Scenarios on complications could be numerous and needs to be handled from the clinical situation.

References

1. Semm K. Endoscopic appendectomy. Endoscopy. 1983;15(2):59–64.
2. Ohtani H, Tamamori Y, Arimoto Y, Nishiguchi Y, Maeda K, Hirakawa K. Meta-analysis of the results of randomized controlled trials that compared laparoscopic and open surgery for acute appendicitis. J Gastrointest Surg. 2012;16(10):1929–39.
3. Markar SR, Blackburn S, Cobb R, Karthikesalingam A, Evans J, Kinross J, Faiz O. Laparoscopic versus open appendectomy for complicated and uncomplicated appendicitis in children. J Gastrointest Surg. 2012;16(10):1993–2004.
4. Southgate E, Vousden N, Karthikesalingam A, Markar SR, Black S. Zaidi A Laparoscopic vs open appendectomy in older patients. Arch Surg. 2012;147(6):557–62.
5. Woodham BL, Cox MR, Eslick GD. Evidence to support the use of laparoscopic over open appendicectomy for obese individuals: a meta-analysis. Surg Endosc. 2012;26(9):2566–70.
6. Korndorffer Jr JR, Fellinger E, Reed W. SAGES guideline for laparoscopic appendectomy. Surg Endosc. 2010;24(4):757–61.
7. Wilasrusmee C, Sukrat B, McEvoy M, Attia J, Thakkinstian A. Systematic review and meta-analysis of safety of laparoscopic versus open appendicectomy for suspected appendicitis in pregnancy. Br J Surg. 2012;99(11):1470–8.
8. Andersson M, Andersson RE. The appendicitis inflammatory response score: a tool for the diagnosis of acute appendicitis that outperforms the Alvarado score. World J Surg. 2008;32:1843–9.
9. Mayol J, Gaarcia-Aguilar J, Ortiz-Oshiro E, De Diego CJ, Fernandex-Represa JA. Risk of the minimal access approach for laparoscopic surgery: multivariate analysis of morbidity related to umbilical trocar insertion. World J Surg. 1997;21:529–33.
10. Moberg AC, Montgomery A. Primary access-related complications with laparoscopy: comparison of blind and open techniques. Surg Endosc. 2005;19(9):1196–9.
11. Moberg AC, Petersson U, Montgomery A. An open access technique to create pneumoperitoneum in laparoscopic surgery. Scand J Surg. 2007;96(4):297–300.
12. Moberg AC, Ahlberg G, Leijonmarck CE, Montgomery A, Reiertsen O, Rosseland AR, Stoerksson R. Diagnostic laparoscopy in 1043 patients with suspected acute appendicitis. Eur J Surg. 1998;164(11):833–40.
13. Van den Broek WT, Bijnen AB, De Riuter P, Gouma DJ. A normal appendix found during laparoscopy should not be removed. Br J Surg. 2001;88:251–3.
14. Vettoretto N, Gogg S, Corradi A, Belli F, Piccolo D, Pernazza G, Mannino L. Italian Association of Hospital Surgeons (Associazione dei Chirurghi Ospedalieri Italiani). Consensus conference on laparoscopic appendectomy: development of guidelines. Colorectal Dis. 2011;13(7):748–54.
15. Pisanu A, Porceddu G, Reccia I, Saba A, Uccheddu A. Meta-analysis of studies comparing single-incision laparoscopic appendectomy and conventional multiport laparoscopic appendectomy. J Surg Res. 2013;183(2):e49–59. doi:pii: S0022-4804(13)00232-1.
16. Arezzo A, Zornig C, Mofid H, Fuchs KH, Breithaupt W, Noguera J, Kaehler G, Magdeburg R, Perretta S, Dallemagne B, Marescaux J, Copaescu C, Graur F, Szasz A, Forgione A, Pugliese R, Buess G, Bhattacharjee HK, Navarra G, Godina M, Shishin K, Morino M. The EURO-NOTES clinical registry for natural orifice transluminal endoscopic surgery: a 2-year activity report. Surg Endosc. 2013;27(9):3073–84. PMID:23519494.

Laparoscopic Right Colectomy

28

Luigi Boni, Giulia David, and Elisa Cassinotti

28.1 Introduction

Jacobs et al. first reported a case of laparoscopic right colectomy was in 1991. Since then several reports, large series and randomized controlled trials proved that laparoscopic right colectomy is equal to open surgery in terms of oncological results. Furthermore, minimally invasive approach to right colon has also been proved safe and feasible for benign disease. Recent data also demonstrated that the laparoscopic approach has several advantages in comparison to open techniques including shorter postoperative stay, lesser use of analgesia, shorter postoperative ileus, reduction in wound related complications and incisional hernia rate and faster return to normal life activities.

28.2 Indications

The indications for laparoscopic right colectomy are the same as for open surgery, including malignant disease, benign polyps not suitable for endoscopic resection, inflammatory bowel disease, bleeding from arterovenous malformations, obstruction and cecal volvulus and diverticular disease of the right colon.

28.3 Contraindications

There are no absolute contraindications to laparoscopic right colectomy other than those related to specific patient's conditions such as advanced pregnancy, uncorrectable coagulopathy, increased intracranial pressure, severe congestive heart failure, respiratory insufficiency, severe chronic liver disease and all the other general contraindications to laparoscopic surgery. Locally advanced stage of disease it is not a contraindication itself unless peritoneal carcinomatosis, suitable for peritonectomy and intraoperative chemotherapy, is present.

28.4 Preoperative Work-Up

During preoperative colonoscopy tattooing of small lesions is recommended especially for tumors located at some distance from the cecum in order to be sure of exact site and the level of lymphadenectomy (see ahead). Contrast enhanced abdominal CT scan has to be performed in order to complete the preoperative staging hence to identify liver metastases and to evaluate the T stage of the tumor, especially to demonstrate duodenal infiltration. Preoperative evaluation will include routine blood test, carcinoembryonic antigen (CEA) in case of malignant disease, electrocardiogram and chest X-ray. Bowel preparation is not recommended but patient has to be on low fiber diet at least 1 week before surgery. Barium enema should be given the night before surgery in case of constipation. Prophylactic IV antibiotics should be administered according local hospital policy. Compressive stocking should be applied to prevent deep venous thrombosis. Foley catheter is placed in a sterile manner and, once oral-tracheal anesthesia is completed, temporary oro-gastric tube should be placed in order to empty the stomach and prevent aspiration. Venous central line is usually not required since fast-track post-operative protocol and early oral intake will be applied.

28.5 General Operative Settings

The patient is placed in supine position with left arm alongside the body. Security devices, such as belts and shoulder holders, will guarantee body position during the procedure

L. Boni, MD, FACS (✉) • E. Cassinotti, MD
Minimally Invasive Surgery Research Center,
University of Insubria, Azienda Ospedaliero Universitaria,
Fondazione Macchi, Varese, Italy
e-mail: luigi.boni@uninsubria.it

G. David, MD
Minimally Invasive Surgery Center, Department of Surgical and Morphological Sciences, University of Insubria, Varese, Italy

H.J. Bonjer (ed.), *Surgical Principles of Minimally Invasive Procedures*, DOI 10.1007/978-3-319-43196-3_28

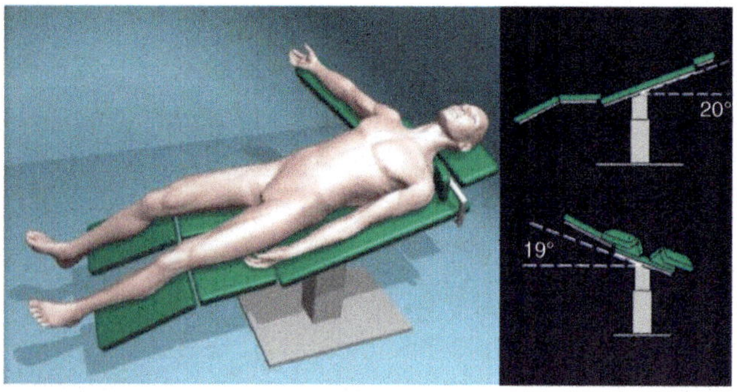

Fig. 28.1 Patient's position for right colectomy

(Fig. 28.1). In selected cases (i.e. female patients where transvaginal specimen extraction is scheduled or patients with hepatic or proximal transverse colon lesions where extensive middle colic artery dissection is recommended) lithotomy position should be preferred.

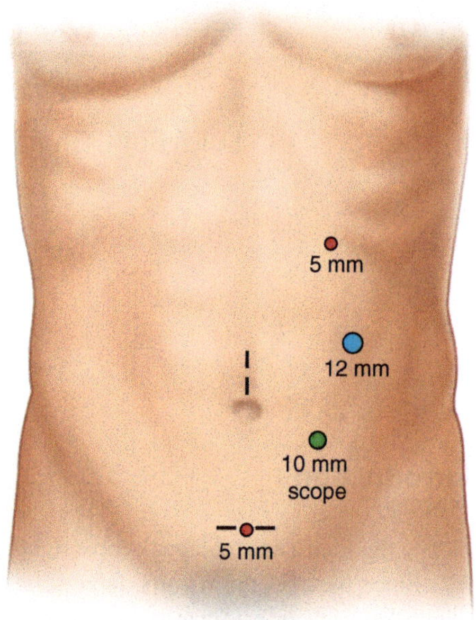

Fig. 28.2 Trocar position

28.6 Instrumentation

Instruments required for laparoscopic right colectomy are:

- 30° 10 or 5 mm scope
- High definition camera
- CO_2 insufflator
- Light source
- High frequency generator
- Advanced energy source (according to surgeon's preference)
- One 12 mm, one 10 mm and two 5 mm trocars
- Atraumatic forceps
- Hook
- Scissors
- Suction and irrigation device
- Clip applier
- 60 mm articulated linear stapler and cartridges
- Needle holders
- Retrieval endoscopic bag
- Wound protector

28.7 Surgical Technique

Patient is prepped with iodine or alcohol based solution from half to the chest to the sovra-pubic abdominal area; sterile drapes are place and secured. The main monitor or the laparoscopic tower is placed on the right side of the bed, towards patient's shoulder and adjusted according to surgeon's preferences.

The operating surgeon, the camera holder as well as the assistant stand on the patient's left side, while the scrub nurse on the right. Pneumoperitoneum is induce either with Veres needle (place in the left subcostal region) or with open approach for the first 10 mm port (or 5 mm in case 5 mm scope is used) that is inserted in the left flank 1 cm below the umbilicus along the left middle clavicular line. The remaining trocars are placed under direct vision as follows (Fig. 28.2):

- 12 mm trocar, for the right hand of the surgeon, in left upper quadrant, along the left mid-clavicular line, 5 cm below the costal margin
- 5 mm trocar, for the left hand of the surgeon, in the sovra-pubic quadrant
- 5 mm trocar, for the assistant, under left costal margin

28.8 Surgical Steps

Once the trocars are placed the patient is placed in mild reverse Trendelenburg position tilted to the left side in order to move most of the small bowel in the left iliac fossa, exposing the mesentery of the right colon. Procedure begins with exploration of the abdominal cavity in order to assess the feasibility of laparoscopic procedure, to identify the tumor (whether it could be located on the caecum, on the ascending colon or on the hepatic flexure) and to search for macroscopic peritoneal deposits or superficial hepatic metastases. The assistant will gently grab the transverse colon and the

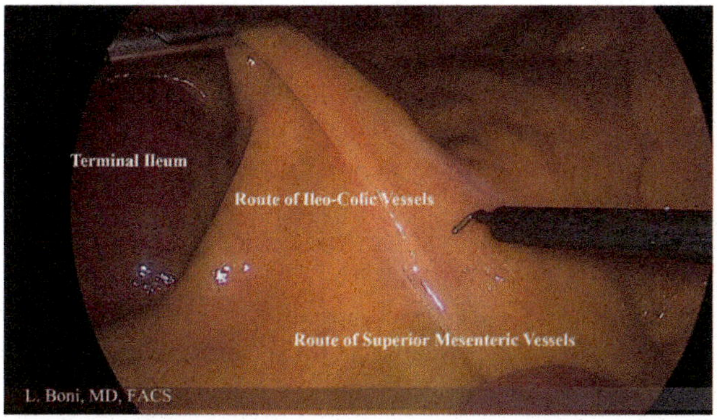

Fig. 28.3 Exposure of the ileo-colic pedicle

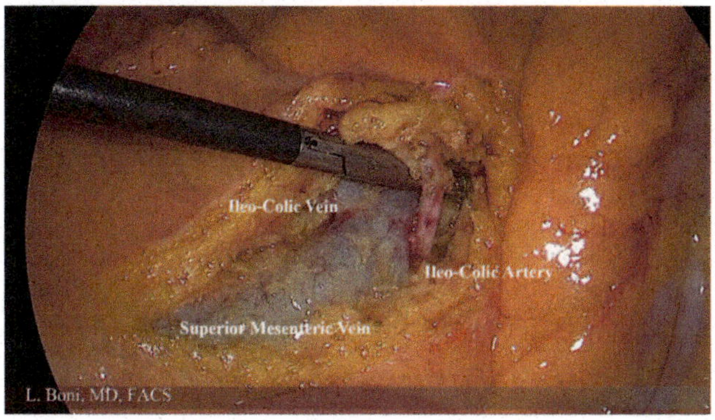

Fig. 28.4 High Ligation of ileo-colic vessels

omentum and will move it upwards exposing the caecum, the terminal ileum and the axis of the superior mesenteric artery which will be an useful landmark for the first part of the procedure. The surgeon, using an atrumatic forceps in his left hand, retracts the mesocolon of the ascending colon anteriorly and laterally in order to lift the pedicle of the ileocolic vessels (Fig. 28.3). At this point using a hook monopolar the peritoneum at the level of the origin of ileocolic vessels from superior mesenteric axis is dissected and ileocolic artery and vein are isolated and divided between clips. During this phase of the procedure, in order to achieve a complete lymphadenectomy, at least the superior mesenteric vein should be partially exposed (Fig. 28.4). After the division of ileocolic vessels, the duodenum is identified and gently detached from the mesentery of the right colon.

At this point, following the route of the superior mesenteric vessels upwards, towards the transverse colon, the lymphadenectomy is completed; during this phase, if present, the right colic vessels can be divided using an advanced energy source. In case of tumor located at the level of the cecum/ascending colon, the main trunk of the middle colic artery can be preserved while its right branch is clipped and divided (Fig. 28.5). On the other hand, for tumor of the hepatic flexure/proximal transverse colon, the middle colic artery should be dissected, clipped and divided at its origin. Procedure carries on with dissection of the

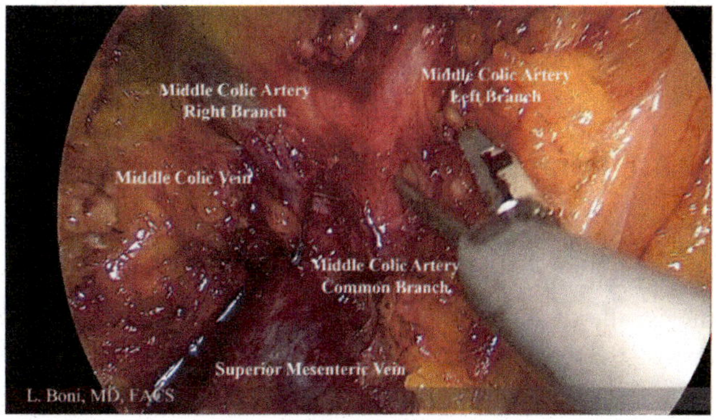

Fig. 28.5 Exposure of the middle colic pedicle

Toldt's fascia that separates the right mesocolon from the retroperitoneal organs. The surgeon, lifting the ileocolic pedicle with his left hand, gently proceeds with dissection along an avascular plane pushing down the Toldt's fascia preserving the retroperitoneal structures such as the second and third duodenal portions, the head of the pancreas and the right kidney. The right ureter and gonadal vessels lie underneath the fascia, so if dissection is made along the correct plane, there is no need to identify them. Following the avascular plane up to the transverse colon, the mesentery is finally opened, exposing the liver surface. At this point the gastrocolic ligament is put under tension by the assistant on one side and by the left hand of the surgeon on the other side and it is divided medial to lateral toward the right colic flexure. Procedure carries on with transection of the transverse colon using an articulated linear stapler choosing the cartridge according to tissue thickness. The assistant gently retracts upwards the ileocolic pedicle in order to expose the mesentery of the terminal ileum; that will be divided approximately 5 cm from the ileo-caecal valve. Marginal arteries are cauterized with advanced energy device. The terminal ileum is then transected using surgical stapler. By applying traction on the divided ileum, full mobilization of the lateral attachments is carried out, from the cecum up to the transverse colon. In case of "difficult" hepatic flexure it might be useful to complete the mobilization starting from the transected transverse colon towards the ascending.

The specimen is then inserted into an endobag and temporarily placed above the liver; the surgical field is checked for hemostasis.

28.9 Anastomosis

The restoration of bowel continuity can be performed intra or extracorporeally depending on surgeon's preferences. Nevertheless intracorporeal approach carries several advantages such as the possibility to choose the most suitable extraction site, including the transvaginal route, reduced risk of torsion of the small bowel, limited tension to the mesentery that could lead to bleeding as well as a smaller abdominal incision.

28.9.1 Intracorporeal Anastomosis

The ileum is approximated to the transverse colon in order to perform an intracorporeal isoperistaltic side to side anastomosis; the assistant will help holding the bowel to better expose the two segments in front of the surgeon. During this phase it is recommended to remove the bed tilting and the reverse Trendelemburg position. Using monopolar hook two small enterotomies are created on the antimesenteric edge of the ileum and on the free taenia of transverse colon. An articulated linear stapler is introduced through the 12 mm port and gently advanced on both sides of the bowel through the enterotomies (Fig. 28.6).

Anastomosis is checked for bleeding and the bowel defect is closed with a two layers running suture with absorbable material. Specimen is then extracted through a sovrapubic mini-Pfannestiel incision (performed including the sovrapubic port site) using a wound protector or, in selected female patients, performing a colpotomy on the posterior aspect of the vagina.

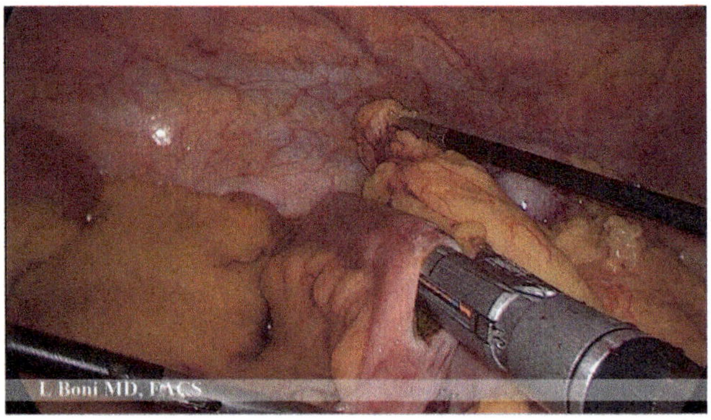

Fig. 28.6 Intracorporeal side to side anastomosis

28.9.2 Extracorporeal Anastomosis

In those cases where extracorporeal anastomosis is performed, the pneumoperitoneum should be reduced gradually in order to choose the most suitable location for the mini-laparotomy according to the position of the transverse colon, that most of the time will be sovraumbilical, along the midline. Since accidental twisting of the small bowel has been reported after extracorporeal anastomosis, the terminal ileum and transverse colon can be approximated intracorporeally and fixed with stay sutures. At this point the mini-laparotomy is carried out, the specimen is extracted after positioning of a wound protector and the ileum and transverse colon previously fixed are exteriorized. Ileo-colic side to side isoperistaltic mechanical anastomosis is then performed according to surgeon's preferences.

Suggested Reading

Zollinger RM, Ellison EC. Zollinger's atlas of surgical operations. 9th ed. Copyright © 2011 by The McGraw-Hill Companies, Inc. – plate 69.

Lee KH, Ho J, Akmal Y, Nelson R, Pigazzi A. Short- and long-term outcomes of intracorporeal versus extracorporeal ileocolic anastomosis in laparoscopic right hemicolectomy for colon cancer. Surg Endosc. 2013;27(6):1986–90.

Cirocchi R, Trastulli S, Farinella E, Guarino S, Desiderio J, Boselli C, Parisi A, Noya G, Slim K. Intracorporeal versus extracorporeal anastomosis during laparoscopic right hemicolectomy-systematic review and meta-analysis. Surg Oncol. 2013;22(1):1–13.

Milone M, Elmore U, Di Salvo E, Delrio P, Bucci L, Ferulano GP, Napolitano C, Angiolini MR, Bracale U, Clemente M, D'ambra M, Luglio G, Musella M, Pace U, Rosati R, Milone F. Intracorporeal versus extracorporeal anastomosis. Results from a multicentre comparative study on 512 right-sided colorectal cancers. Surg Endosc. 2015;29(8):2314–20. doi:10.1007/s00464-014-3950-7. Epub 2014 Nov 21.

Young-Fadok TM, Nelson H. Laparoscopic right colectomy: five-step procedure. Dis Colon Rectum. 2000;43(2):267–71.

Boni L, Dionigi G, Cassinotti E, Di Giuseppe M, Diurni M, Rausei S, Cantore F, Dionigi R. Single incision laparoscopic right colectomy. Surg Endosc. 2010;24(12):3233–6.

Left Colectomy and Sigmoidectomy

29

A.M. Lacy and M. Fernández-Hevia

29.1 Introduction

Laparoscopic surgery has emerged as the procedure of choice for many intrabdominal disease processes. At the beginning laparoscopy was used for diagnostic purposes. Surgical technology development allowed to perform therapeutic procedures as laparoscopic appendectomy was originally described by Semm in the early 1980s.

It was not until, Muhe in Germany in 1985 and Mouret in France in 1987 described laparoscopic cholecystectomy that this approach did not acquire more interest. Next years other procedures were performed by laparoscopy as anti-reflux surgery, adrenalectomy, splenectomy, pancreatic surgery, liver resection or intestinal surgery. Fifteen years after first laparoscopic cholecystectomy, minimally invasive surgery became the preferred approach for treatment of symptomatic cholecystolithiasis, gastro- oesophageal reflux and morbid obesity.

Laparoscopic surgery offers numerous advantages when compared with the open procedures, including less postoperative pain and ileus, reduced perioperative immunosuppression, decreased hospital stay, improved cosmesis and earlier return to normal activity.

The development of laparoscopic techniques in colorectal surgery represents try to decrease the morbidity associated with colorectal procedures. In 1991, Jacobs et al reported a successful laparoscopic sigmoidectomy for cancer. Laparoscopic colectomy for cancer was not readily accepted: the safety of the procedure was questioned because of early reports of port-site metastases. Trials randomizing patients with colon cancer to laparoscopic assisted surgery or open resection have evaluated the oncological safety of this approach. Different trials as COLOR, COST, CLASSIC or Barcelona trials have shown short and long-term outcomes and have demonstrated colectomy by laparoscopy for cancer is oncologically safe. Laparoscopic colectomy is associated with improved convalescence and decreased morbidity compared with open resection [1–5].

29.2 Indications

The indications of laparoscopic sigmoidectomy/left colectomy are the same as open surgery. It exists different issues that can affect this part of the colon as tumors, diverticulosis, inflammatory disease, sigmoid volvulus (Table 29.1).

It could be divided into two groups elective and emergency events. In emergency procedures the incidence of stoma increases. In patients with stenosant tumors that have an occlusion an alternative could be to use a stent, as a bridge to an elective surgery. If the stent is not possible, an emergency colostomy or a resection, depending on the extension of the lesion, could be performed.

29.3 Preoperative Work-Up

A detailed history and physical examination is required, it is important to know familiar history. Special value has previous surgery as well as previous pathology that can limit laparoscopic surgery, as cardiac or pulmonary problems.

Complementary studies:

- *Colonoscopy*. Represents the optimal method of diagnosis, giving information about the location, allowing to perform biopsies and if it is necessary doing an ink tattoo. If the colonoscopy is not complete, a virtual colonoscopy can be done (colono-CT), because it helps us to dismiss injuries in proximal colon bigger than 6 mm–1 cm. In small lesions, (i.e. tumor occupying less than a half of the circumference) it is recommended to perform an ink tattoo for intraoperative location. Other possibility is perform the colonoscopy intraoperatively if the injury is not detected

A.M. Lacy (✉) • M. Fernández-Hevia
Department of Surgery, Hospital Clinic, University of Barcelona, Barcelona, Spain
e-mail: alacy@clinic.ub.es

H.J. Bonjer (ed.), *Surgical Principles of Minimally Invasive Procedures*, DOI 10.1007/978-3-319-43196-3_29

Table 29.1 Indications of left hemicolectomy/sigmoidectomy

Colorectal cancer
Diverticulitis and diverticular disease
Inflammatory bowel disease (ulcerative, Crohn's disease)
Ischaemic colitis
Iatrogenic (perforation after colonoscopy, surgery…)
Sigmoid volvulus
Trauma
Other tumors (GIST)
Endometriosis

during the procedure, but we considerer that the best option is having the lesion located previously. In the case of benign disease it is necessary to discard malignancy.

- Thorax and abdominal computed tomography (CT). They must be performed to complete extension study in malignant lesions. It is useful to evaluate possible distance metastasis, local organ invasion and the situation of the tumor. In colitis or diverticulitis, it will help us to evaluate acute complications (abscesses, pneumoperitoneum, fistula, pneumatosis, peritonitis).
- Liver MRI. If there is any suspicious lesion in the CT scan.
- PET. Only if there is any doubt of possible metastasis.
- Contrast enema: It can be useful to localizing the lesion or extension in diverticular disease. It is not indispensable.
- Preoperative study. Blood test (liver function, coagulation test and carcinoembryonic antigen-CEA), electrocardiogram, chest radiography and anaesthesiologist evaluation are necessary. Other tests will be performed if anaesthesiologist considers them.

In occluded patients with stenosant tumors, if possible, we consider using a stent to resolve the acute problem offering a posterior elective surgery. Insomuch as it is an option that decreases the need of stoma.

The day previous surgery, anterograde lavage can be performed although there are multiple reports against this procedure. It is commendatory administrate prophylactic antibiotics (i.e. cefoxitin 2 g) intravenously 1 h before beginning surgery.

29.4 Operating Room

Patient will be place in supine position, both arms adjusted at the body and both legs are open, stirrups can be use but there are not necessary. Lower extremity pneumatic compression stockings are used in all cases and in high-risk patients they will be maintained during postoperative period. The patient will be fixed to the table to try to avoid displacements of the patient during the procedure. An orogastric tube and a Foley catheter are used in all cases. Peripheral intravenous lines are used and a central catheter will be used in relation with patient's morbidity. General endotracheal anaesthesia with pharmacologic paralysis is required.

The rectum is irrigated with 1 % diluted iodine solution. The patient is prepared and drapped sterile.

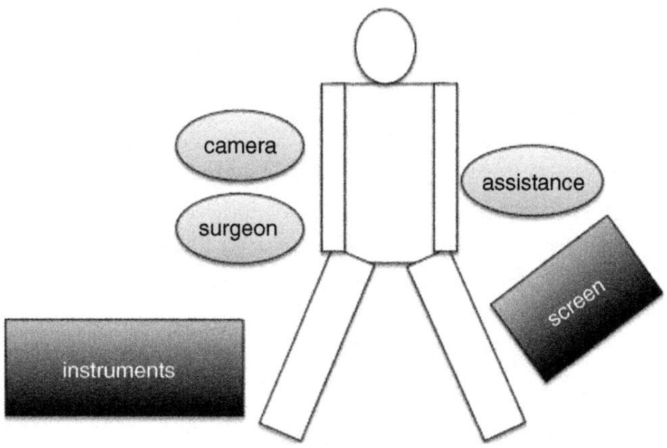

Fig. 29.1 Position in the operating room during sigmoidectomy

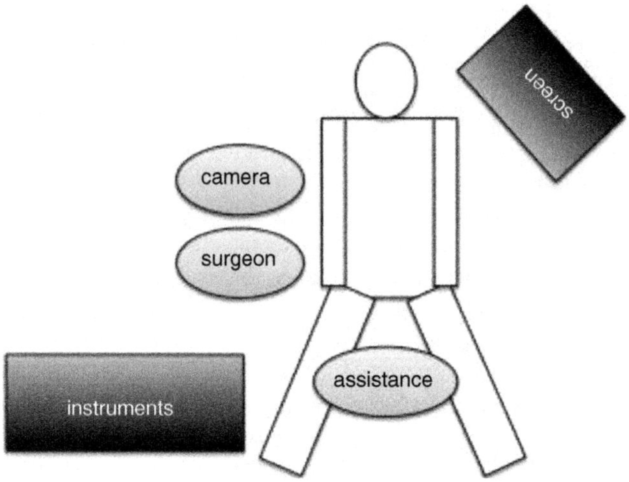

Fig. 29.2 Position in the operating room during splenic flexure mobilization

29.5 Surgical Technique

The screen will be positioned next to left leg of the patient. In Fig. 29.1 we can see the disposition of the surgeon, camera, assistance and the nurse in the operating room. Figure 29.2 shows the disposition if it is necessary mobilization of splenic flexure.

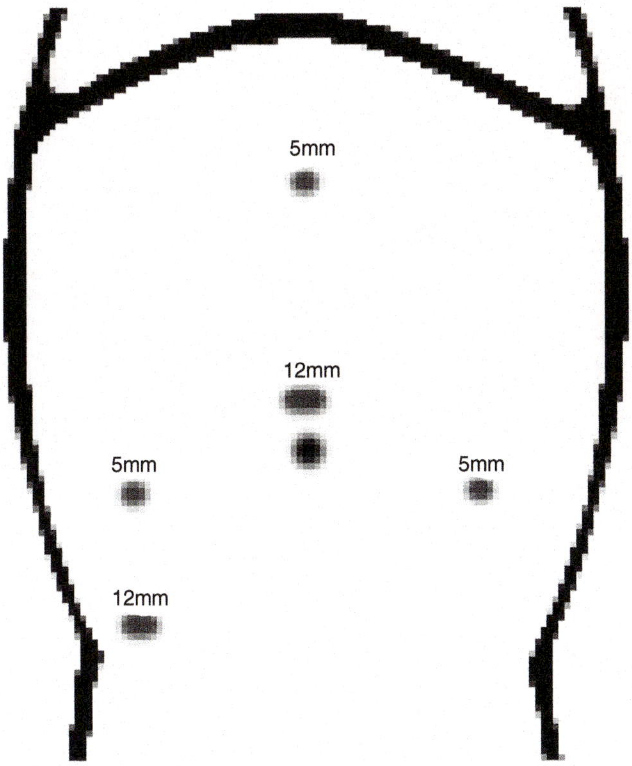

Fig. 29.3 Placement of the ports during sigmoidectomy

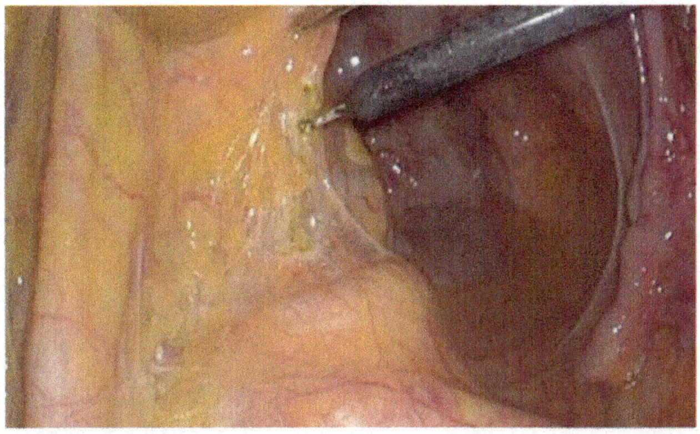

Fig. 29.4 Opening peritoneum of the mesosigma

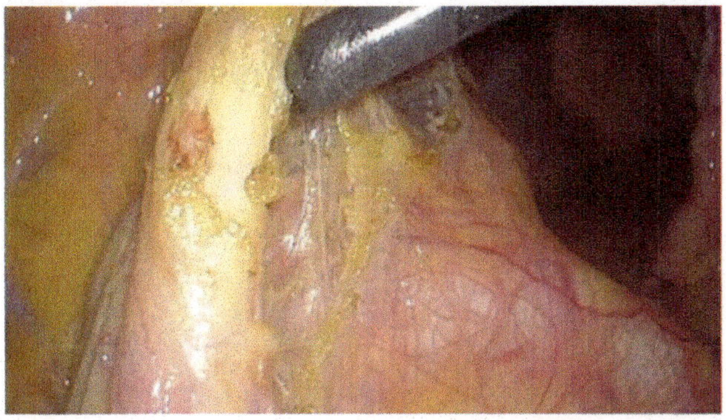

Fig. 29.5 Dissection of inferior mesenteric artery (IMA). In malignant disease a high ligation will be performed, though it is not necessary in benign processes

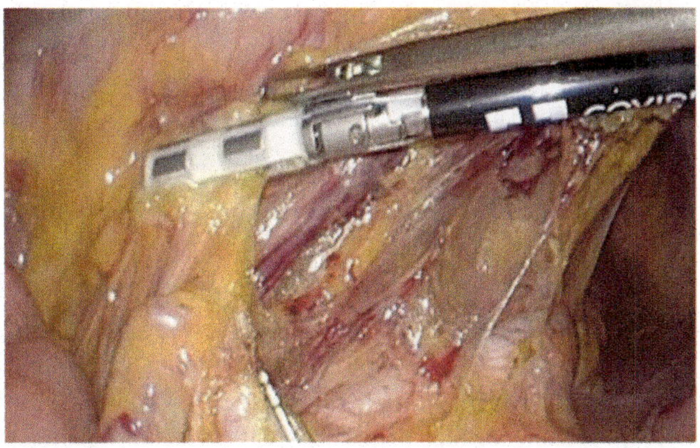

Fig. 29.6 In the image it is possible appreciate the section of IMA between clips and the section of the vein using a coagulation device (LigaSure, Covidien, Ireland)

29.5.1 Operative Technique

The abdomen is insufflated to a pressure of 15 mmHg via a Veres needle inserted through the umbilicus or left upper quadrant. A 12 mm port is inserted through the umbilicus, 0° or 30° angled scope can be used, preferring last one if it is needed mobilization of splenic flexure. Abdominal exploration is compulsory to discard disease progression or other processes.

After that the other ports will be inserted under direct view. A 12 mm port is inserted in the lower right quadrants, a 5 mm port at right side and a 5 mm port at low left quadrant. If it is necessary mobilize the splenic flexure, it could be used a 5 mm port at epigastrium. The position of the ports can be seen in Fig. 29.3. Patients are placed in Trendelenburg position and right side, which facilitates exposure of the pelvis and low left quadrant.

- Releasing adhesions between sigmoid colon and other organs or the wall.
- Identify inferior mesenteric vessels (IMV). Sigmoid and left colon mobilization can be performed medial to lateral or lateral to medial how it is performed usually in open left colectomy. In the medial to lateral mobilization we start with the section of IMV (Fig. 29.4).
- Laparoscopic graspers (port low left quadrant) are used to retract and aid the dissection of the rectosigmoid and expose the vascular pedicle. Once IMV are identified, the peritoneum of sigmoid mesocolon is opened distally to them progressing the dissection. The IMV are transected closest to the base to respect oncologic principles. The vessels can be divided with vascular endostapler, ligation, clips, or a coagulator device (Figs. 29.5 and 29.6). Previous the transection it is recommended

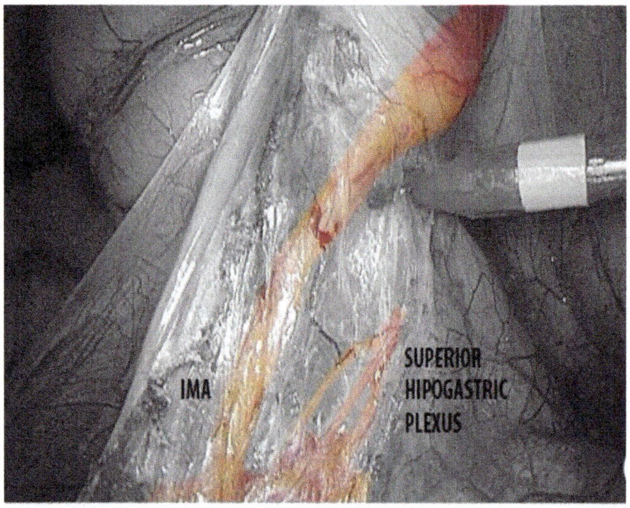

Fig. 29.7 Relation between the inferior mesentery artery (IMA) and the superior hipogastric plexus

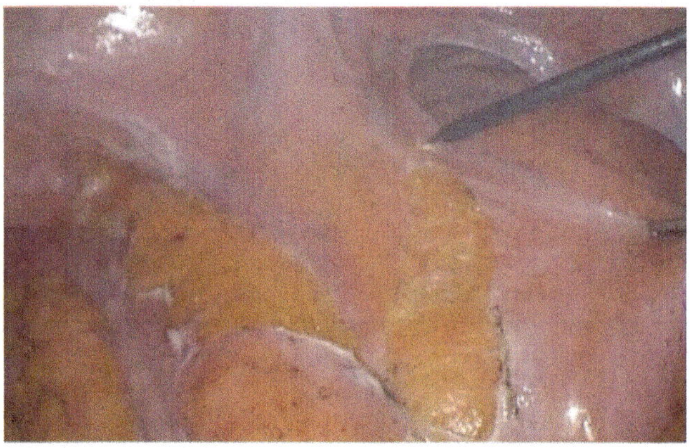

Fig. 29.8 The left paracolic gutter opens to complete the mobilization initiated from medial

identify left gonadal vessels and the ureter if the retroperitoneum has not been respected. It is important be careful during a high dissection of inferior mesentery artery (IMA) to avoid injuries in the superior hipogastric plexus (Fig. 29.7). In benign disease vascular ligation could be performed distally.

- A tip is using a gauze in this step putting it over the ureter and retroperitoneum, when left paracolic gutter will be opened we will find the gauze that will be protecting retroperitoneum. The remaining mesentery is dissected and sectioned by a coagulation device. The dissection progresses by an avascular plane until splenic flexure. In this plane we can find in the posterior part Gerota's fascia, superior part mesocolon and medially the ligament of TReitz and Aorta. The inferior mesenteric vein can be transected in its base if it is necessary.
- The left paracolic gutter opens to complete the mobilization initiated from medial (Fig. 29.8).

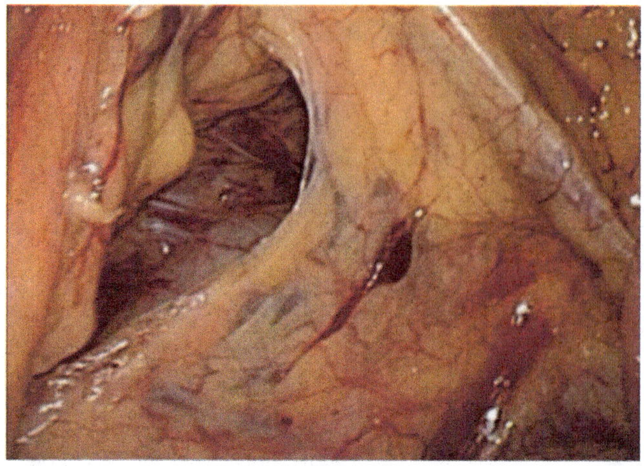

Fig. 29.9 Dissection of transverse mesocolon, through the hole of the mesocolon it is possible see posterior side of the greater curvature and the lesser sac

- Distally, sigmoid colon will be mobilized until promontory where the colon will be prepared to the transection with endostapler. Sometimes reticulating linear staplers can be used, some surgeons use a suprapubic port which can facilitate division of the rectosigmoid.
- If the length of the colon is not enough to perform the anastomosis, it will be required mobilization of splenic flexure.
- If the lesion is near splenic flexure or its mobilization is needed, a 5 mm port is inserted in the epigastrium. Patient has to be positioned in anti-Trendelenburg and the surgeon and assistants as Fig. 29.2. If a segmentary resection can be performed, retraction of the left colon to the left and transverse colon cranially, will help us to start to show mesocolon at the level of the ligament of Treitz, we can identify inferior mesenteric vein and artery and their branches and decide which section. After section it, continuing the dissection medial to lateral in an avascular plane. If the dissection enters too deeply, it will have increased risk of bleeding. The cephalic border of the dissection is the caudal edge of the pancreas. One mistake can be dissection the posterior surface of the pancreas at this level. Once mesocolon is dissected, it is necessary access to the lesser sac, so grasper in epigastric trocar separates greater omentum cephalic and low right quadrant grasper pulls the transverse colon caudally, with a coagulation device open gastrocolic ligament and access to lesser sac. The dissection progresses to the spleen. Opening paracolic left gutter and communicating retroperitoneal dissection with lesser sac (Figs. 29.9 and 29.10).
- Exteriorization of the colon. An assistance incision can be used to exteriorize the colon, it can be a Pfannestiel incision, previous incisions as inferior laparotomy or

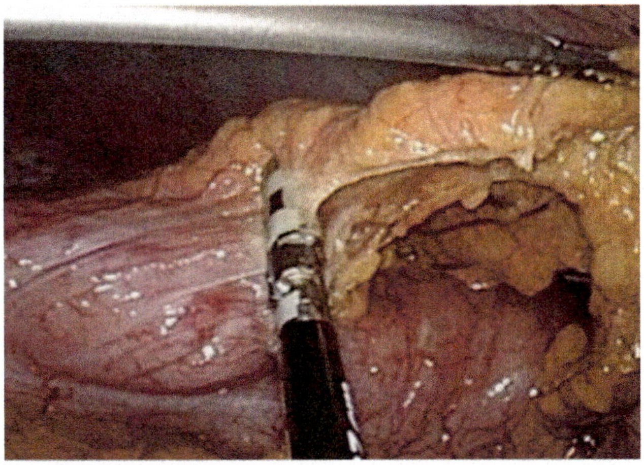

Fig. 29.10 Section of the omentum

extension of one of the ports. A wound protector is used to help prevent tumor cell implantation and possibly reduce the risk of post-operative wound infection. The colon is fixed with a grasper to facilitate the extraction. Once the colon is out, it is necessary decide where the transection will be performed, it depends on the ethiology. Protection of the operative field during the transection is mandatory to avoid gross contamination. After transection of the bowel, the specimen will be removed from the field. In function of the diameter of the colon, the size of the circular stapler will decide. A purse-string suture will be performed in proximal colon and the anvil will be inserted. After introducing the colon into the abdomen and removing wound protector, the closure of assistance incision is accomplished.

- In segmentation resection of the descending colon, extracorporeal anastomosis end-to-end or side-to-side can be performed.
- Re-establishing pneumoperitoneum. The patient is placed the patient in the Trendelenburg position, and bring the proximal colon with the anvil into the pelvis.
- Introduction of the circular stapler into the rectum if it is necessary dilate the anus. The progression and the opening of the circular stapler can be controlled by laparoscopy. Previous performing the anastomosis, it is required to confirm the colon is not twisted (by inspecting the cut edge of the mesocolon and by following the tenia libera) and there is not tension in the anastomosis after joining the anvil with the stapler, if it is satisfied the stapler can fire it. Extract the stapler and evaluate of the two anastomotic rings. The integrity of the anastomosis can be tested with saline or air while occluding the descending colon proximally.
- During all the procedure it has to be mandatory try to respect the marginal artery of the mesentery to avoid its injury, which can compromise the blood supply of the colon.
- A low-pressure aspirative drain can be placed next to the anastomosis.
- Careful review of the haemostasis and trocars under direct view. Aponeurosis will be closed in 12 mm trocars.

29.6 Postoperative Care

Nasogastric tube will be removed in the operating room. Low risk patients spend few hours in postoperative recovery unit and if there is no incidence after that will pass a hospitalization room. High risk patients must go to ICU. Mobilization is initiated the day after operation. Foley catheter will be remove first postoperative day. The drain will be removed second or third day in function of the output. Oral intake will begin after presenting peristaltism, remaining on a liquid diet for 24 h and progressing to hospital discharge with tolerance of a soft diet, it usually begins in the first 24 h. Analgesic will be taken by mouth when the diet is tolerated and in function of the level of pain. All previous drugs will be reintroduced before discharge. Ambulatory control will be performed 7–10 days after discharge.

The most common complication in these patients is ileus and catheter infection.

The most frightening complication is an anastomotic leak and could be necessary performing a stoma. One of the principles of colonic surgery to try to avoid anastomotic leak is perform an anastomosis with good vascularization and without tension. It is very important detect it early and treat it adequately. Another complication is bleeding.

References

1. Lacy AM, García-Valdecasas JC, Delgado S, Castells A, Taurá P, Piqué JM, Visa J. Laparoscopy-assisted colectomy versus open colectomy for treatment of non-metastatic colon cancer: a randomised trial. Lancet. 2002;359(9325):2224–9.
2. Lacy AM, Delgado S, Castells A, Prins HA, Arroyo V, Ibarzabal A, Pique JM. The long-term results of a randomized clinical trial of laparoscopy-assisted versus open surgery for colon cancer. Ann Surg. 2008;248(1):1–7.
3. Panis Y. Laparoscopic surgery for benign colorectal diseases. J Chir (Paris). 2000;137(5):261–7.
4. Franklin ME, Ramos R, Rosenthal D, Schussler W. Laparoscopic colonic procedures. World J Surg. 1993;17:51–6.
5. Leroy J. Laparoscopic colorectal resection. Technical aspects after 150 operations. Ops Maggiore. 1993;88:262–6.

Total Colectomy

30

Willem A. Bemelman

30.1 Introduction

The best laparoscopic approach to perform a total (procto) colectomy depends largely on patient characteristics, disease characteristics and the skill and experience of the surgeon. These three factors together direct towards the safest and most efficient procedure to remove the (procto)colon. There are a number of techniques that all resort under laparoscopic surgery ie. hand-assisted (procto)colectomy, total laparoscopic multiport (procto)colectomy, total laparoscopic single port (procto)colectomy. Specimen extraction can be done via a minilaparotomy (split incision, Pfannenstiehl incision, a vertical up and down transumbilical incision, transrectal/vaginal (Natural Orifice Specimen Extraction) and the future stoma site). If an anastomosis is performed ie. ileorectal or ileoanal, this can be done open via the minilaparotomy or laparoscopically. The hand-assisted and Single Port approaches are essentially dissections from lateral to medial making the procedures less suitable for oncologic indications. Multiport approaches are more suitable for medial to lateral dissection facilitating central vascular ligation with optimal lymphnode harvest and complete mesocolonic dissection aiming for an optimal oncologic specimen.

It need not to be emphasized that the more is done laparoscopically or with fewer ports, the difficulty of the procedure increases demanding more advanced skills from the surgeon. At the same time the required operating time and costs are rising. The available literature data point towards similar functional outcome of all these different types of laparoscopic procedures as long the incision to retrieve the specimen is limited. Converted patients, particularly the reactive as opposed to the strategic conversions do worse. It must be appreciated that the more complex the procedure the more sensitive the operation will be to complications.

W.A. Bemelman
Academic Medical Center, University of Amsterdam, Amsterdam, The Netherlands
e-mail: w.a.bemelman@amc.uva.nl

There are *various indications and circumstances* to perform a total colectomy or proctocolectomy. Emergency colectomy is mostly done for toxic colitis in inflammatory bowel disease (IBD), elective indications for (procto)colectomy are poliposis coli, heriditary non-poliposis syndromes and functional disorders like slow transit (colonic) obstipation. Most indications are therefore for benign disease, but malignancy might have developed in longstanding IBD, in hereditary cancer syndromes or sometimes a double colon cancer is present.

Lastly, but not the least, the *patients characteristics* will determine the type of laparoscopic approach. In an emergent setting, the procedure needs to be fast, efficient and safe. A hand-assist procedure is therefore advised. In an elective setting, the BMI and intra-abdominal fat dictates the most suitable procedure [1]. suggested to taper the type of procedure to the BMI of the patients; single port BMI<25, multiport colectomy 25<BMI<30, and hand-assist (procto)colectomy BMI>30.

This chapter will guide the reader in a stepwise approach of a hand-assist (procto)colectomy, multiport medial to lateral total laparoscopic (procto)colectomy and a Single Port total laparoscopic (procto)colectomy.

30.1.1 Choice and Rationale of the Minimal Invasive Approach

1. Hand-assist colectomy: emergency procedures, benign indications, limited time available, troublesome exposure (distended small bowel, abdominal obesity), in learning curve.
2. Multiport laparoscopic: elective surgery, oncologic procedures (medial to lateral), planned extraction via rectum or stoma site.
3. Single port: elective surgery, benign indications, good exposure (lean patient), future stoma site available for single port insertion and specimen extraction, required skills present.

H.J. Bonjer (ed.), *Surgical Principles of Minimally Invasive Procedures*, DOI 10.1007/978-3-319-43196-3_30

30.1.2 Preoperative Work-Up

Preoperative work-up is of particular importance in oncologic indications. The colorectal cancer need to be tattooed colonoscopically in order to identify the tumor during surgery. The draining mesentery of the tumour must be taken out completely in contrast to other parts of the colon that will removed. The abdomen and thorax have to be scanned to screen for distant disease.

30.1.3 Preoperative Preparations

It is for debate how to prepare the bowel. Since the total (procto)colon is taken out, a laxative enema will suffice to clean the distal bowel in case a ileosigmoidal/rectal or ileoanal anastomosis is planned. If a single port procedure is planned with extraction via a relatively small incision, bowel preparation is mandatory. A stool loaded bowel is difficult to extract. Others would prefer a full bowel preparation to increase exposure during the laparoscopic procedure.

30.1.4 Stepwise Approach

A. Hand-assisted colectomy:

1. Positioning: French position on a short beanbag. Left arm alongside the body (Fig. 30.1a)
2. Trocar and hand-port positioning: supraumbilical 10 mm (camera), left lower quadrant 11–12 mm (dissection, clip applier, endostapler) and 5 mm epigastrio (ultracision, grasper)
3. Suprapubic Pfannenstiehl incision with a length according to glove size (transverse incision skin, subcutis and anterior rectus sheet, mobilization anterior sheet from the rectus muscle, midline incision fascia transversalis, preperitoneal fat and peritoneum). Placement of the Alexis ring of the Applied Handport ™.
4. Open mobilization sigmoid: Slight Trendelenburg position. Removal of the small bowel out of the pelvis using a large gauze to keep it in the right upper abdomen. Mobilisation of the sigmoid via the Alexis ring as far as possible using diathermia, pick-ups and specula.
5. Insertion of trocars, pneumoperitoneum: Removal of the gauze. Placement of the supraumbilical trocar. Placement of the handport. Insufflation 12–15 mmHg pneumoperitoneum. Insertion of the non dominant hand and 30° videoscope. Insertion of the two additional trocars under direct vision.
6. Exposure: Lateral tilt to the right. With the hand the small bowel is removed to the right. The left colon is grasped with the left hand. The assistant inserts a 5 mm grasper via the epigastric trocar to retract the upper part of the left colon and later on the omentum.
7. Mobilisation left colon: Surgeon in between the legs. The assistant on the right side of the table. The left colon is mobilized from lateral to medial up to the flexure using ultracision inserted via the left lower trocar. It is important to stay on the mesentery and close to the bowel particularly at the splenic flexure.

   Pitfalls: (1). Damage to the ureter (2). The duodenum/jejunum at Treitz can easily be damaged because the colonic mesentery is very thin at that level. (3). It is important to stay on the bowel/colonic mesentery at the level of the left flexure in order to enter the lesser sac safely without damaging the pancreatic tail (Fig. 30.2).
8. Mobilization transverse colon. The assistant retracts the omentum. The omentum is dissected from the colon close to the colon. As long the colon is not perforated, there is no need to be very careful, because the colon will be taken out. Dissection is continued as far as possible from this position.

   Pitfalls: Due to adhesions in the lesser sac the greater curvature vessels are quite close to the colon. They might be damaged. If the patient is very thin, there is a danger taking all layers (omentum and transverse colon mesentery) at the same time.
9. Mobilisation right part of the transverse colon and right colon: The surgeon is now positioned on the left of the patient. The assistant stands in between the legs of the patient. Left lateral tilt. The small bowel is positioned in the left part of the abdomen. The dissection on the colon is continued on the right part of the transverse colon. It is important to visualize the duodenum by blunt dissection. The lateral attachments are taken close to the bowel in order to avoid the gonadal vessels and the right ureter. The left hand retracts the transverse colon/right colon and protects at the same time the small bowel. The hand guides safe dissection with the ultracision. The tip of the device can become very hot!
10. Vascular ligation:

    Once the right colon is mobilized the transverse colon is grasped with the four fingers and thumb. The fingers under the mesentery push the mesentery up thereby exposing the branches of the middle colics (Fig. 30.1). Using 5 mm clips and ultracision the vessels can be taken one by one starting at the window in the mesentery of the transverse colon left to the left branch of the middle colic artery. The mesentery of the right colon must be secured close to the bowel particularly at

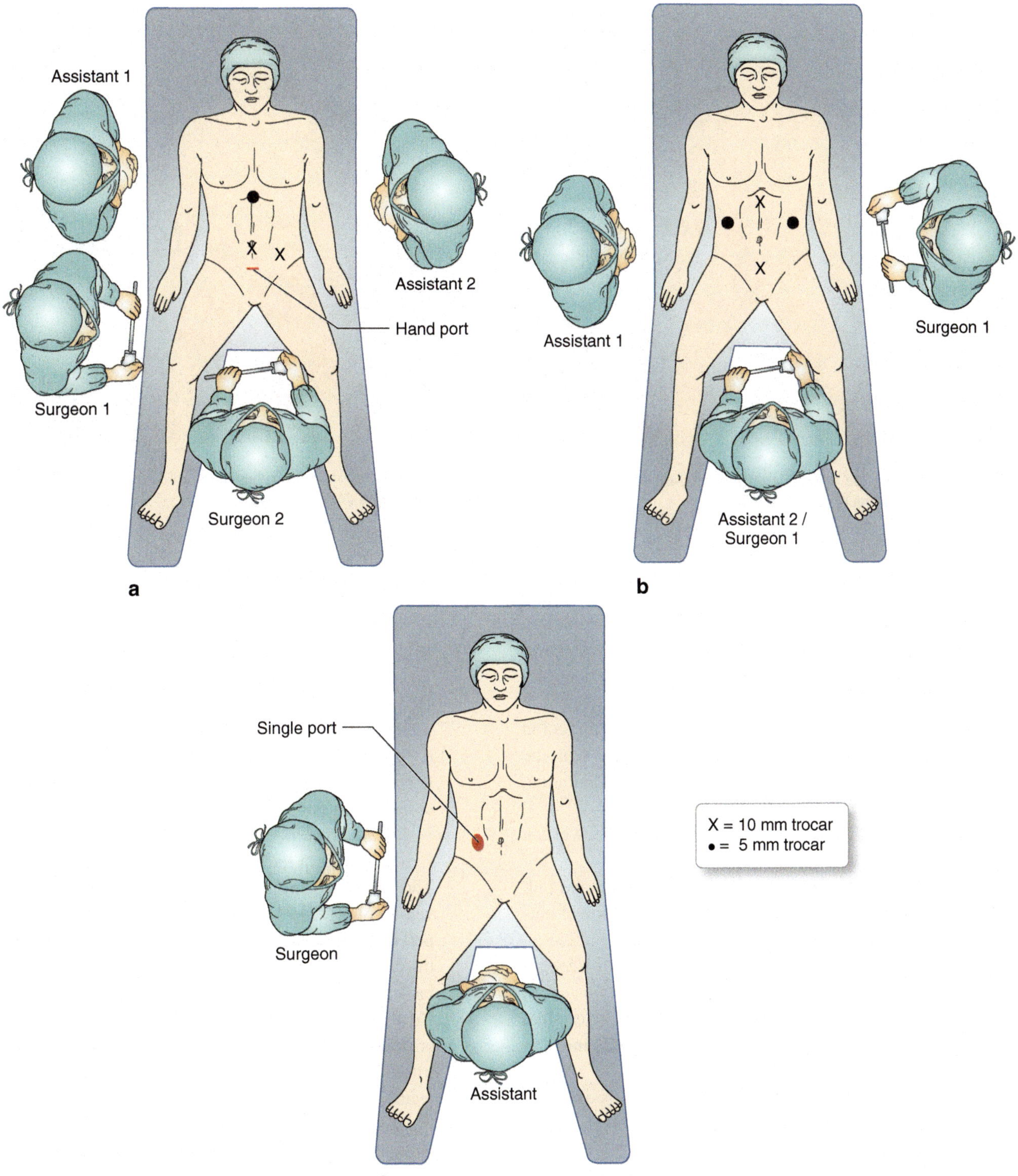

Fig. 30.1 Patient position and trocars (**a**) Handport, (**b**) Multiport, (**c**) Single port

the ileocolic junction. Here a number of large terminal branches are mostly present. Close to the bowel the vessels are easily taken by the ultracision. The terminal ileum is cleaned from its mesentery and transected with an endostapler (blue cartridge).

11. The position of the team is once more changed in order to deal with the mesentery of the left colon. The surgeon moves back to the position between the legs. The assistant to the right of the patient. The table is tilted back to the right to remove the small bowel from the left to the right. The mesentery is

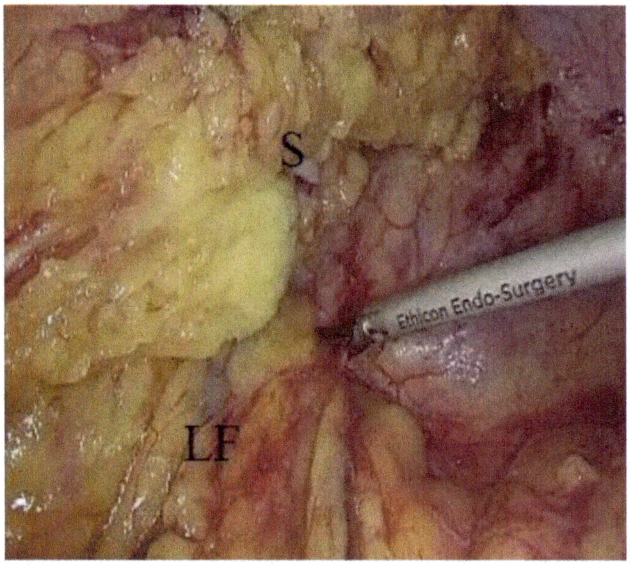

Fig. 30.2 Entering the lesser sac during hand-assist mobilisation of the left colon (*S* stomach, *LF* left flexure)

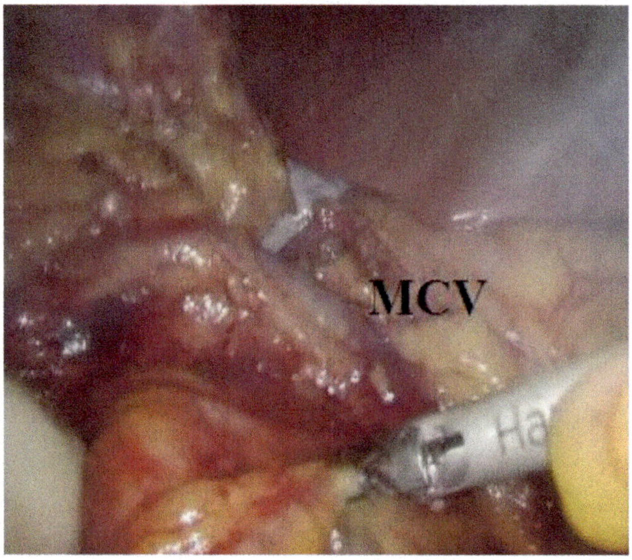

Fig. 30.3 Exposure of the branches of the middle colic vessels using the hand (*MCV* mid colic vessels)

taken starting at the rectosigmoid junction working towards the mesentery of the left transverse colon to complete the vascular ligation. Close to the bowel the ultracision is generally sufficient, more centrally clips can be placed to have more security.

12. Extraction. It is important before pulling the colon out to be sure the colon is not intermingled with the small bowel. The cut end at the terminal ileum and coecum must be freed and pulled out first.

    De handport is removed, and the whole bowel can be exteriorized.

    Pitfall: It is important to free the cecum and pull the cecum out first. Otherwise the large bowel gets stuck in between the small bowel loops.

    End ileostomy/ileorectal anastomosis or ileoanal anastomosis

13. End-ileostomy: After cross-stapling of the terminal ileum, the terminal ileum is matured into an ileostomy.
14. Ileorectal anastomosis. Using the Alexis ring for exposure, a handsewn side to end colorectal anastomosis can be made.
15. Proctectomy and ileoanal anastomosis. The rectal dissection can be proceeded via the Alexis ring in an open fashion. The rectal dissection can be done close rectal using vessel sealing devices or as a total mesorectal excision. Cross stapling of the very distal rectum is done using an open TA-30 linear stapler. The ileoanal anastomosis can be double stapled as done in open surgery. Defunctioning ileostomy is created at the discretion of the surgeon.

B. Multiport medial to lateral total laparoscopic (procto) colectomy

1. Positioning: French position on a short beanbag. Right arm parallel to the body (Fig. 30.1b)
2. Trocar positioning (Fig. 30.1b): infraumbilical 10 mm (camera), left pararectal below umbilus 5 mm (grasper for exposure, dissection of left flexure), right pararectal below umbilicus 5 mm (grasper for exposure) and 11–12 mm right lower abdomen (dissection, clipping, endostapling).

   Left hemicolon

3. Exposure: Right lateral tilt and steep Trendelenburg. The greater omentum is placed cranially to the transverse colon. The small bowel is moved out of the pelvis. If necessary, a gauze is put at the entrance of the pelvic floor to prevent the small bowel of falling back
4. Creation of the submesenteric tunnel. The dissection is started on the left. The assistant lifts the vascular trunk of the sigmoid to expose the arc of the superior rectal artery. The peritoneum is incised to start with the creation of the submesenteric tunnel down to the lateral attachments at the rectosigmoid junction and up to the pancreatic tails. Downwards creation of the submesenteric tunnel is done below the level of the inferior mesenteric artery (IMA). After dissection of the root of the inferior mesenteric artery, the peritoneum is incised cranial to the IMA towards Treitz ligament. Upward creation of the submesenteric space up to the pancreatic tail is done via this window.

   Pitfalls: Take care not to end up underneath the gonadal vessels and ureter. There should not be any

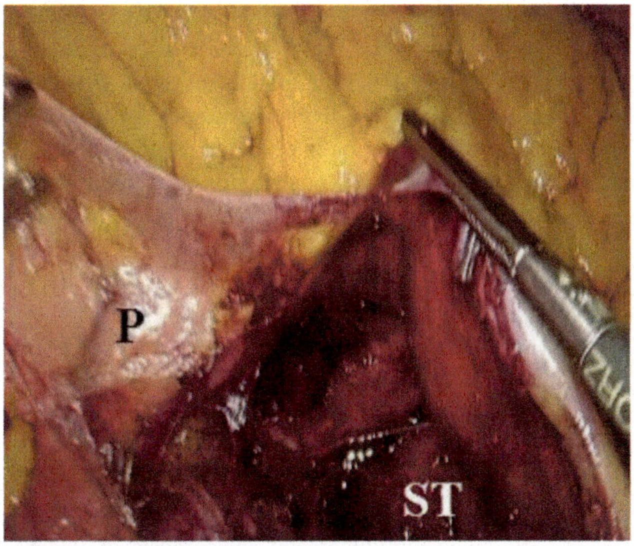

Fig. 30.4 Transbursal mobilisation of the left flexure (*P* pancreas, *ST* submesenteric tunnel)

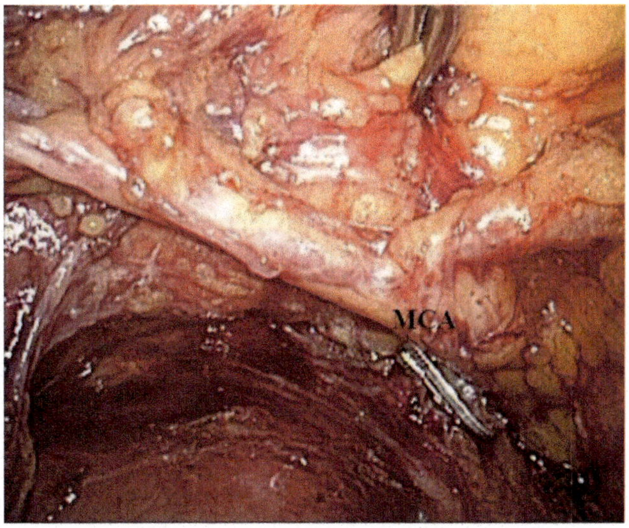

Fig. 30.5 Dissected central branches of the middle colics (*MCA* middle colic artery)

structure attached to the left colonic mesentery in the roof of the submesenteric tunnel.

Care must be taken not to end up underneath the pancreas. With anterior traction to expose the mesenteric tunnel, the pancreas rotates exposing the backside of the pancreas and the splenic vein

5. Ligation the vessels. The IMA can be ligated with vessel sealing devices, clips or vascular endostaplers. It should not be done to close to the aorta in order to prevent damage to the autonomic orthosympatic plexus. The inferior mesenteric vein must be clipped at the lower border of the pancreas proximal to the branching of the left colonic vein.
6. Transbursal mobilization of the left flexure. The assistant grasps the middle colics exposing the avascular window in the mesentery of the transverse colon. The peritoneum is incised left to the left branch of the middle colics. The lower and anterior border of the pancreas is followed until the lesser sac is opened. The mesentery of the transverse colon is now dissected from the pancreas (Fig. 30.4). If the left flexure is reached, the next step is to dissect the omentum from the colon. The assistant grasps the transverse colon and pulls it down. The omentum is now dissected from the transverse colon from the middle towards the left flexure. Now only the lateral attachments need to be taken to free the left colon.

Right hemicolon

7. Exposure. The surgeon moves towards the position in between the legs, the assistant stands on the left of the patient. An additional 10 mm trocar is inserted suprapubically at the site of the future minilaparotomy to facilitate the videoscope. The patient is put in a slight Trendelenburg and left lateral tilt. The small bowel is moved to the left part of the abdomen. The assistant lifts the terminal ileum to expose the lower border of the small bowel mesentery.
8. Creation of the submesenteric tunnel. The peritoneum is incised below the terminal ileum. The submesenteric tunnel is created starting at the level of the terminal ileum to avoid injury to the duodenum. Sometimes the duodenum is positioned quite low in the abdomen. The tunnel is dissected over the duodenum and head of the pancreas exposing the venous plexus originating from the portal vein. When in the right plane the ureter is still covered with a fibrous sheet.

   Pitfalls: Care should be taken not to damage the duodenum or end up below the duodenum.
9. Ligation the vessels. By pulling at the cecum, the fold of the ileocolic vessels is easily identified. The ileocolic vessels are dissected by entering the submesnteric tunnel below the fold. They can be safely dissected in this way and secured with clips or vascular endostaplers. Following the superior mesenteric vein towards the pancreatic head the right branches of the middle colics are encountered (Fig. 30.5). They can be secured using clips or endostaplers. Next the dissection is continued towards the earlier dissection plane from the left at the Treitz ligament. The left branches of the middle colics have to be secured to finalize the vascular division of the transverse colon.

It is very **important** to understand exactly the anatomy. If this is unclear, one should first complete the dissection of the omentum from the transverse colon. If the lesser sac adhesions disturb the anatomy, they should be taken care of.

Pitfalls:
- Injury to the venous plexus on the pancreatic head
- Erroneous ligation of the gastroduodenal vessels

10. Transection of the terminal ileum. Using an endostapler with blue cartridge, the terminal ileum is cross-stapled.
11. Extraction: The colon can be exteriorized via a 4 cm Pfannenstiehl incision.

    End ileostomy/ileorectal anastomosis or ileoanal anastomosis
12. End-ileostomy: After cross-stapling of the terminal ileum, the terminal ileum is matured into an ileostomy.
13. Ileorectal anastomosis. Using the Alexis ring for exposure, a handsewn side to end colorectal anastomosis can be made. Alternatively, the proximal rectum is cross-stapled and a double stapled side to end ileorectal anastomosis can be made advancing the circular stapler transanally
14. Proctectomy and ileoanal anastomosis. The rectal dissection can be continued laparoscopically. The rectal dissection can be done close rectal using vessel sealing devices or as a total mesorectal excision. Cross stapling of the rectum is done using laparoscopic endostaplers. It must be clear that the more cartridges are needed to secure the distal rectum, the more unreliable the cross stapling line is and the higher the chance of redundant remaining rectum. The ileoanal anastomosis can be double stapled laparoscopically. Defunctioning ileostomy is generally advised.

C. Single port colectomy
1. Positioning: French position on a short beanbag. Right arm parallel to the body (Fig. 30.1c)
2. The Single Port is positioned transumbilical or in the future stoma site.
3. **Notes:** It might be more convenient that the assistant takes the grasper and the surgeon the videoscope and the dissecting instrument. In this way crossing of the instruments does not pose a big problem, and the handles of the instruments stay separated. Since the bowel must be exteriorized via the stoma site it is important to keep the specimen as slim as possible. This requires dissection close to the bowel leaving as much mesentery in place.

   Left hemicolon
4. Exposure: Right lateral tilt and steep Trendelenburg. The greater omentum is placed cranially to the transverse colon. The small bowel is moved out of the pelvis. If necessary, a gauze is put at the entrance of the pelvis floor to prevent the small bowel of falling back.
5. The first step is to mobilize the sigmoid in order to transsect the bowel at the level of the rectosigmoid. The mesentery is dissected and a linear endocutter is used to transsect the rectosigmoid. While retracting the cut end with the grasper, the bowel is mobilized from lateral to medial and the mesentery is transsected step by step. It is important to stay close to the bowel in order to have optimal hemostasis using the vessel sealing devices. Lateral mobilization is done just enough to be able to divide the mesentery close to the bowel. The dissection is proceeded until halfway the transverse colon. The omentum is dissected from the transverse colon and is preserved.

   Right hemicolon
6. Starting at the level of the appendix, the right colon is mobilized from lateral to medial just far enough to ligate the mesentery close to the bowel with vessel sealing devices. Following the ascending colon, the right colon is resected in an antegrad fashion until the previously dissected part of the transverse colon is reached. If the colon is now completely freed, it can be exteriorized via the Single Port picking up the cut-end at the sigmoid first.

   End ileostomy/ileorectal anastomosis or ileoanal anastomosis
7. After cross-stapling of the terminal ileum, the terminal ileum is matured into an ileostomy. If the opening in the fascia is too wide to facilitate the ileostomy, the edges need to be approximated using PDS sutures.
8. Ileorectal anastomosis. After cross stapling of the terminal ileum, the anvil can be inserted extracorporeally. A double stapled side to end ileorectal anastomosis can be made advancing the circular stapler transanally.
9. Proctectomy and ileoanal anastomosis. The rectal dissection can be continued laparoscopically. The rectal dissection can be done close rectal using vessel sealing devices or as a total mesorectal excision. Cross stapling of the rectum is done using laparoscopic endostaplers. Coming from the Single Port it can be troublesome to make a straight low cross stapling line. It must be clear that the more cartridges are needed to secure the distal rectum, the more unreliable the cross stapling is and the higher the chance is of redundant remaining rectum. The ileoanal anastomosis can be double stapled laparoscopically. A defunctioning ileostomy is generally advised.

30.2 Postoperative Care

It is advised that if an anastomosis is created the CRP level is measured the fourth postoperate day. If the CRP level is < 150 mg/l the chance of having a septic complication is very low. If the CRP level is > 150 mg/l it should be either repeated or a CT scan must be made to diagnose or rule out anastomotic leakage or abscesses.

Reference

1. Holubar SD, Privitera A, Cima RR, Dozois EJ et al. Minimal Invasive Total Proctocolectomy with Brooke Ilesotomy for Ulverative Colitis. Inflammatory Bowel Disease 2009;15:1337–42.

Part XII

Rectum

31 Laparoscopic Resection of the Rectum

Timothy A. Rockall and Bruce F. Levy

31.1 Indications and Contra-indications

The principal indication for rectal resection is rectal cancer but benign lesions, prolapse, endometriosis and inflammatory bowel disease are also common. Broadly four operations are routinely performed both at open surgery and laparoscopically. These are:

1. The high anterior resection where the proximal rectum is removed necessitating transection of the mesorectum and rectum at a defined point distal to the pathology.
2. The total mesorectal excision (TME) of the rectum with primary anastomosis at the level of the pelvic floor.
3. TME with inter-sphincteric resection of the anal canal.
4. Abdomino-perineal resection with inter-sphincteric, extra-sphincteric or extra levator resection.

All of these procedures can be undertaken laparoscopically and there are no specific pathological contraindications.

The standard laparoscopic approach involves dissection of the mesorectum from the abdomen. There is a relatively new concept of trans-anal TME, which is in evolution and is a technique whereby a variable amount of the distal rectal dissection is performed transanally using a single port device placed in the anal canal. There is inevitably an abdominal component to achieve the proximal dissection and mobilization which can be performed sequentially or simultaneously with two teams. The technique avoids the laparoscopic transection of the distal rectum with a stapler and may be an easier approach to a difficult distal dissection.

31.1.1 Relative Contraindications

Certain situations make the laparoscopic approach more challenging and so represent relative contraindications depending on the skill and experience of the operator. These include

- Adhesions
- Inflammatory conditions such as Crohn's disease (with complex fistulating disease) and endometriosis
- Previous left sided colorectal resection
- Locally advanced malignancy
- Severe radiotherapy changes
- Morbid obesity

31.1.2 Absolute Contraindications

There are a few situations that many would regard as more absolute contraindications:

- Patients who are unable to tolerate a prolonged pneumoperitoneum in a head down position. With good anaesthetic input this represents a small minority of patients and is usually confined to patients with significant cardiac failure.
- Patient choice
- Any situation where oncological treatment might be compromised

In many of these cases however the patients may benefit from a laparoscopic mobilization of the splenic flexure and left colon prior to conversion to complete the pelvic dissection.

T.A. Rockall, MBBS, FRCS, MD (✉) • B.F. Levy, MBChB, MRCS
Minimal Access Therapy Training Unit, Post Graduate Medical School, University of Surrey, Guildford, Surrey, UK
e-mail: tim.rockall@btinternet.com

H.J. Bonjer (ed.), *Surgical Principles of Minimally Invasive Procedures*, DOI 10.1007/978-3-319-43196-3_31

31.2 Patient and Surgical Team Set-Up

Preoperative preparation and patient set-up is critically important to the successful completion of the surgery and for patient safety.

31.2.1 Bowel Preparation

There remains some debate about the benefits or otherwise of bowel preparation. For rectal surgery we have a policy of a simple enema preoperatively to ensure the rectum is empty. If the enema has been unsuccessful an on-table rectal washout is easily accomplished. In cases where a primary anastomosis with a defunctioning ileostomy is planned we have a policy of full bowel preparation to ensure that the colon proximal to the anastomosis is empty.

Variations in the surgical approach exist. Our preference for all left sided and rectal resections is for the personnel to be positioned as demonstrated.

31.2.2 Patient Set-Up

A tilting operating table is mandatory as a steep Trendellenburg position is required to perform rectal resections.

The anaesthetized patient is placed supine with skin in direct contact with a gel mat or a non-slip mattress. This prevents the patient slipping down the table (see Fig. 31.1).

Bilateral shoulder and right lateral supports are required. Additional gel padding is required to help prevent neuropraxia arising from pressure against the supports.

Both arms are bound in at the sides and protected to avoid contact with the metallic part of the table and to prevent pressure related trauma.

The legs are placed in extending supports with the knees flexed and the thighs parallel to abdomen. Sequential pressure stockings are applied.

A urinary catheter is placed.

Nasogastric tubes are not necessary. In the event of inadvertent gastric insufflation during induction of anaesthesia, a temporary naso or oro-gastric tube is placed preoperatively and removed at the end of the procedure.

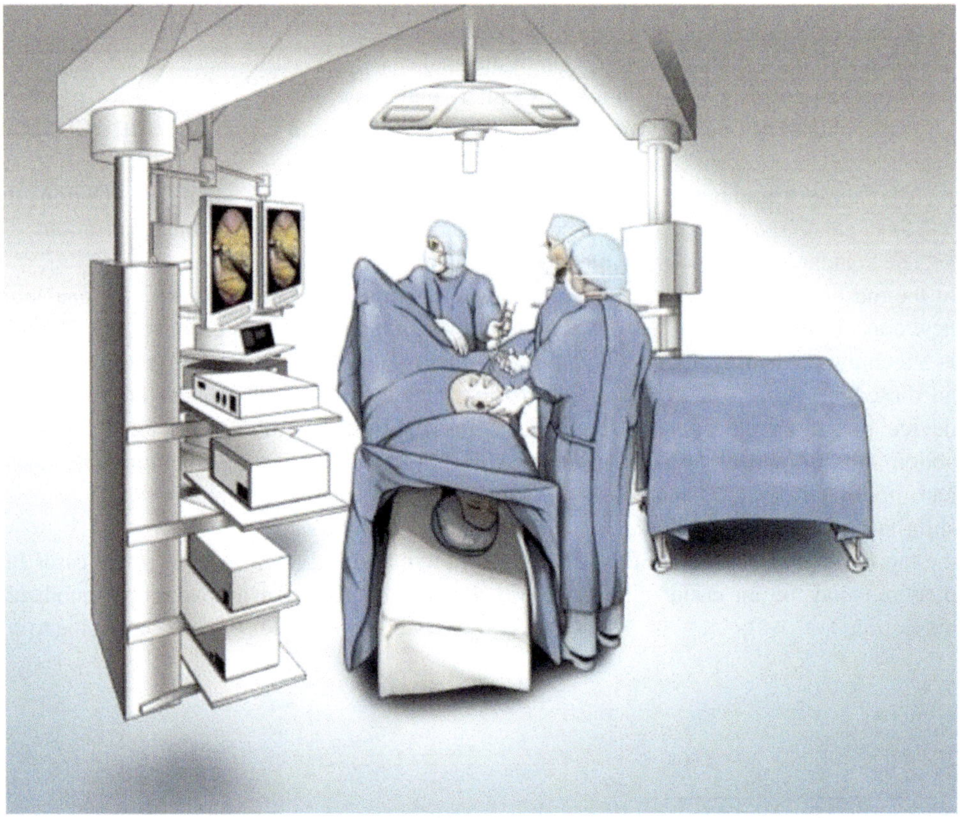

Fig. 31.1 Patient positioning. (Reproduced with permission of Prof. Guy-Bernard Cadière, illustrator: Massimiliano Crespi)

31.3 Instrument Checklist

31.3.1 Hardware

A single high quality monitor and a standard laparoscopic stack is sufficient although there are benefits to operating within an integrated operating theatre environment. Either 5 or 10 mm laparoscopes may be used. Similarly, a 0° and 30° lens can be used depending on the surgeons preference and the nature of the procedure. Our preference is for a 10 mm 0° laparoscope just above the umbilicus.

31.3.2 Ports and Instruments

In terms of ports, the following will be required:

- 12 mm blunt tipped Hasson trocar
- 12 mm trocar
- One to four 5 mm trocars

Once the pneumoperitoneum has been established by the preferred method and the ports inserted, the following instruments, which can be re-usable or disposable, will be required to perform the surgery:

- 2 Johann forceps or equivalent (preferably 1 short and 1 long)
- Angled dissecting forceps
- 1 or a pair of needle holders

Angled dissecting forceps and needle holders are relatively rarely used but need to be available.

The energy sources that will be required include:

- Ultrasonic dissection device or a bipolar vessel sealer/tissue dissector.
- Diathermy

Devices that are required to transect the vessels, transect the rectum, assist with safe removal of the specimen and restore continuity include:

- 60 mm flexible stapler with white/blue/gold/green refills
- Optional 45 mm stapler
- Large clip applicator
- Wound protector/retractor
- Circular stapler for colo-rectal/colo-anal anastomosis

31.3.2.1 Additional Equipment

- Vaginal probe to elevate the vagina anteriorly in cases of previous hysterectomy. For patients with a uterus that falls back into the surgical field, suturing the uterus to the anterior abdominal wall using a monofilament suture placed through the abdominal wall is effective.
- Tonsil swabs
- Suction-irrigation device
- Rigid sigmoidoscope used to delineate the height of a lesion/the point of transection and also to check the integrity of the anastomosis. Some surgeons like to perform an air-leak test by air insufflation.
- Endo-close device may be used to close the larger 10 or 12 mm port sites.

31.4 Surgical Anatomy

This is discussed in section e as the anatomy is encountered.

31.5 Technique(s), Step by Step

31.5.1 Primary Port Placement

This is generally placed above the umbilicus using the Hasson technique. Two stay sutures inserted into the fascia are used to secure the 12 mm blunt tipped Hasson trocar by wrapping the stay sutures around the locking supports which helps to maintain an air tight seal and prevents accidental trocar removal as the camera/instruments/swabs are inserted and removed.

31.5.2 Secondary Port Placement

The insertion of the secondary ports is done under vision to ensure their safe placement. For laparoscopic rectal surgery, we place our secondary ports as shown below (see Fig. 31.2).

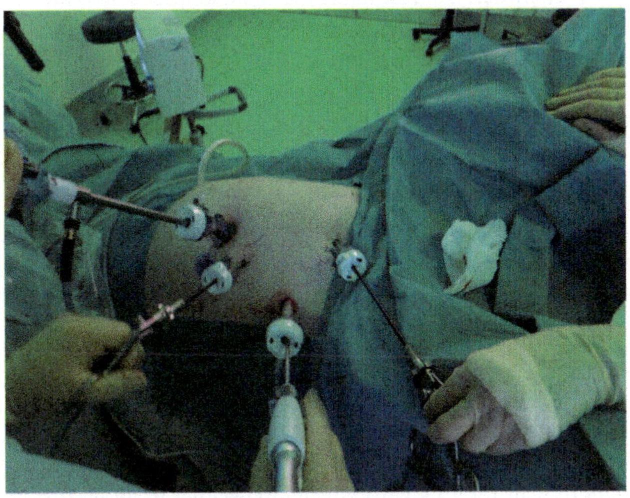

Fig. 31.2 Port placement

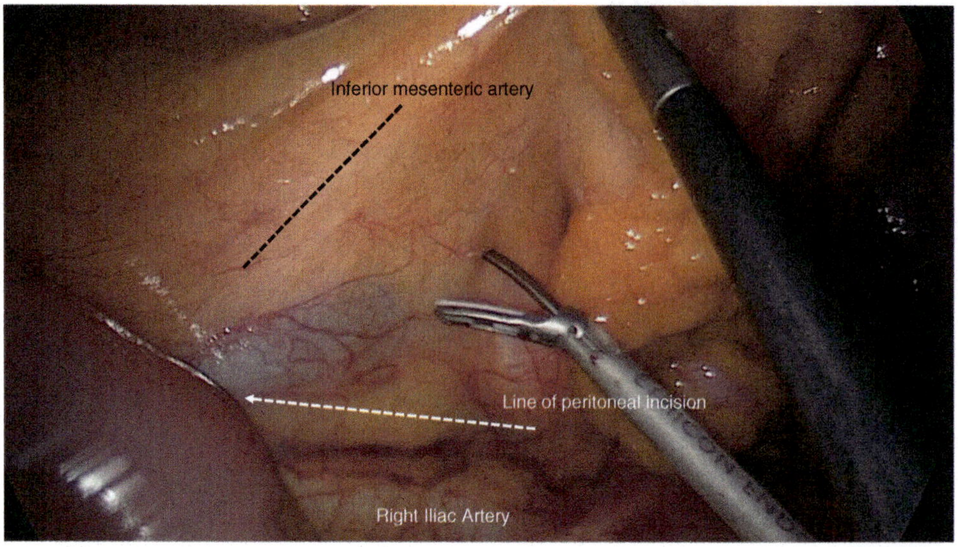

Fig. 31.3 Landmarks for initial dissection of IMA

31.5.3 Initial Positioning and Operative Set-Up

Following the insertion of the secondary ports, the patient is placed into the steep Trendelenburg position with right lateral tilt. The first step is to divide any adhesions. The omentum is placed above the transverse colon and the small bowel positioned in the right upper quadrant.

31.5.4 Initial Dissection and Division of IMA

The landmarks that will guide the initial dissection of the inferior mesenteric artery (IMA) are the sacral promontory, the aorta and the right common Iliac artery. To assist with orientation, the aorta is kept horizontal on the screen (see Fig. 31.3).

With the left hand elevating the sigmoid mesocolon, the initial incision of the peritoneum is made anterior to the right common iliac artery extending cranially towards the origin of the IMA. After making the initial peritoneal incision, the left hand instrument is used to elevate the IMA away from the aorta and the plane of dissection is developed anterior to the hypogastric nerves, left ureter and left gonadal vessels (see Fig. 31.4).

After careful dissection has exposed the IMA, and having ensured that the left ureter is safe, the IMA can be ligated. A technical decision based on the operation being performed needs to be made whether to divide the IMA above or below the left colic branch. Ligation of the IMA may be accomplished using a number of different techniques such as a suitable energy device, clips or a laparoscopic linear stapler with a vascular cartridge (white). When using a stapler it is important to wait for 15 s before firing the stapler to allow for tissue compression. If there is some oozing after firing the stapler, placing a tonsil swab on the vessel will absorb the blood and in a short time this usually stops. (see Sect. 31.11 for tips and tricks if it continues). Energy devices such as the Harmonic scalpel are effective and cost effective. They require some skeletalisation of the vessels of appropriate size (<5 mm). The energy source is activated on the low power setting without pressure on the active blade and with no tension on the vessel. This ensures a good and safe vascular seal. Newer devices are able to seal vessels up to 7 mm in diameter. Our preference for dividing the IMA and inferior mesenteric vein (IMV) is to use the Harmonic ACE 7. Advanced bipolar diathermy devices are equally effective.

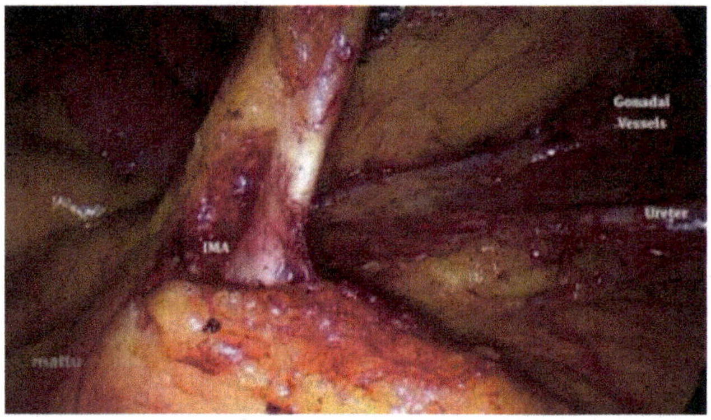

Fig. 31.4 Plane of dissection anterior to hypogastric nerves, left ureter and left gonadal vessels

31.5.5 Dissection and Division of IMV

Having divided the IMA, there is the option at this point to divide the IMV. In some cases though, it is helpful to leave the IMV intact whilst the medial to lateral dissection is performed as the continuous IMV helps tent up all of the mesentery, which assists, with the medial to lateral dissection.

In cases where it is necessary to mobilize the splenic flexure it is better to divide the IMV proximally. The IMV can be divided with an energy source or with clips. Usually we place two large clips above and two below the point where the IMV will be transected or use the harmonic ACE 7. In circumstances where splenic flexure mobilization is not required the IMV may also be divided at the same level as the IMA using a single stapler firing across the pedicle.

31.5.6 Medial to Lateral Dissection

The divided IMA in the mesentery is elevated with the left hand whilst the dissecting tool in the right hand is used to dissect Toldt's fascia posteriorly (see Fig. 31.5). At appropriate times, the left hand is advanced, and elevated to increase exposure and maintain tension whilst the right hand continues to push the fascia posteriorly. The dissection is continued to beyond the gonadal vessels in what is an avascular plane. Once this has been achieved, attention is paid to the lateral sigmoid attachments.

31.5.7 Lateral Division of Sigmoid Attachments

The lateral attachments are divided to free the sigmoid colon from the lateral wall. This then allows the lateral dissection plane to be united with the medial to lateral dissection plane.

31.5.8 Elevating Sigmoid Out of Pelvis and Dissection in Mesorectal Plane

The free sigmoid is then elevated to allow dissection at the level of the sacral promontory. Dissection at this point is then continued to enter the mesorectal plane. Anterior retraction/elevation of the rectum with the left hand exposes the plane and allows rapid development. The right and left hypogastric nerves begin at the point where superior hypogastric plexus divides. These nerves descend in the avascular plane between the mesorectum and sacral fascia (see Fig. 31.6). The dissec-

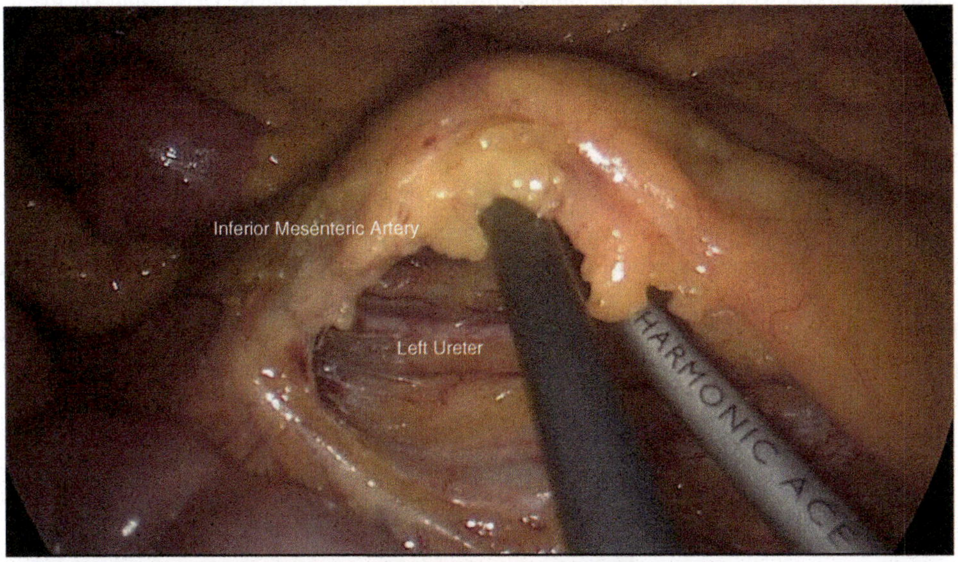

Fig. 31.5 Elevation of IMA

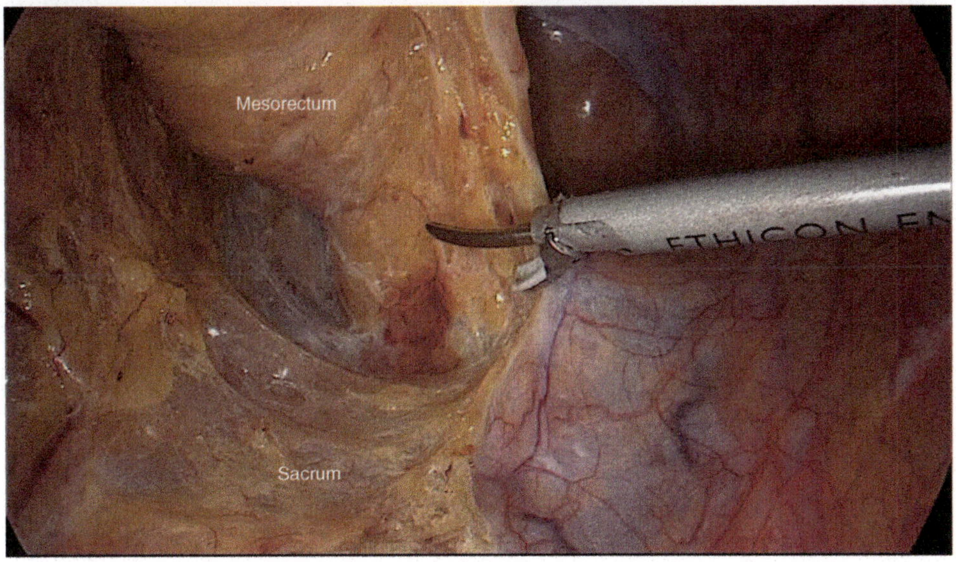

Fig. 31.6 Avascular plane between mesorectum and sacral fascia

tion needs to be kept to this plane so that the mesorectal fascia is not breached and the nerve continuity maintained. The dissection is continued to the point where rectal division is planned. Most of the dissection is performed from the right side. Using an atraumatic grasper through the suprapubic port it is possible to move the rectum over to the right to gain access the peritoneal reflection on the left.

Anterior to the upper part of the rectum is the recto-vesical pouch in men and the recto-uterine pouch in women. An incision of the peritoneum just above the lowest point of the pouch will lead to a plane between the seminal vesicles and the anterior mesorectum in males and a plane between the vagina and the anterior mesorectum in females. To assist with the dissection at this point, the assistant can insert an instrument to elevate the prostate or vagina, creating counter traction.

Denonvilliers fascia is the retroprostatic fascia that separates the prostate from the rectum. Its presence is important for anterior rectal tumours where this fibrous layer often contains the tumour. Therefore, for anterior tumours, dissection must be anterior to this to prevent tumour disruption. The plane anterior to Denonvilliers fascia is entered by dissecting just posterior to the seminal vesicles.

31.5.9 Division of Mesorectum

In cases being performed for rectal cancer, it may be clear where the rectal tumour is whilst in others, it can be difficult to be sure, especially if it is only a small lesion. However, it is always prudent for the assistant to check the position of the rectal tumour with a rigid sigmoidoscope to ascertain its lowest level of the lesion whilst the surgeon holds the laparoscope and notes an oncologically safe position for division. Digital rectal examination by the operating surgeon is also helpful. Once the point of rectal division has been identified, the mesorectum is then divided in a manner that approaches the rectum at right angles. Whatever dissecting/haemostatic instrument is used, caution must be taken that the heat of the instrument does not injure the rectum.

31.5.10 Division of Rectum

The rectum is then divided at the designated point using the flexible stapler. This part of the operation, which can be difficult, must be done well as errors here will predispose to anastomotic leaks. The stapler is inserted through the 12 mm right iliac fossa port. If access from this port is difficult, the 5 mm suprapubic port can be exchanged for a 12 mm port and the stapler inserted through here. Elevating the rectum helps to get the stapler at a better angle as discussed in section K. Depending on the level of transection and the size and thickness of the rectum it may not be possible to transect with one firing of even a 60 mm stapler. Often, two cartridges of a 45 mm or 60 mm stapler are required to transect the rectum and careful placement of the staple lines relative to each others is important (see Fig. 31.7).

31.5.11 Splenic Flexure Mobilization

There are a number of approaches to the splenic flexure. This can be performed at the beginning of the procedure or following pelvic dissection and rectal transection. The lateral

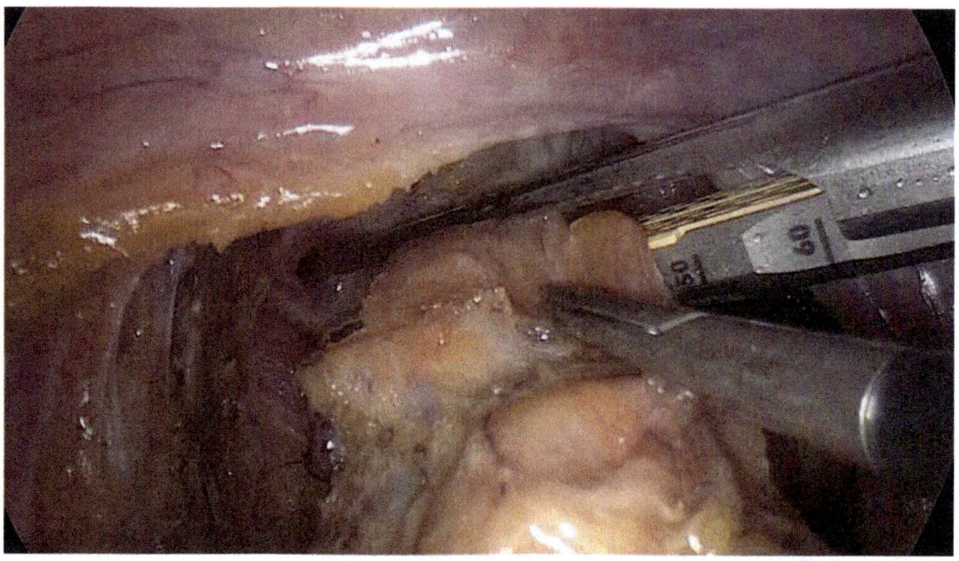

Fig. 31.7 Placement of staple line

attachments of the descending colon are dissected in a caudal to cranial direction. If full mobilization is required, a further port will be required in the epigastrium. Having divided the IMV proximally, the medial to lateral dissection is continued up to the lower border of the pancreas over the right kidney towards the spleen. The patient is positioned flat or head-up, removing the head down tilt. Using the left hand to lift the omentum and the assistant to provide traction on the transverse colon the greater omentum is separated from the transverse colon by dissection to enter the lesser sac, exposing the anterior aspect of the pancreas. The superior leaf of the transverse mesocolon is then incised at the lower border of the pancreas to join with the previous retroperitoneal dissection and the splenic flexure mobilization is then completed.

31.5.12 Extraction of Specimen, Transaction of Colon and Placement of Anvil

Prior to commencing with the skin extraction site, a grasper must be applied to the terminal end of the rectum to assist with its extraction. A Pfannenstiel incision is the made on either side of the 5 mm port that is in the lower midline. The fascia is divided transversely. The rectus abdominae muscles are retracted laterally and the peritoneum is entered. After applying gentle traction to open the wound, the wound protector is then inserted. The grasper with the end of the colon is brought to the extraction site and the colon is removed. The marginal vessels in the mesentery are divided in a conventional manner extra-corporeally up to the edge of the colon at the planned transection point. Vascularity can be tested at this point by observing arterial flow in the marginal vessel. We use a purse string applicator although conventional suturing to create a purse string is also an option. After the specimen has been removed, the anvil of the colorectal gun is inserted and the purse string tightened. The colon is then returned into the abdomen. An airtight seal is then created as described in section K or a cap placed, and the pneumoperitoneum re-created.

31.5.13 Stapled Anastomosis

The circular stapling gun is carefully inserted through the anus and advanced cautiously. If two firings have been required to transect the rectum, then the aim is for the pin of the gun to come through just anterior or posterior to the staple line in a position that will incorporate the area of cross stapling in the area of the anastomosis that will be excised. If it is very difficult to advance the gun to the end of the rectal stump, bringing the pin of the gun out through the anterior rectum to create an end to side anastomosis is acceptable. This is not possible if a TME has been performed. The position of the left colon must be checked prior to firing the stapler to ensure that the colon is not twisted. For a TME our preference is to perform a side to end anastomosis.

31.5.14 Wound Closure

The peritoneum is closed with an absorbable suture followed by closure of the fascia using an appropriate suture according to the surgeons preference. All port sites larger than 5 mm are closed directly. The skin is closed with sutures or clips.

31.6 Specific Complications of the Technique(s) and How to Avoid Them

31.6.1 Small Bowel Injury

- Use a blunt entry technique, especially in the presence of previous surgery or known adhesions.
- Avoid activation of energy sources outside of the field of view and always allow time for instruments to cool before using them as dissection instruments.

31.6.2 Pelvic Nerve Injury

Accurate dissection to stay in the mesorectal plane.

31.6.3 Ureteric Injury

Dissect medial to lateral and identify the left ureter beneath an intact Toldts fascia prior to division of the IMA. If the ureter is obstructed or potentially involved by pathology consider pre-operative stenting.

31.6.4 Vaginal Injury

Use a Valchev retractor or probe or uterine elevation helps to identify the recto-vaginal septum. If in doubt, digital examination can be very useful.

31.6.5 Haemorrhage

- Use energy sources appropriate to the size of vessel.
- Use clips or ties where indicated.

- Keep in the correct plane anterior to the gonadal vessels.
- Avoid traction on the spleen

31.6.6 Anastomotic Leak

The anastomotic leak rate has not been shown to be higher in laparoscopic surgery than open surgery. Points to consider to help reduce this are:

- When the colon is divided extra-corporially, check the flow in the marginal artery of Drummond before ligating the vessel.
- The use of indocyanine green (ICG) to confirm vascularity of the colonic conduit has not yet been of proven benefit.
- Ensure that there is adequate length of the colon to reach the rectum so that the anastomosis is not under tension, and always mobilize the splenic flexure if tension exists.
- We frequently place interrupted sutures across the anastomosis

31.7 Management of Complications (What Can Be Done Laparoscopically, When to Convert)

The extent to which complications can be managed laparoscopically is dependant on the individual's laparoscopic abilities and the severity of the problem. Complications that arise include:

31.7.1 Intraoperative

Haemorrhage
Bowel injury
Staple failure
Leak test positive
Ureteric injury
Splenic injury

31.7.2 Postoperative

Haemorrhage
Anastomotic leak
Adhesional bowel obstruction
Delayed perforation of thermal injuries

Where complications occur or are suspected, many can be diagnosed and indeed managed by further laparoscopy. The main determinant of whether further laparoscopic management is feasible is the clinical state of the patient and the presence or otherwise of bowel obstruction/distension. Where it is technically possible to safely re-establish a pneumo-peritoneum, this is the preferred option. Laparoscopic washout and drainage of sepsis/anastomotic repair/conversion to Hartmann's/defunctioning/division of adhesions can all be accomplished without resorting to laparotomy. Having said that in the absence of appropriate expertise or when safe laparoscopic management cannot be undertaken laparotomy is appropriate.

31.8 Limitations and Problems

The dissection for a total mesorectal excision can be difficult in males with a narrow pelvis. For the low rectal resection in these circumstances, getting the flexible stapler across the rectum in this confined space can be a significant challenge. Inability to staple distally however is usually a sign of insufficient dissection and mobilization. Options here include open conversion via a Pfannenstiel or low midline to complete the dissection and to apply an open stapler or transanal resection and colo-anal anastomosis. The development of Transanal TME (taTME) may help resolve some of these problems but has complications of its own and remains a technique in evolution that has not yet been subject to a trial.

The planes in obese patients can be difficult to identify. Equally the dissection in very thin patients can be difficult. When identifying potential laparoscopic cases in the early part of ones learning curve, it is best to choose people of intermediate build.

31.9 Polemic Points of the Technique(s)

The dissection of the rectum in laparoscopic surgery must follow all the same principals that have been developed over many years in open surgery and there is no place for any alteration in approach that might impact on the oncological safety of the procedure. The operation whether done open or laparoscopically should produce the identical pathological specimen. All decisions pertaining to operability, level of rectal division, anastomotic technique, sphincter preservation and defunctioning should be unchanged.

The decision to mobilize the splenic flexure is more controversial (especially in laparoscopic surgery as it can be difficult) but is essentially a question of vascularity. The only end point of importance is that, following an oncologically safe procedure, the anastomosis is technically well formed, tension free and well vascularised. If any of these criteria are not met then the splenic flexure must be mobilized.

31.10 Results

Up to 95 % of all patients are potentially suitable for laparoscopic resection in centres with experience and advanced skills. Difficult cases with higher conversion rates include those with obesity, android pelvis, locally advanced tumours and post radiotherapy and previous pelvic surgery.

Large case series and randomized controlled trials have consistently shown similar oncological results to open surgery with respect to surgical resection margins, lymph node yield and recurrence rates. Complications related to the anastomosis are also similar in open and laparoscopic groups but blood loss and complications related to the wounds are all consistently less. Hospital stay and early recovery are consistently improved by laparoscopic surgery

31.11 Specific "Tips and Tricks"

If there is ongoing bleeding when the IMA has been divided, two options exist. The first is to use the energy device to obtain haemostasis or to apply clips. The second method, which is particularly useful if there is significant haemorrhage is to place an endo-loop over the stump of the IMA to get control. It is a mistake to divide the IMA flush with the Aorta. Direct suturing of the IMA stump is also possible.

When it comes to firing the flexible staple gun across the rectum, the jaws of the gun can be partially closed on the rectum. This can then act as a retractor to gently elevate the rectum and allow the Johan grasper to hold further down the rectum. This then allows for a better angle of the stapler across the rectum and fewer firings of the staple gun. This can be combined with pressure on the perineum.

To recreate an air-tight seal after having inserted the anvil into the colon and returned it to the abdomen, elevate the wound retractor so that it is under some tension and twist it. Then wrap a small swab around the base of the twisted plastic and secure with a large clip. Some products are supplied with a cap that allows an air-tight seal and the possibility of reinserting the port through the cap.

Try and predict if there is going to be tension at the anastomosis as it is a lot easier to mobilise the splenic flexure before the anastomosis has been created. Mobilising the splenic flexure after the resection has been performed may jeopardize the vascularity at the anastomosis.

Laparoscopic Rectopexy with or without Resection for Full Thickness Rectal Prolapse

32

Syed Abbas and Roberto Bergamaschi

32.1 Introduction and Historical Perspective

Approaches to the management of rectal prolapse have been the subject of discussion for more than a century. Described operations for rectal prolapse are myriad and include well-recognized eponymous associations. The literature on this rather uncommon condition has stimulated a disproportionate number of diverse operations, which include those directed at narrowing the anal orifice, obliteration of the pouch of Douglas, restoration of the pelvic floor, bowel resection by a number of routes, and suspension by various means. All have their advocates, especially when the procedure is to be used under limited circumstances. It is prudent for surgeons to have knowledge of history when selecting an operation for the treatment of rectal prolapse.

Suspension of the redundant colon to the anterior abdominal wall had been advocated by Quénu [1] as early as 1882 and Ball [2] in 1910. Suspension of the rectum to the sacrum and the sigmoid colon to the psoas muscle has been performed for more than 100 years. In 1934 Carrasco [3], reported suturing the rectum to the sacrum, a concept resurrected by Cutait [4] in 1959. The addition of a mesh for suspension of the rectum to the sacrum was proposed by Wells [5] in his work on the polyvinyl alcohol sponge in 1959, whereas Ripstein [6] employed Teflon in 1965. An anterior suspension of the rectum to the posterior vaginal wall with sutures was described by Lloyd-Davies [7] in 1949, whereas the term ventral rectopexy used by Deucher [8] in 1960. An anterior suspension was also reported by Nigro [9] in 1970 as he designed a sling-shaped mesh that suspended the rectum from the pubis. An anteroposterior rectopexy was also suggested by Nicholls [10].

S. Abbas, MD • R. Bergamaschi, MD, PhD, FACS, FRCS, FACRS (✉)
Division of Colon and Rectal Surgery, State University of New York, Stony Brook, NY, USA
e-mail: rcmbergamaschi@gmail.com

Up to that point, the addition of an adjective indicated the anatomical organ to which the rectum was suspended: the sacrum posteriorly, the vagina or pubis anteriorly. However, no reference was made as to where on the rectum the mesh was sutured. In fact, with the exception of the Lloyd-Davies and Deucher techniques, the mesh was sutured to the posterior mesorectum. In more recent years, the adjective ventral has been utilized to indicate that a mesh was sutured to the anterior rectal wall, yet suspended posteriorly to the sacrum.

This chapter will focus only on laparoscopic rectopexy with or without resection for full thickness rectal prolapse.

32.2 Indications and Treatment Options

32.2.1 Rectopexy vs. Mobilization Only

Controversies have not yet been resolved as to which step of an abdominal operation for rectal prolapse contributes the most to containment of recurrence. For decades there has not been any evidence to support the opinion that the addition of rectopexy to mobilization of the rectum would decrease recurrences Bachoo [11]. Moreover, the additional rectopexy may have disadvantages such as added operating time, implantation of foreign material, bleeding from the sacral veins, and nerve injury to the presacral plexus. On the other hand, the data on rectal mobilization without rectopexy have been very limited, and published recurrence rates have often been unreliable. In a meta-analysis on individual patient data, published recurrence rates differed by as much as 47 % from recurrence rates re-estimated by actuarial analysis DiGiuro [12]. A recent randomized controlled trial (RCT) concluded that rectopexy significantly decreases recurrence rates at 5-year follow-up when compared to mobilization without rectopexy Karas [13].

The extent of rectal mobilization has also been a controversial subject including the option of anterior, posterior, circumferential mobilization. In a recent pooled analysis of 532

H.J. Bonjer (ed.), *Surgical Principles of Minimally Invasive Procedures*, DOI 10.1007/978-3-319-43196-3_32

patients with a median follow-up of 60 (12–235) months, circumferential mobilization of the rectum was independently associated with significantly decreased recurrence rates at multivariate regression Bishawi [14].

32.2.2 Suture vs. Mesh Rectopexy

Due to Karas et al. failure to standardize the rectopexy study arm in their RCT, which included patients undergoing suture and mesh rectopexy, we can only rely on retrospective data. In fact, a pooled analysis of 643 patients showed no difference in recurrence rates between suture and mesh rectopexy at a median follow-up of 43 (1–235) months Raftopoulos [15]. The critical concern is whether mesh rectopexy will withstand the test of time, especially when data on adverse event rates emerge. In addition to the increased risk of infection, posterior rectopexy may increase the rates of postoperative constipation, whereas erosion of the mesh resulting in perforation of the posterior vaginal wall is a devastating complication of ventral rectopexy. The rationale of using sutures has been to keep the rectum in its new position to allow its eventual fixation to the sacrum by scar tissue Khanna [16]. There are a few technical details about the surgical technique of suture rectopexy that need our attention. Most authors would suture the posterior mesorectum to the presacral fascia Khanna [16] Graf [17] Heah [18]. However, some authors would also include a partial thickness of the posterior rectal wall Khanna [16]. Some authors Heah [18] favor placing the sutures on the sacral promontory as initially described by Cutait [4]. Alternative sites on the sacrum below its promontory have been suggested Graf [17]. Most authors would agree that two sutures are adequate Khanna [16] Heah [18].

32.2.3 Sigmoid Resection

Sigmoid resection should be considered only in cases of preexisting constipation and should be strictly avoided in incontinent patients. Adding resection to rectopexy does not seem to decrease recurrence rates as compared to rectopexy alone Bachoo [11]. In a recent pooled analysis of 532 patients with a median follow-up of 60 (12–235) months, resection was not independently associated with recurrence at multivariate regression Bishawi [14]. In addition to a significant history of constipation well documented using validated scoring systems, clustering of rings in the sigmoid should be demonstrated at colorectal transit time. If resection is indicated, it should be kept at a minimum without mobilizing the proximal colon. The superior rectal artery should be spared Bergamaschi [19], since preserving the blood supply to the rectal stump may in fact minimize the risk of anastomotic leak and its related morbidity. Therefore, by obviating the need to divide the mesorectum at the rectosigmoid junction, this may prove to have a favorable impact on anastomotic leak rates. Moreover, avoiding dissection of the inferior mesenteric artery is particularly relevant in male patients undergoing resection for rectal prolapse due to potential damage to the sympathetic nerves.

32.3 Pre-operative Work-Up

32.3.1 Risk Assessment

Patients with FTRP are a heterogeneous group with a variety of additional symptoms. Hence, a single treatment would not be appropriate, and treatment options should be selected. The first step of the algorithm is to evaluate the risk of death for a specific individual undergoing surgery. This evaluation should be based on the colorectal Physiologic and Operative Severity Score for the enUmeration of Mortality (POSSUM) score [20], rather than on the American Society of Anesthesiologists (ASA) score. The colorectal POSSUM score can be quickly evaluated online, entering four physiological and four operative data. If the patient is unfit for abdominal surgery under general anesthesia, a perineal procedure under spinal anesthesia can be offered. All patients who are fit for general anesthesia should be offered an abdominal procedure, regardless of chronological age. One exception to this rule is the occasional male patient with true FTRP. The risk of iatrogenic impotence in abdominal surgery should be thoroughly explained to male patients, and the advantages and disadvantages of perineal procedures considered individually. There are four risk areas of autonomic nerve damage during rectal dissection. Damage to the sympathetic nerves may occur when dissecting the inferior mesenteric artery, and during posterior rectal mobilization at the promontory close to the hypogastric nerves. Damage to the parasympathetic nerves may occur during dissection of the lateral stalks of the rectum and anterior rectal mobilization from the seminal vesicles and prostate.

32.3.2 Functional Evaluation

The patient with rectal prolapse may present with a myriad of different symptoms that range from constipation and straining to fecal incontinence. Therefore, it is of utmost importance that all patients undergo a complete preoperative workup before surgery. Upon physical examination, inspection may reveal an obvious rectal prolapse, especially during straining. However, FTRP must be differentiated from mucosal prolapse. The mucosal prolapse can be differentiated from the full-thickness presentation because of the radially oriented grooves, while the FTRP has concentric grooves. In order to measure the prolapse adequately, the patient is asked to position themself in a squatting position. The patient is then asked to increase straining and the prolapse enlarges and lengthens. While the patient is straining, the distance from the perianal skin to the top of the prolapse is measured. Digital rectal examination may also add valuable information by detecting anal pathology and assessing sphincter tone and squeeze pressures. This information is important and aids the surgeon to choose the appropriate procedure for each individual patient. As standard test ordered for the evaluation of patients with rectal prolapse, defecography provides valuable anatomic and functional information for pelvic floor abnormalities. In addition, the results may indicate the presence of sigmoidocoele or enterocoele. The colorectal transit time provides essential information when con- fronted with a patient with concomitant constipation. Among the different methods for establishing the colorectal transit time, the authors recommend the method where The patient receives six numbered daypacks. The five first packs contain 10 rings and the sixth contains 10 rings and 20 cylinders. Each day, at the same time, a pack is ingested. A plain abdominal radiography is taken on day 7. Rings are counted and the transit time is measured by the hospital's radiology department protocol. Colonoscopy must be performed in order to rule out any mucosal abnormality, especially in patients with a prior diagnosis of diverticulitis, inflammatory bowel disease, or cancer. Anal manometry evaluates the patient with a longstanding history of rectal prolapse and incontinence. Patients with pudendal nerve damage, from either obstetric trauma, diabetes, or neoplasms, must also undergo manometric evaluation prior to surgery.

32.4 Operating Room

The day before the planned surgical intervention, the patient should be restricted to a clear diet. It is the author's preference to administer a bowel preparation the day before surgery. The patient is instructed to take nothing by mouth as of midnight before surgery, to evacuate the rectum with an enema, and have a chlorhexidine neck-down shower prior to traveling to the hospital. In the preoperative area, the patient should receive intravenous fluids, as the bowel preparation often contributes to dehydration. Epidural analgesia should also be offered to the patient, especially if the surgery entails a bowel resection. General endotracheal anesthesia is administered by the anesthesiologist, and a Foley catheter and oral-gastric tube are inserted. The patient is positioned in lithotomy (Fig 32.1). It is important that the height of the knee and the torso is at the same level, to avoid any impediment while the surgeon is operating. For obese patients, the surgeon may want to consider strapping the patient to the operating table at the chest. Prior to creating a sterile field, the surgeon must verify that the patient is secured to the table. This is accomplished by maneuvering the remote control of the operating room table and positioning the patient in a steep Trendelenburg position. Antibiotics should be administered intravenously within the hour prior to the planned incision.

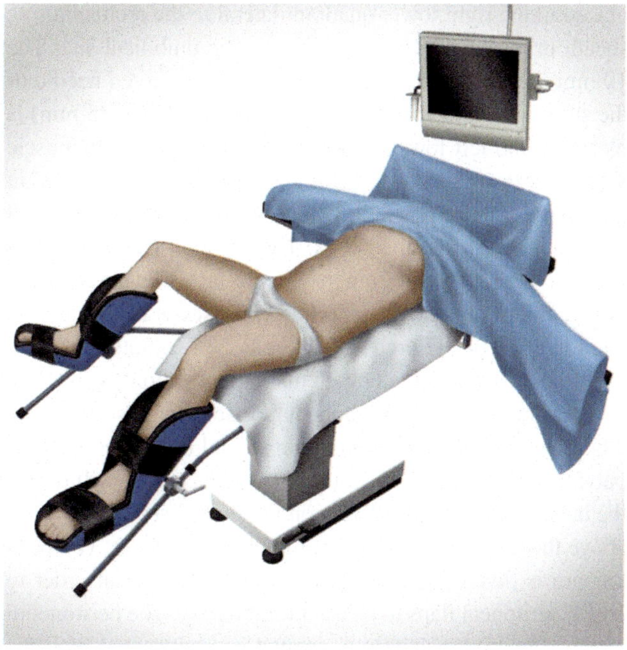

Fig. 32.1 Set up of the operation room. Position of patient

32.5 Surgical Technique

32.5.1 Laparoscopic Suture Rectopexy

We prefer to suture the right and left peritoneal flaps to the presacral fascia. The exact location on the promontory is lateral to the hypogastric nerves and medial to the ureter on both sides of the rectum. If the rectum is prolapsed it should be reduced prior to starting the procedure. The abdomen and perineum is then prepped and draped in a sterile fashion. The stirrups securing the patient's legs are also draped. Prior to the incision, the identity of the patient and the scheduled procedure are verified in a time out with reconciliation of medications and allergies. It is the authors' preference to achieve the pneumoperitoneum through an open technique. A 10 mm incision is made just below the umbilicus, and its stalk is dissected and lifted with a Kocher clamp. The fascia is incised with a knife longitudinally along the midline under direct visual control. A Hasson trocar is then inserted into the peritoneal cavity. The port is secured in place by two sutures placed on each side of the incision. It is not necessary to exceed 11 mmHg since most of the procedure will be performed with in the bony structure of the pelvis. Two ports (10 mm and 5 mm) are placed in the right lower quadrant lateral to the rectus muscle sheath in a triangulating fashion with the umbilical site. The 10 mm port allows the surgeon to insert the curved needle of the suture into the abdominal cavity. A fourth port (5 mm) is placed in the left lower quadrant lateral to the rectus muscle sheath for the assistant's instruments. The patient is placed in the Trendelenburg position, which facilitates the small bowel and omentum out of the pelvis. The assistant proceeds to lift the rectosigmoid colon from the epiploic appendages. The sigmoid colon should not be mobilized. The second step includes identification of the ureters. This may be facilitated by prior insertion of lighted ureteral stents. Visualization of the iliac bifurcation as well as the gonadal vessels can also facilitate this identification. The peritoneum should be incised into the pelvic sulcus, toward the pouch of Douglas. This will define the lateral extent of the dissection. Medial dissection is begun above the level of the sacral promontory (Fig 32.2). The peritoneum is divided at least 2 cm from the rectum in order to create peritoneal flaps to be used for the pexy. The peritoneum of the sigmoid mesentery is opened and connected with the lateral dissection just posterior to the inferior mesenteric pedicle, which is elevated as the rectosigmoid colon is maintained on stretch. The medial peritoneal dissection is extended over the sacral promontory along the sulcus toward the pouch of Douglas, to mirror the lateral dissection. At the level of the sacral promontory, the hypogastric nerves are amenable to injury (Fig 32.2).

To avoid such an injury, the dissection is kept close to the fascia propria of the rectum. The surgeon continues to lift and provide appropriate traction to the rectosigmoid colon. This dissection is often facilitated by the abnormal lack of fixation in this area, which has contributed to the prolapse. The presacral fascia and hypogastric nerves should remain away from the area of dissection. It is important to be mindful of the presacral vessels as the dissection approaches the pelvic floor. As the levator ani muscles become visible, the rectum will be—come parallel to the pelvic floor and the angle of dissection should be adjusted to avoid injury to the presacral vessels. Diffuse bleeding may occur if these vessels are inadvertently injured. The posterior dissection is completed to the level of the coccyx. The lateral dissection includes division of the lateral stalks (ligaments). The rectum is lifted by the assistant and a point is selected for the rectopexy. The rectum should not be placed on tension, but the prolapse defect should be reduced. Non-absorbable 2–0 silk sutures are secured to the right and left sacral promontory. The site on the promontory is lateral to the hypogastric nerves and medial to the ureter on both sides of the rectum (Fig. 32.3). Attention to the position of the hypogastric nerves and the presacral vessels will guide the suture placement. The surgical assistant will maintain the anatomic posi-

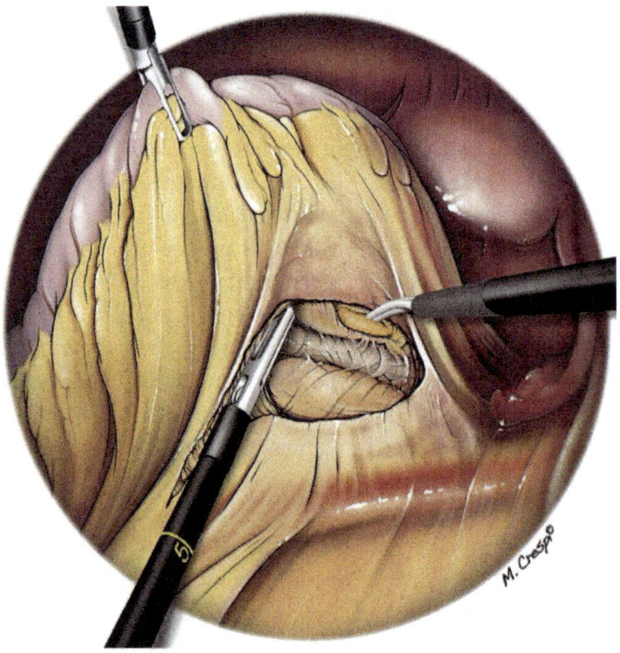

Fig. 32.2 Dissection of the rectum, promontory and creation of peritoneal flaps. (Reproduced with permission of Prof. Guy-Bernard Cadière, illustrator: Massimiliano Crespi)

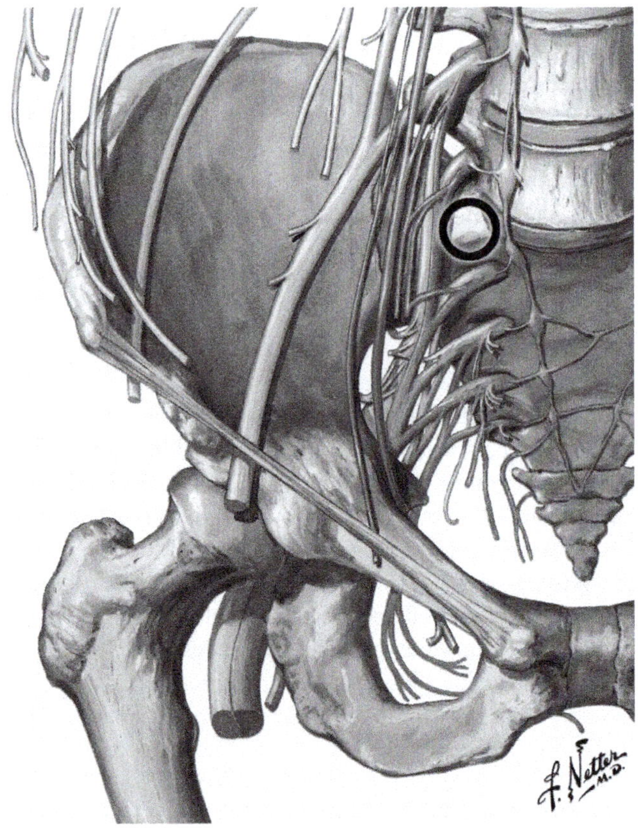

Fig. 32.3 The sites of sutures on the promontory are lateral to the hypogastric nerves and medial to the ureter on both sides of the rectum (Reprinted with permission from Netter Images, Elsevier Health Sciences, Philadelphia, PA)

tion of the rectum while the surgeon secures the two previously placed sutures to the peritoneal flaps. Once the mobilization and rectopexy are completed, hemostasis should be reaffirmed. The pelvis is irrigated with saline. There should be no reason to place a drain in the pelvis. All port sites are closed layer by layer using non-absorbable sutures on a UR6 needle. The wounds are cleaned and dressed, and the patient is extubated and transported to recovery. The Foley catheter should be left in place, but the oral-gastric tube will be discontinued on leaving the operating room.

The previously mentioned technical steps remain the same, yet there are some important points worth describing. While performing the circumferential rectal mobilization, the posterior mesorectum is dissected off the posterior wall of the rectum at approximately 14 cm from the anal verge. This distance is verified by an intraoperative rigid sigmoidoscopy. The sigmoid colon is then divided by a laparoscopic linear stapler that is positioned perpendicular to the axis of the sigmoid colon. The mesentery of the sigmoid colon is divided close to the bowel, and the mesorectum is not divided, therefore sparing the superior rectal artery (Fig. 32.4). The specimen is retrieved through a Pfannenstiel incision with a disposable wound retractor. We then proceed to perform a double-stapled colorectal anastomosis without the need to re-establish pneumoperitoneum.

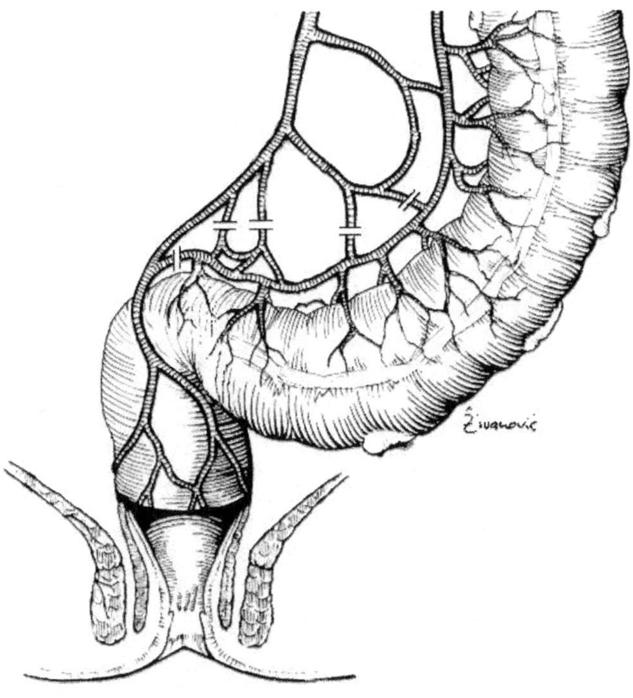

Fig. 32.4 The sigmoid arteries are divided preserving the superior rectal artery (Reprinted with permission from Bergamaschi et al. [19])

32.6 Postoperative Care

Postoperatively, early activity and incentive spirometry are encouraged. Pain is initially controlled with an epidural catheter with local anesthetic or intravenous NSAID. Diet is advanced with the return of bowel function, and the pain medication is transitioned to oral NSAID formulations. The Foley catheter can be removed on the postoperative day one unless other co- morbidities are present. Upon discharge, the patient is instructed to avoid heavy lifting. Dietary goals should be addressed. Avoidance of constipation or overly loose stool should be discussed. The patient should be seen in the office within 1–2 weeks of discharge. Continued follow-up will assist the surgeon in his or her evaluation of the success of the repair

References

1. Quenu E. Rev Chir. Spontaneous rupture of the rectum 1882;2:173–88.
2. Ball C. The rectum. London: Oxford Medical Publications; 1910.
3. Carrasco AB. Contribution a l Etude du Prolapsus du Rectum. Paris: Masson; 1934.
4. Cutait D. Sacro-promontory fixation of the rectum for complete rectal prolapse. Proc R Soc Med. 1959;52(suppl):105.
5. Wells C. New operation for rectal prolapse. Proc R Soc Med. 1959;52:602.
6. Ripstein CB. The repair of massive rectal prolapse. Surg Proc. 1965;2:2.
7. Lloyd-Davies OV. Rectal prolapse: President's address. J R Soc Med. 1955;48:33–44.
8. Deucher F. Ventral rectopexy in the treatment of rectal prolapse. Helv Chir Acta. 1960;27:240–6.
9. Nigro ND. A sling operation for rectal prolapse. Proc R Soc Med. 1970;63 Suppl 1:106–7.
10. Nicholls RJ, Simson JN. Anteroposterior rectopexy in the treatment of solitary rectal ulcer syndrome without overt rectal prolapse. Br J Surg. 1986;73:222–4.
11. Bachoo P, Brazzelli M, Grant A. Surgery for complete rectal prolapse in adults. Cochrane Database Syst Rev. 2000;2, CD001758.
12. DiGiuro G, Ignjatovic D, Brogger J, Bergamaschi R. Rectal Prolapse Recurrence Study Group. How accurate are published recurrence rates after rectal prolapse surgery? A meta-analysis of individual patient data. Am J Surg. 2006;191:773–8.
13. Karas JR, Uranues S, Altomare DF, Sokmen S, Krivokapic Z, Hoch J, Bartha I, Bergamaschi R. Rectal Prolapse Recurrence Study Group. No rectopexy versus rectopexy following rectal mobilization for full-thickness rectal prolapse: a randomized controlled trial. Dis Colon Rectum. 2011;54(1):29–34.
14. Bishawi M, Foppa C, Tou S, Bergamaschi R. Recurrence of rectal prolapse following rectopexy: pooled analysis of 532 patients. Colorectal Dis. 2016;18(8):779–84.
15. Raftopoulos Y, Senagore AJ, Di Giuro G, Bergamaschi R. Rectal Prolapse Recurrence Study Group. Recurrence rates after abdominal surgery for complete rectal prolapse: a mul- ticenter pooled analysis of 643 individual patient data. Dis Colon Rectum. 2005;48:1200–6.
16. Khanna AK, Misra MK, Kumar K. Simplified sutured sacral rectopexy for complete rectal prolapse in adults. Eur J Surg. 1996;162:143–6.

17. Graf W, Stefansson T, Arvidsson D, Pahlman L. Laparoscopic suture rectopexy. Dis Colon Rectum. 1995;38:211–2.
18. Heah SM, Hartley JE, Hurley J, et al. Laparoscopic suture rectopexy without resection is effective treatment for full- thickness rectal prolapse. Dis Colon Rectum. 2000;43:638–43.
19. Bergamaschi R, Lovvik K, Marvik R. Preserving the superior rectal artery in laparoscopic sigmoid resection for complete rectal prolapse. Surg Laparosc Endosc Percutan Tech. 2003;13:374–6.
20. Constantinides VA, Tekkis PP, Senapati A. Association of Coloproctology of Great Britain and Ireland. Comparison of POSSUM scoring systems and the surgical risk scale in patients undergoing surgery for complicated diverticular disease. Dis Colon Rectum. 2006;49(9):1322–31.

33 Transanal Endoscopic Microsurgery

Mario Morino and Marco E. Allaix

33.1 Introduction

The last three decades have witnessed significant improvements in the diagnosis, staging and treatment modalities of rectal tumors leading to a more tailored approach. One of the most clinically relevant advances is the development and diffusion of Transanal Endoscopic Microsurgery (TEM) [1]. TEM is a minimally invasive procedure that allows to perform a full thickness en bloc local excision of a rectal tumor down to the perirectal fatty tissue and to suture the rectal defect. It is performed under general or spinal anesthesia with very limited postoperative morbidity and mortality.

Even though TEM was initially conceived for the treatment of tumors located in the extraperitoneal rectum, there is increasing evidence that a full thickness TEM can be offered also to patients with intraperitoneal rectal cancers, with no increased morbidity and cancer-related mortality.

The current evidence supports the use of TEM with a curative intent only for rectal adenomas and selected T1 rectal cancers [2, 3], while TEM alone for the treatment of more advanced rectal cancers should be considered with palliative intent only. Recently, several reports have shown that neoadjuvant (chemo)radiation therapy followed by TEM in selected T2 N0 rectal cancer reproduces the results of radical total mesorectal excision (TME) [4].

This chapter discusses the indications and the technical aspects of a TEM procedure for the treatment of rectal tumors.

M. Morino, MD (✉) • M.E. Allaix, MD, PhD
Department of Surgical Sciences, University of Torino, Torino, Italy
e-mail: mario.morino@unito.it

33.2 Indications

At our institution, rectal adenomas that are judged unsuitable for endoscopic removal and staged uT0 N0 by preoperative transanal endoscopic ultrasound (EUS), or rectal adenocarcinomas preoperatively staged uT1 N0 M0 are the indications for TEM with a radical intent. TEM alone is a compromise procedure for the treatment of more invasive or metastatic rectal cancers. Recently, we have expanded the indications for TEM to selected uT2 N0 M0 adenocarcinomas with either down-staging or down-sizing of the lesion following neoadjuvant radiotherapy after informed consent of the patient.

While in the past we considered rectal lesions suitable for TEM only when the proximal extent is located within 12 cm from the anal verge on the anterior wall, 15 cm from the anal verge on the lateral walls and 18 cm from the anal verge on the posterior wall, to date we perform a TEM procedure even for intraperitoneal rectal tumors. Although technically demanding, a TEM procedure with an end-to-end anastomosis can be performed also for circumferential rectal adenomas.

33.2.1 Rectal Adenomas

We consider a full thickness TEM procedure as the current standard of care for rectal adenomas judged unsuitable for endoscopic removal, even larger than 5 cm.

Conventional endoscopic mucosal resection (EMR) cannot provide an *en-bloc* resection in case of large lesions, and incomplete or piecemeal resection may occur in up to 50 % of cases. In addition, EMR does not provide a submucosal dissection, therefore precluding an accurate staging in case of malignancy. Since up to 26 % of the adenomas endoscopically resected are found to be invasive adenocarcinoma at the definitive pathologic examination, a full-thickness excision should be offered to all patients with rectal neoplasm, even in case of benign preoperative histology instead of a partial

H.J. Bonjer (ed.), *Surgical Principles of Minimally Invasive Procedures*, DOI 10.1007/978-3-319-43196-3_33

wall piecemeal endoscopic resection. The endoscopic submucosal dissection (ESD) was introduced to overcome these difficulties and to allow *en bloc* resection of specimens, especially in case of lesions larger than 20 mm. However, compared to conventional EMR, ESD is technically more challenging and time consuming than EMR. As a result, ESD has not gained wide acceptance in the Western countries, and transanal surgery is still the approach of choice for the excision of large rectal adenomas [5].

Conventional transanal excision with retractors is burdened by higher specimen fragmentation rates, and positive margins rates than TEM. Positive surgical margins are independent risk factors for local recurrence after TEM, along with the tumor size [6]. In our experience of 293 large rectal adenomas treated by TEM, 21 % of adenomas with a diameter ≥5 cm were removed with positive margins versus 9 % of adenomas <5 cm ($p = 0.047$). Tumor diameter ≥5 cm was found to be a predictive factor for local recurrence ($p = 0.007$) [7].

Since a local recurrence is relatively common after excision of adenomas larger than 5 cm, we recommend a strict clinical and endoscopic follow-up in these cases. TEM has been shown to be an important therapeutic option even in the treatment of recurrent adenomas, when the endoscopic resection is not feasible.

33.2.2 Rectal Cancer

The absence of perirectal lymph node involvement at the preoperative staging, a submucosal tumor invasion less than 1000 μ (T1 sm1), and negative resection margins are the strongest prognostic factors for long-term survival in rectal cancer patients treated by local excision. The incidence of lymph node metastasis is very low for T1 sm1, but for T1 sm2-3 and for T2 it increases up to 25 %.

There is increasing evidence that TEM can be safely performed in selected T1 N0 rectal cancer patients [3]. While “low risk” T1 rectal cancer patients treated by TEM have excellent oncologic outcomes, the survival of “high risk” T1 and T2 rectal cancer patients after TEM alone is significantly poorer than after rectal resection and TME. To reduce postoperative morbidity and mortality associated with rectal resection and TME without jeopardizing long term survival, a multimodal organ-preserving approach including TEM and neoadjuvant (chemo)radiation therapy has been recently proposed in selected patients [8].

33.3 Preoperative Work-Up

The preoperative work-up includes:

- clinical evaluation
- complete colonoscopy to rule out the presence of synchronous colonic lesions
- rigid proctoscopy to locate the lesion along the circumference and to measure the distance of the upper and lower limits from the anal verge
- EUS to assess the depth of invasion of the rectal wall.
- A pelvic magnetic resonance imaging (MRI) aiming to detect potential lymph node metastases, a chest and abdominal computed tomography to exclude distant metastases, and serum carcinoembrionyc antigen (CEA) assay are obtained in the presence of cancer.

The accurate preoperative evaluation of both depth of tumor invasion and perirectal lymph nodes is crucial to obtain satisfactory oncologic results, since a lymphadenectomy is not performed with TEM. Recent technological improvements in EUS probes have led to a progressive reduction in staging discrepancies from a rate of almost 50 % in the early 1990s to less than 15 % in the last 5 years. If there is a discrepancy between clinical evaluation (soft and mobile lesion) and EUS staging (uT2) of a large adenoma, TEM should be considered as a means to assess the exact pathologic diagnosis and depth of wall penetration.

33.4 Patient Preparation

All patients are told to take a low fiber diet the week before TEM. A rectal enema is performed 12 and 2 h preoperatively. Intravenous antibiotics, such as a second-generation cephalosporin and metronidazole, are administered before insertion of the proctoscope and continued for 24 h postoperatively. Deep venous thrombosis prophylaxis is not routinely administered.

33.5 Equipment

Since 2008 we perform the TEM procedures with TEO (Transanal Endoscopic Operation) Instrumentation by Karl Storz GmbH (Tuttlingen, Germany), according to the standard technique described by Buess. TEO instrumentation consists of a 7 or 15 cm rectal tube (4 cm in diameter) with 3 working channels (12, 5 and 5 mm) for dedicated or conventional laparoscopic instruments, and a 5 mm channel for a 30° 2D optic (Fig. 33.1). A holding arm consisting of three joints and a single screw connects the proctoscope to the operating table via (Fig. 33.2). A standard laparoscopic unit is used in combination with this system. Camera imaging is projected on screen; insufflation is obtained by a conventional CO_2 thermo-insufflator which is connected to the proctoscope through a luer lock connector.

Recently, the use of equipment for single incision laparoscopic surgery (SILS) has been proposed. The single disposable SILS equipment is cheaper than each single reusable TEM proctoscope. However, large comparative studies are

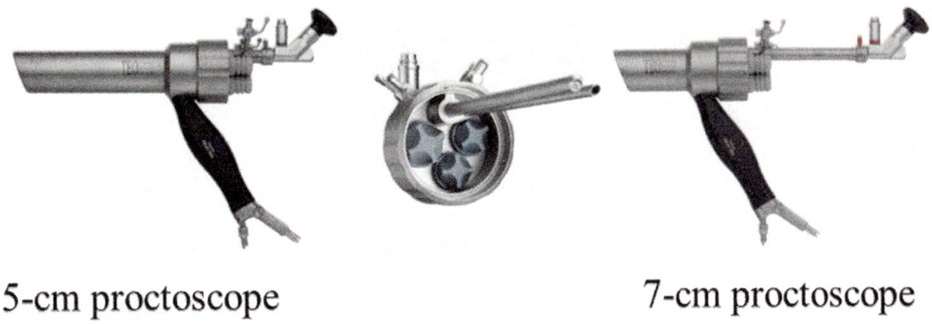

Fig. 33.1 Long (*left*) and short (*right*) proctoscope with 3 working channels

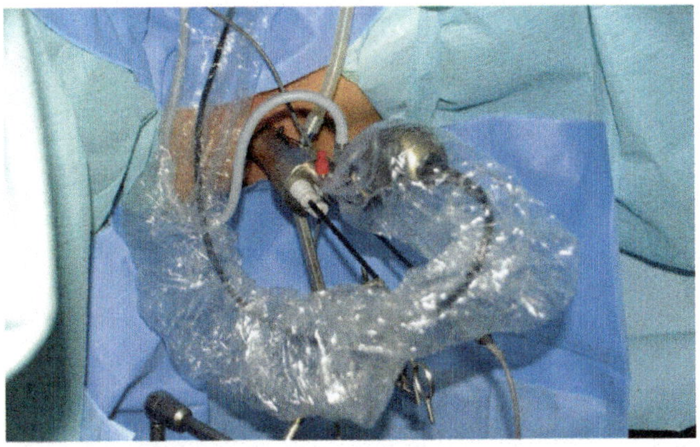

Fig. 33.2 TEO instrumentation in place

needed to evaluate the real benefits and the disadvantages of SILS equipment compared to TEM in the treatment of rectal tumors.

33.6 Positioning of the Patient on the Operating Table

The TEM procedure can be performed either under general or spinal anesthesia. The patient is placed either prone or supine in order to keep the lesion as close to the 6 o'clock position as possible, even with lateral lesions. However, since the shape of the proctoscope tip allows manipulation and suturing of the rectal wall on a 360° surface, most patients are kept in a supine position. Patients with lateral lesions are usually placed in the supine position unless the lesion is predominantly located in 12–3 o'clock position or 9–12 o'clock position. We do not place the patient in the lateral decubitus position as the benefit is minimal. Patients affected by circumferential lesions are at higher risk of entering the peritoneal cavity. Therefore, they are always positioned in a prone position to reduce the descent of small bowel loops into the surgical field while suturing the peritoneal opening.

A Foley catheter is inserted before starting the procedure and is usually removed on postoperative day 1.

33.7 Surgical Technique

Step 1: Dissection

The surgeon is seated between the patient's legs, while the assistant is to the left of the surgeon. The monitor is placed in front of the surgeon.

The proctoscope is inserted into the rectum and fixed after identification of the rectal lesion. However, the position of the proctoscope might be adjusted during the procedure in order to ensure optimal visualization and access to the margins of the lesion. Carbon dioxide (CO_2) is inflated to maintain an 8-mmHg endorectal pressure that in some cases might be increased up to 16 mmHg. The surgeon usually starts the dissection at the right lower border of the tumor (Fig. 33.3a). Due to the uncertainty of the preoperative diagnosis and staging, a full-thickness excision with adequate margins of clearance should be performed. Macroscopic clear margins of at least 5 mm from the neoplasm should be obtained with both benign and malignant lesions. Tumor excision is usually performed by using monopolar hook cautery. In difficult cases, ultrasonic shears or a Electrothermal Bipolar Vessel Sealing System may be helpful to complete the dissection circumferentially around the lesion down to the perirectal fat (Fig. 33.3b, c). The specimen is then retrieved transanally and is pinned on a corkboard before fixation in 10 % buffered formalin to preserve the margins of normal mucosa surrounding the tumor.

Troubleshooting Intraoperative peritoneal perforation (PP) is a challenging event that may occur during TEM for high or anterior rectal lesions. It is frequently reported as a complication and therefore tumors of the upper rectum, especially those located on the anterior or lateral wall, are considered a contraindication to TEM. The learning curve and the case volume of the surgeon are two main factors that influence the treatment strategy (direct suturing, conversion to open surgery or stoma

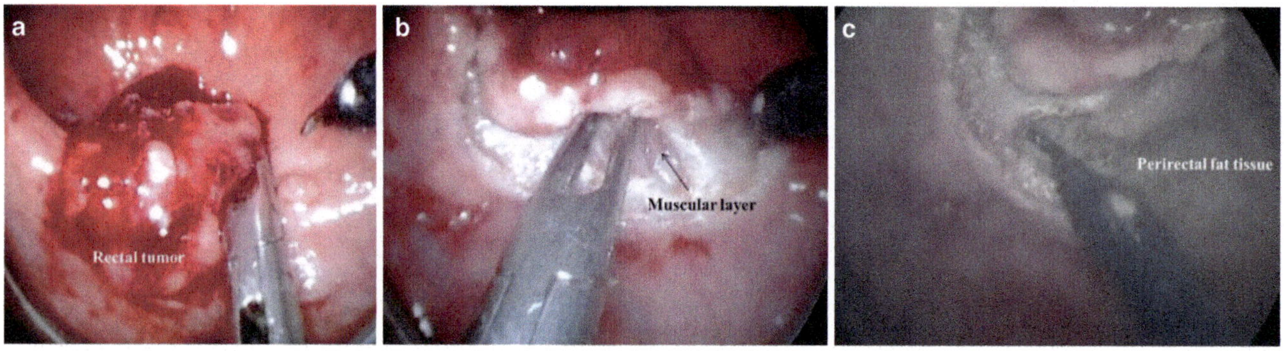

Fig. 33.3 (**a**) Start of dissection at the right lower border of the tumor, (**b**, **c**) Circumferential dissection

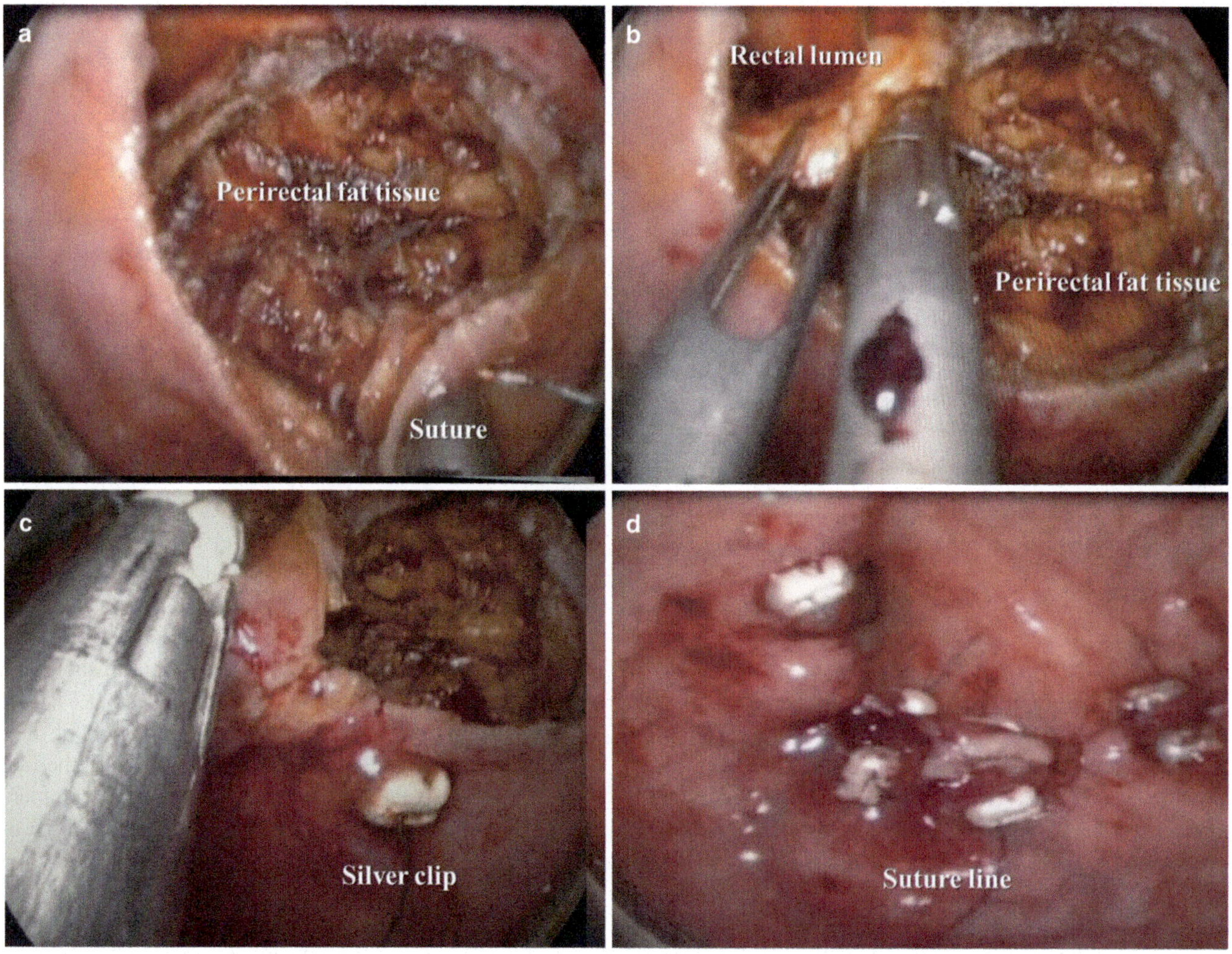

Fig. 33.4 Suture of the rectal wall defect

creation) adopted when PP occurs. In our experience, the prone position of the patient on the operating table and the particular shape of the tip of the TEO proctoscope help suture the rectal wall on a 360° surface, thus minimizing the risk of conversion to open surgery or the need for a stoma [9].

Special care is mandatory when performing a TEM procedure for an anterior rectal tumor in female patients, due to the risk of developing postoperative rectovaginal fistulas. In those cases we suggest to perform a mucosectomy instead of a full-thickness excision.

Step 2: Wall Defect Suturing
After the parietal defect is disinfected with iodopovidone solution, the surgeons closes the rectal wall defect with one or more long-term monofilament absorbable running sutures. Dedicated silver clips are used to secure the suture since knot tying during TEM is challenging. As an alternative, the single use suturing device like Endo Stitch™ can be used to suture the rectal wall.

Reduction of the endorectal pressure increases compliance of the rectal wall. In case of large wall defects, a midline stitch is placed to approximate proximal and distal margins (Fig. 33.4); at the end of the procedure, patency of the rectal lumen is carefully checked through the TEM proctoscope.

Troubleshooting One controversial technical aspect of full thickness TEM concerns the management of the rectal wall defect. Even though there is no strong evidence supporting the suture of the defect, the closure of the wall represents one of the technical advantages of TEM compared to classical transanal excision and might reduce the risks of postoperative local infection and sepsis, and complications in case of later rectal resection with total mesorectal excision.

33.8 Post-operative Care

Patient's mobilization occurs immediately after surgery. The urinary catheter placed intraoperatively is removed on postoperative day 1 (postoperative day 2 if the anterior rectal wall was involved). Intravenous paracetamol is administered for 24 h postoperatively. Oral intake is allowed on postoperative day 1.

Postoperative complication rates range between 2 and 15 %. Most frequent local complications are rectal bleeding and suture dehiscence.

Rectal bleeding is self-limiting in most cases. Treatment options include blood transfusions and endoscopic clipping.

Suture dehiscence occurs more frequently after neoadjuvant radiation therapy [10]. Patients with suture dehiscence experience severe rectal pain that may be associated with tenesmus and fever. An endoscopy is always obtained to check the suture line and the size of the perirectal collection. Conservative treatment include intravenous antibiotics and 10 % iodine solution enemas. A further treatment to control sepsis such as a diverting stoma creation is rarely necessary.

References

1. Buess G, Hutterer F, Theiss J, Böbel M, Isselhard W, Pichlmaier H. A system for a transanal endoscopic rectum operation. Chirurg. 1984;55:677–80.
2. Suppiah A, Maslekar S, Alabi A, Hartley JE, Monson JR. Transanal endoscopic microsurgery in early rectal cancer: time for a trial? Colorectal Dis. 2008;10:314–27.
3. Bach SP, Hill J, Monson JR, et al. Association of Coloproctology of Great Britain and Ireland Transanal Endoscopic Microsurgery (TEM) Collaboration. A predictive model for local recurrence after transanal endoscopic microsurgery for rectal cancer. Br J Surg. 2009;96:280–90.
4. Lezoche E, Baldarelli M, Lezoche G, Paganini AM, Gesuita R, Guerrieri M. Randomized clinical trial of endoluminal locoregional resection versus laparoscopic total mesorectal excision for T2 rectal cancer after neoadjuvant therapy. Br J Surg. 2012;99(9):1211–8.
5. Arezzo A, Passera R, Saito Y, Sakamoto T, Kobayashi N, Sakamoto N, Yoshida N, Naito Y, Fujishiro M, Niimi K, Ohya T, Ohata K, Okamura S, Iizuka S, Takeuchi Y, Uedo N, Fusaroli P, Bonino MA, Verra M, Morino M. Systematic review and meta-analysis of endoscopic submucosal dissection versus transanal endoscopic microsurgery for large noninvasive rectal lesions. Surg Endosc. 2014;28:427–38.
6. Christoforidis D, Cho HM, Dixon MR, Mellgren AF, Madoff RD, Finne CO. Transanal endoscopic microsurgery versus conventional transanal excision for patients with early rectal cancer. Ann Surg. 2009;249(5):776–82.
7. Allaix ME, Arezzo A, Cassoni P, Famiglietti F, Morino M. Recurrence after transanal endoscopic microsurgery for large rectal adenomas. Surg Endosc. 2012;26:2594–600.
8. Morino M, Risio M, Bach S, Beets-Tan R, Bujko K, Panis Y, Quirke P, Rembacken B, Rullier E, Saito Y, Young-Fadok T, Allaix ME. Early rectal cancer: the European Association for Endoscopic Surgery (EAES) clinical consensus conference. Surg Endosc. 2015;29(4):755–73.
9. Morino M, Allaix ME, Famiglietti F, Caldart M, Arezzo A. Does peritoneal perforation affect short- and long-term outcomes after transanal endoscopic microsurgery? Surg Endosc. 2013;27(1):181–8.
10. Arezzo A, Arolfo S, Allaix ME, Munoz F, Cassoni P, Monagheddu C, Ricardi U, Ciccone G, Morino M. Results of Neoadjuvant Short-Course Radiation Therapy Followed by Transanal Endoscopic Microsurgery for T1-T2 N0 Extraperitoneal Rectal Cancer. Int J Radiat Oncol Biol Phys. 2015;92(2):299–306. pii: S0360-3016(15)00097-8. doi:10.1016/j.ijrobp.2015.01.024. [Epub ahead of print].

34 TransAnal Minimally Invasive Surgery (TAMIS)

A.M. Lacy and M. Fernández-Hevia

34.1 Introduction

Transanal endoscopic microsurgery (TEM) was first described by Buess et al in 1983, as a procedure of minimally invasive surgery for full-thickness resection of benign rectal lesions. The advantages of this approach, compared with transanal excision, were superior visualization, improved access to proximal lesions, increased rates of negative margins, decreased fragmentation of specimens and lower recurrence rates. The indications quickly expanded and nowadays T1 N0 rectal tumors can be performed using this approach, furthermore it can be an alternative in patients with advanced lesions with contraindication for radical resection. Benefits of a TEM procedure are reducing the adverse effects of radical rectal surgery, minor postoperative complications, lower rates of anorectal, urinary and sexual dysfunction.

TEM system have got limited widespread adoption, one of its limitations is the need for specialized expensive instruments and a steep learning curve. Popularity of single-port system in abdominal surgery last years has facilitated to introduce these platforms in transanal surgery. Single-port devices are introduced into anal canal and allow performing transanal excision using standard laparoscopic instruments. The colocation in the anal canal is easier with these new devices. One problem with TEM is the complexity of the TEM setup, it was essential to know exactly where was the lesion to adapt the position of the patient in the table (i.e. lesion at 6 h, patient would be positioned in prono), with new devices it is not essential, the patient may always be placed in the dorsal lithotomy position. New devices are more ergonomic, allowing wider range of movement. Preliminary studies using these devices have demonstrated technical feasibility, low morbidity and its oncological safety. Many different platforms have been used and different nomenclatures have been appeared, including different acronyms such as Transanal Mini-Invasive Surgery (TAMIS), Transanal Single-Port Microsurgery (TSPM), Transanal Endoscopic Video-Assisted surgery (TEVA) and SILSTEM. This TEM alternative could reduce cost and allow extend transanal surgical endoscopic resection for rectal pathologies in centres nor equipped with TEM system.

34.2 Indications

Transanal minimally invasive surgery (TAMIS) indications are initially the same as TEM (Table 34.1). The endoscopic approach avoids the need of anterior resection, preserving sphincters and allowing access to rectal tumors located up to 20 cm from the anal verge, using the better vision provided through the rectoscope and the creation of a pneumorectum.

It is typically used for the treatment for benign polyps that are not amenable to flexible endoscopic excision and for early rectal cancers, specially to low risk T1. Patients with T1 without adverse pathologic factors (i.e., high grade, blood or lymphatic vessel invasion, sm3) can be adequately treated with local excision alone, preferably a TEM procedure. This approach allows accurate assessment of histopathological parameters such as margin, differentiation, vascular involvement and depth of penetration Furthermore there are currently different trials comparing rectal anterior resection vs chemoradiotherapy plus transanal miniinvasive surgery in T2 and T3a N0. In just some cases, it can be an alternative in patients with advanced rectal lesions with contraindication for radical resection.

TEM and TAMIS have the same limitations as traditional endoanal resection (high recurrence rates for more advanced tumors and tumors with high-risk histological features). Nevertheless in patients with T1 rectal cancer, local recurrence rates are similar between TEM/TAMIS and TME. (0–5 % in T1 sm1/sm2 cancers, but up to 10–12 % in T1 sm3

A.M. Lacy (✉) M. Fernández-Hevia
Department of Surgery, Hospital Clinic de Barcelona, Barcelona, Spain
e-mail: alacy@clinic.ub.es

H.J. Bonjer (ed.), *Surgical Principles of Minimally Invasive Procedures*, DOI 10.1007/978-3-319-43196-3_34

Table 34.1 Indications for TAMIS

Benign rectal polyps
Low risk rectal cancer (T1)
Trials comparing with TME in T2–T3a after ChR
Palliative surgery
Other possibilities:
Total mesorectal excision
Drainage of pelvic and perirectal abscesses
Colorectal anastomotic stenosis.
Rectourethral fistula. Rectovaginal fistulas.
Condylomas in rectal ampulla.
Retrorectal tumors. Rectal duplication. Rectal GIST.
Conservative treatment for the leaks in low colorectal anastomoses.
Haemorrhage in rectal anastomoses.

cancers). Furthermore it is associated with lower mortality (<0.5 %) and morbidity (3–12 %) compared with radical resection.

Other additional criteria are tumor size (less than 4 cm) and histology (well- or moderately well-differentiated tumors). The probability of lymph node metastases is modified based on the above factors, thereby a T1 G1 (well-differentiated) tumor has a lymph node metastases risk around 0 % compared with more than 10 % for a T1 G3 (poorly differentiated) tumor.

In last years TAMIS indications have extended, using this approach in natural orifice transluminal endoscopic surgery (NOTES). TAMIS total mesorectal excision in rectal cancer assisted by laparoscopy is a new procedure that have earned popularity in recent years, there are a case of pure NOTES published using this approach.

Atypical:

- Drainage of pelvic and perirectal abscesses above the levator muscles of the anus. It can be an alternative in patients in which transanal access or radiological guided drainage is unsuccessful.
- Colorectal anastomotic stenosis. The initial treatment of choice in these cases is endoscopic dilatation, but a possible alternative in middle-high rectal anastomoses could be stricturoplasty, if endoscopic dilatations fail.
- Rectourethral fistula after laparoscopic radical prostatectomy. Recent publications have reported successful interventions in these cases.
- Gastrointestinal stromal tumors (GIST), less than 2 cm in size with a pathology result of low mitotic activity (less than 5 mitoses per 50 HPF), are considered to have good prognosis, and so local surgery is the treatment of choice.
- The excision of condylomas in the anal canal and their extension toward the rectal ampulla.
- An alternative to failure laparoscopic ventral rectopexy. In this situation, after endoanal resection of the prolapsed rectal cylinder and the reconstruction of the rectum by attaching it to the wall of the pelvis, the fibrosis produced impedes relapse of the prolapse.
- Rectal foreign bodies. Depending on the anatomical location of the lesion, time of evolution and severity on the rectal organ injury scale. In extraperitoneal rectal lesions, the primary suture can be performed without faecal derivation, provided (a) the rectal injury scale is below II, (b) fewer than 8 h have passed since the trauma occurred, and (c) the lesion is accessible.
- Retrorectal tumors.
- Rectovaginal fistulas
- Rectal duplication
- Pyogenic granuloma
- Conservative treatment for the leaks in low colorectal anastomoses.
- Treatment of anastomotic haemorrhage in high and middle rectal anastomoses.
- The association with laparoscopic techniques:
  - Synchronous colonic neoplasm with rectal lesions.
  - TAMIS-TME assisted by laparoscopy in the treatment with bloc resection in rectal neoplasm.

34.3 Preoperative Work-Up

We are to focus in patients with benign polyps or early rectal cancer. Preoperative study will englobe the next tests.

1. Detailed history and physical examination. Familiar history. Previous pathology. Digital rectal examination will facilitate important information about distance to the anal verge, location (anterior, posterior, right/left side), percentage of circumference affected or kind of lesion (pediculate, sessile).
2. Rigid rectoscopy. Easy test to perform ambulatory, just need a simple preparation and is the most reliable test to define the distance to the anal verge, moreover in the highest rectal lesions.
3. Colonoscopy. Allowing to explore all colon and dismissing other synchronous lesions.
4. Biopsy of the lesion. Essential to know malignancy. Polyps resected by flexible endoscopy with doubtous deep margin can be tributaries of performing TAMIS.
5. In malignant or doubtous lesions must be perform:
   (a) Endorectal ultrasound to study deepness of the invasion and possibility of suspicious lymph nodes.

(b) Pelvic MRI to complete T and N staging.
(c) Thorax and abdominal computed tomography to discard possible distance metastases.

6. Preoperative study.
   - Blood test with carcinoembryonic antigen-CEA, liver function and coagulation test.
   - Electrocardiogram.
   - Chest radiography.
   - Anaesthesiologist evaluation.

34.4 Operating Room

Mechanical bowel preparation or rectal enemas will be administered preoperatively. Prophylactic antibiotics (i.e. cefoxitin 2 g) intravenously 1 h before beginning surgery will be administrated.

Patient will be placed in modified lithotomy position. Both legs are place in adjustable stirrups, both arms are tucked, padded and protected along the each side. The patient is positioned so that the perineum is reachable from between the legs. Lower extremity pneumatic compression stockings are used in all cases and in high-risk patients they will be maintained during postoperative period. The patient will be fixed to the table to try to avoid displacements of the patient during the procedure.

Peripheral intravenous lines are used and a central catheter can be used in function patients' comorbidities.

The rectum was irrigated with 1 % diluted iodine solution. A rigid rectoscopy will be performed to control the place of the lesion.

The patient is prepared and drapped sterile.

Surgical material: single-port device, 30 degrees angled scope will be used in these surgery, an alternative is a flexible scope but one limitation is reduced space to work and triangulation during surgery specially in high rectal lesions. Standard laparoscopic material (forceps, needle holder). Coagulation device.

The surgeons and the camera are placed between legs and the screen will be place over the patient's head.

34.5 Surgical Technique

Lone star® retractor is positioned before inserting transanal single-port (Fig. 34.1) and posteriorly it can be removed. Pneumorectum will be established by using CO2 insufflation with an initial pressure set at 12–15 mmHg and flow set at 40 mmHg per minute. High-definition laparoscopic cameras and a 30° will be used for visualization. Standard laparoscopic instruments will be used to perform excision. Full-thickness excision will be performed respecting TEM principles resection, with the objective of obtaining a 1 cm minimum negative lateral margin and a clear margin to the perirectal tissue without tumor fragmentation.

The line of section around the lesion will be marked with the hook and once the circumference is completed, all points will be connected (Fig. 34.2). Coagulation device will be used to complete the resection (Figs. 34.3 and 34.4). All defects will be closed completely with absorbable suture material by use a variety of suturing techniques (Figs. 34.5 and 34.6). This is the most critical issue. Many authors reported difficulties in repairing the excision defect so different methods have been proposed, as endoGIA stapler, intracorporeal suture-tying or interrupted sutures with/without extracorporeal knots that are secured with a knot-pusher.

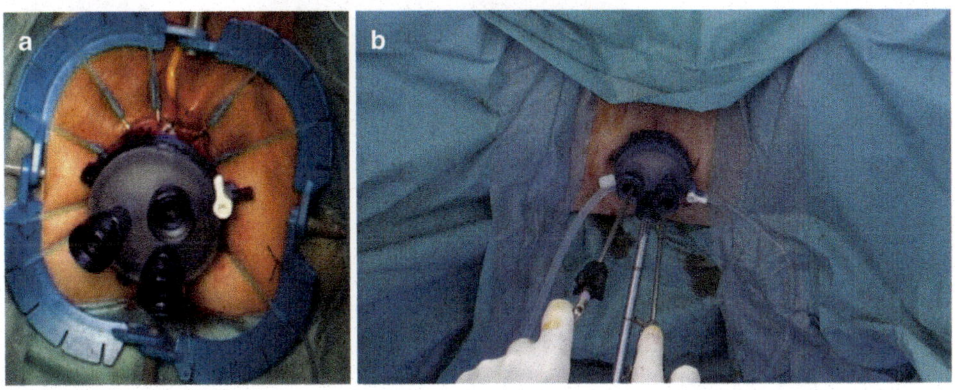

Fig. 34.1 (**a**) Position Lone star® retractor and insert transanal platform. (**b**) External vision of the team during the surgery (Gelpoint platform – Applied medical)

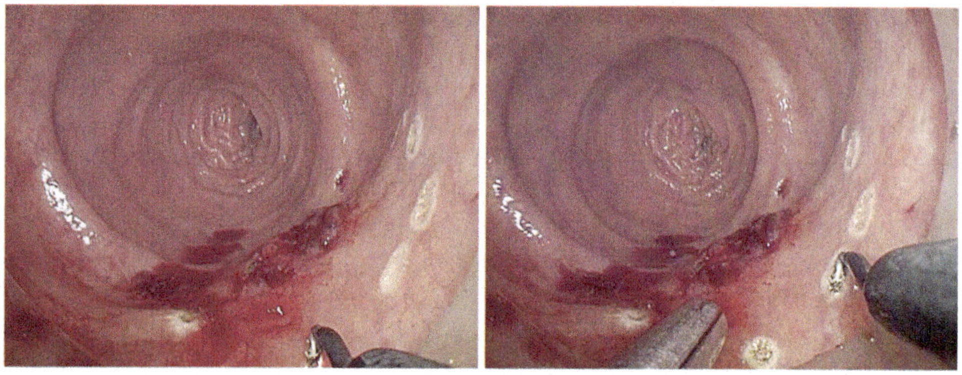

Fig. 34.2 Lesion indification and marking around it

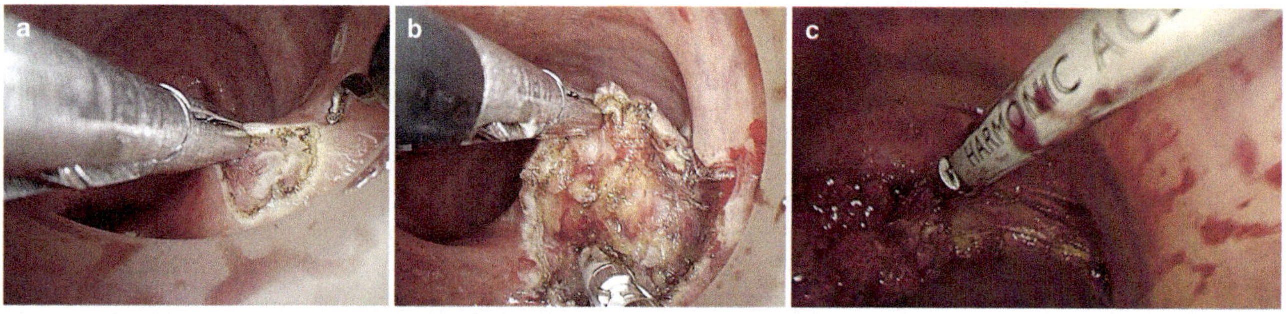

Fig. 34.3 Different images performing tumor resection, (**a**) Connecting all the points marked previously. (**b**) Performing the resection with electrocautery. (**c**) Using Harmonic to complete tumor resection

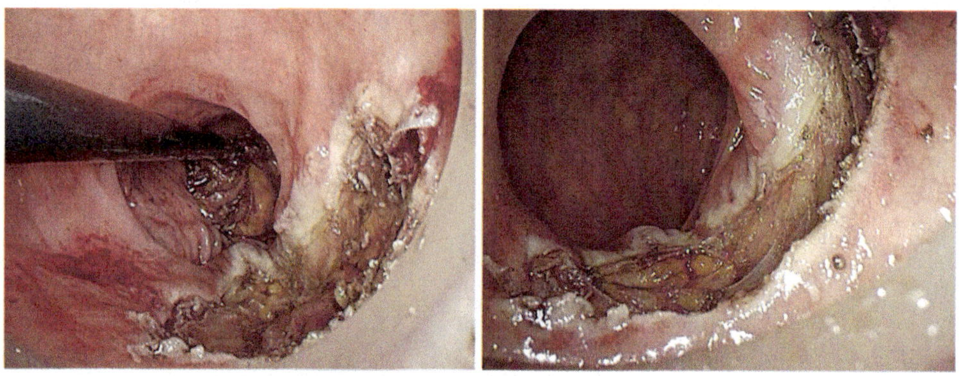

Fig. 34.4 Defect in rectal wall after complete tumor resection

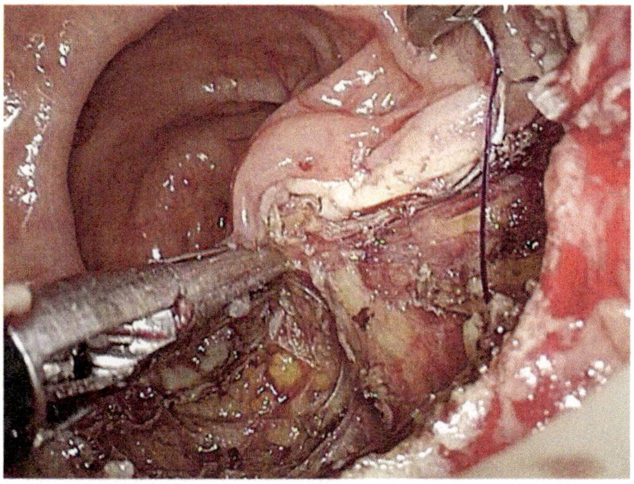

Fig. 34.5 Suturing the wall defect using standard laparoscopic instruments

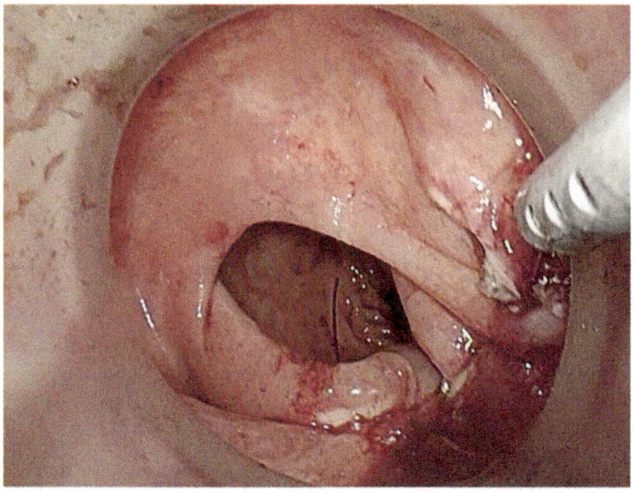

Fig. 34.6 Final vision after suturing defect

34.6 Postoperative Care

Low risk patients spend few hours in postoperative recovery unit and if there is no incidence after that will pass a hospitalization room and can be discharged the same day or 24 h after surgery. Diet will be reintroduced some hours after surgery and discharged with low residue diet. Foley catheter will be removed in operating room. Fever after surgery can appear in these patients so prophylactic antibiotics are usually held at discharge.

Bibliography

1. Buess G, Theiss R, Günther M, Hutterer F, Pichlmaier H. Transanal endoscopic microsurgery [in German]. Leber MagenDarm. 1985;15:271–9.
2. Serra-Aracil X, Mora-Lopez L, Alcantara-Moral M, Corredera-Cantarin C, Gomez-Diaz C, Navarro-Soto S. Atypical indications for transanal endoscopic microsurgery to avoid major surgery. Tech Coloproctol. 2013;18(2):157–64.
3. Lee W, Lee D, Choi S, Chun H. Transanal endoscopic microsurgery and radical surgery for T1 and T2 rectal cancer. Surg Endosc. 2003;17(8):1283–7.
4. Wick EC. Techniques, and outcomes of transanal excision and. Early diagnosis and treatment of cancer: colorectal cancer. Elsevier Inc. 2011; p. 127–33. doi:10.1016/B978-1-4160-4686-8.50017-8.
5. Albert MR, Atallah SB, deBeche-Adams TC, Izfar S, Larach SW. Transanal minimally invasive surgery (TAMIS) for local excision of benign neoplasms and early-stage rectal cancer: efficacy and outcomes in the first 50 patients. Dis Colon Rectum. 2013;56(3):301–7.

Part XIII

Thyroid and Parathyroid

Thyroid and Parathyroid (MIVAT and MIVAP)

35

Paolo Miccoli and Gabriele Materazzi

35.1 Introduction

The first endoscopic procedure in the cervical area was performed by M. Gagner who operated on a patient presenting with a primary hyperparathyroidism (PHPT) caused by a hyperplasia of four glands. PHPT seemed immediately to be an ideal disease to be approached endoscopically for several reasons: (1) the tumor giving rise to the hyperfunction is almost always benign (2) it rarely exceeds 2–3 of cm size (3) there is no need for any surgical reconstruction after the small mass removal. Not much later, also thyroid gland started to be approached endoscopically, although thyroid diseases more often present with a pathologic pattern which makes difficult to operate on them via an endoscopic access. In fact large goiters and invasive tumors are still common indications for thyroid surgery and the size of the mass to remove from the neck strongly limits the prospects of endoscopic thyroidectomy.

In 1998 we ideated and developed in Pisa MIVAT (Minimally Invasive Video Assisted Thyroidectomy) and MIVAP (Minimally Invasive Video Assisted Parathyroidectomy).

At present we might assume that MIVAP and MIVAT are to be considered a valid option for most of the cases of PHPT and thyroid disease and they are widely performed in several Centres as the first option. In spite of the initial caution though, the introduction of new technologies and instrumentation facilitated very much these procedures shortening significantly the operative time and enlarging the indications.

P. Miccoli, MD
Department of Surgery, University of Pisa, Pisa, Italy.

G. Materazzi, MD (✉)
Dipartimento di Chirurgia, Rome, Italy
e-mail: gmaterazzi@yahoo.com

35.2 Indications

35.2.1 Parathyroid

No doubt this is a surgery mostly indicated only for a sporadic disease characterized by the presence of a single, well localized adenoma harbored in a virgin neck This should imply a positive imaging that should be concordant for both ultrasonography and sestamibi scintiscan. Some contraindications are shown in Table 35.1.

35.2.2 Thyroid

The inclusion criteria and the main contraindications are summarized in Table 35.2. The most relevant limit is represented by the size of both the nodule and the gland as measured by means of an accurate ultrasonographic study to be performed pre-operatively. Ultrasonography can also be useful to exclude the presence of a thyroiditis, which might make the dissection troublesome. In case ultrasonography only gives the suspicion of thyroiditis, of course autoantibodies should be measured in the serum.

One of the most controversial aspects in terms of indications is the opportunity of treating malignancies. No doubt "low risk" papillary carcinomas constitute an ideal

Table 35.1 MIVAP: contraindications

Relative contraindications	Absolute contraindications
Adenomas larger than 3 cm	Large goiters
Lack of pre operative localization[a]	Recurrent disease
Neck surgery on the opposite side of the suspected adenoma[b]	Extensive previous neck surgery
Previous neck irradiation or small thyroid nodules[c]	MEN and familial PHPT
	Parathyroid carcinoma

Depending upon their shape, even larger adenomas can be removed
[a]A bilateral exploration can be performed through a central incision
[b]A lateral access can be used
[c]Concurrent thyroidectomy is possible

H.J. Bonjer (ed.), *Surgical Principles of Minimally Invasive Procedures*, DOI 10.1007/978-3-319-43196-3_35

Table 35.2 MIVAT Indications and contraindications

INDICATIONS

1. Thyroid nodules smaller than 3-3.5 cm in their largest diameter:
   - indeterminate cytology
   - follicular tumors
   - small symptomatic goiters

   } ***diagnostic surgery***
2. "Low risk" papillary carcinoma
3. Graves' disease presenting with small volume glands (not over 20 mL)
4. Prophylactic thyroidectomy in RET gene mutation carriers (early diagnosis)

indication for MIVAT but a good selection has to take into account the exact profile of possible lymph node involvement in the neck. In fact, although the completeness of a total thyroidectomy achievable with video assisted procedures is beyond debate, the greatest caution should be taken when approaching a disease involving either metastatic lymph nodes or an extracapsular invasion of the gland. In these cases an endoscopic approach might be inadequate to obtain a full clearance of the nodes or the complete removal of the neoplastic tissue (infiltration of the trachea or the oesophagus) [1–5].

35.3 Contraindications

1. History of thyroiditis (positive autoantibodies)
2. History of neck irradiation
3. Previous thyroid or parathyroid surgery

35.3.1 Preoperative Work-Up

Patients will undergo routine examinations for general anaesthesia.

Before attempting a minimally invasive approach by MIVAT or MIVAP the following examinations are very useful to the surgeon:

- Ultrasonography of the thyroid gland in order to evaluate total gland volume, diameter of the largest nodule, position and diameter of the parathyroid adenoma.
- Blood test to ascertain the euthyroidism and exclude a thyroiditis
- A fine needle aspiration biopsy on the suspicious nodule
- X ray examination of the trachea
- A laryngoscopic examination by an otolaryngologist.

The patient is given detailed written consent, prophylactic antibiotic therapy before surgery and pre-anaesthesia are administered before going to the operating room.

35.3.2 Operating Room

35.3.2.1 Patient

- Supine position without neck hyperextension
- Conventional neck preparation and draping
- A sterile drape covering the skin (Bioclusive © 2003 Johnson&Johnson, Gargrave, Skipton, UK).

35.3.2.2 Team

- The surgeon is on the right side of the table.
- The first assistant is on the left side of the table (opposite the surgeon)
- The second assistant is at the head of the table.
- The third assistant is on the left side of the table
- The scrub nurse is behind the surgeon on the right side of the table.

35.3.3 MIVAT/MIVAP Kit

1. Forward-oblique telescope 30°, diameter 5 mm, length 30 cm
2. Suction dissector with cut-off hole, with stylet, blunt, length 21 cm

3. Ear forceps, very thin, serrated, working length 12.5 cm
4. Conventional tissue retractor army navy type
5. Small tissue retractor, double-ended, length 12 cm
6. Clip applier for vascular clips
7. Straight scissors, length 12.5 cm

35.3.4 Surgical Technique

35.3.4.1 MIVAT Operative Technique

Preparation of the Operative Space

The patient, under general endotracheal anaesthesia, is positioned in supine position with his neck not extended. Hyperextension must be avoided because it would reduce the operative space. The skin is protected by means of a sterile film (Bioclusive © 2003 Johnson&Johnson, Gargrave, Skipton, UK). A 1,5 cm horizontal skin incision is performed 2 cm above the sternal notch in the central cervical area. Subcutaneous fat and platysma are carefully dissected so as to avoid any minimum bleeding. Two small retractors are used to expose the midline which has to be incised for 2–3 cm on an absolutely bloodless plane (Fig. 35.1).

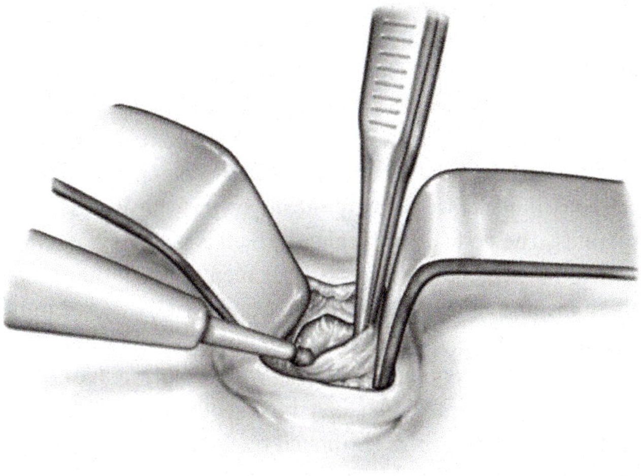

Fig. 35.1 Use of two small retractors to expose midline

The blunt dissection of the thyroid lobe from the strap muscles is completely carried out through the skin incision by gentle retraction and using tiny spatulas. When the thyroid lobe is almost completely dissected from the strap muscles, larger and deeper retractors (army navy-type) can be inserted and they will maintain the operative space during all the endoscopic part of the procedure (Fig. 35.2). Then, a 30° 5 mm or 7 mm endoscope is introduced through the skin incision: from this moment on, the procedure is entirely endoscopic until the extraction of the lobe of the gland. Preparation of the thyro-tracheal groove is completed under endoscopic vision by using small (2 mm in diameter) instruments like spatulas, forceps, spatula-sucker, scissors.

Ligature of the Main Thyroid Vessels

Harmonic® device is utilized for almost all the vascular structures but, if the vessel to be coagulated is running particularly close to the inferior laryngeal nerve, then haemostasis is achieved by means of small vascular clips applied by a disposable or reusable clip applier.

The first vessel to be ligated is the middle vein, when present, or the small veins between jugular vein and thyroid capsule. This step allows a better preparation of the thyrotracheal groove where the recurrent nerve will be later searched.

A further step is represented by the exposure of the upper pedicle, which must be carefully prepared, until an optimal visualization of the different branches is achieved. During this step the endoscope should be rotated of 180° with the 30° degrees tip looking up-ward and hold in a parallel direction with the thyroid lobe and trachea, in order to better visualize the upper portion of the operative camera where the superior thyroid vein and artery are running (Fig. 35.3).

Inferior Laryngeal Nerve and Parathyroid Glands Identification and Dissection

After retracting medially and lifting up the thyroid lobe, the fascia can be opened by a gentle spatula retraction. During this step the endoscope should be re-positioned in a orthogonal axis with the thyroid lobe and trachea, looking downward with its 30° degrees angle (Fig. 35.4). The recurrent

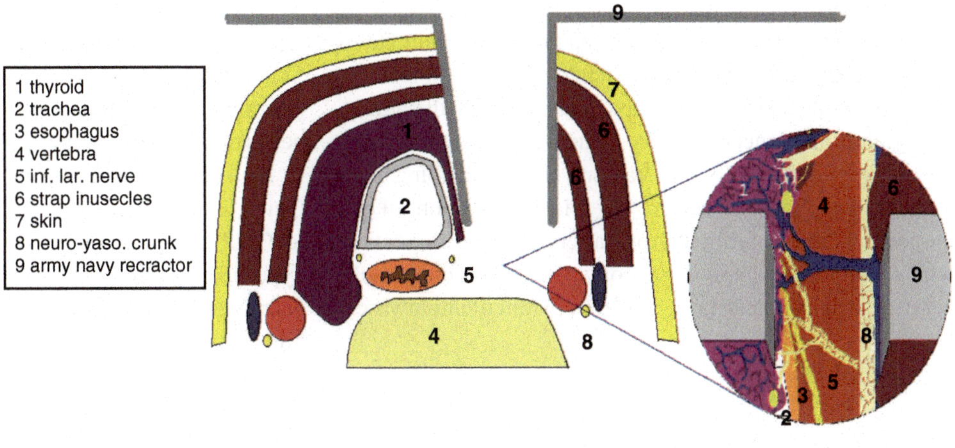

Fig. 35.2 Retractors in operative space

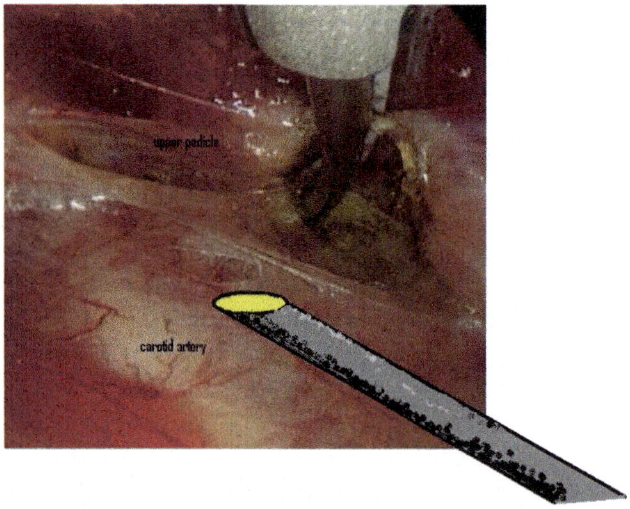

Fig. 35.3 Position of endoscope for visualization of upper portion of operative camera where the superior thyroid vein and artery are running

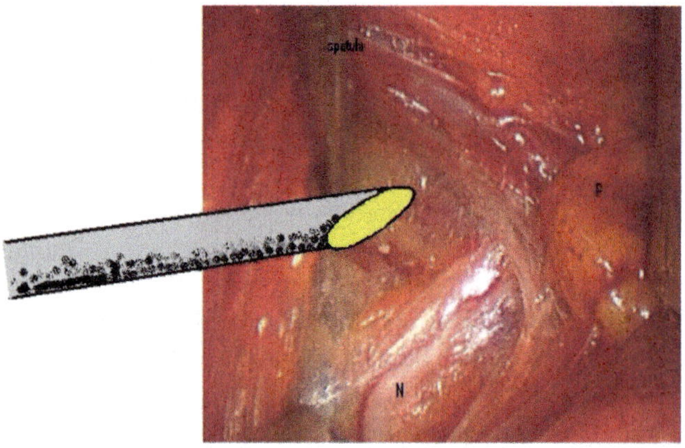

Fig. 35.4 Position of endoscope in orthogonal axis with the thyroid lobe and trachea

laryngeal nerve appears generally at this point in time, lying in the thyrotracheal groove, posterior to the Zuckerkandl tuberculum (posterior lobe) which constitutes an important landmark in this phase. This way the recurrent nerve and the parathyroid glands are dissected and freed from the thyroid (Fig. 35.5).

Dissection of the entire nerve from the mediastinum to its entrance into the larynx is not mandatory and might result in a time waste during the endoscopic phase. Also both parathyroid glands are generally easily visualized during the endoscopic step thanks to the camera magnification. Their vascular supply is preserved by selective section of the branches of the inferior thyroid artery. During dissection, when dealing with large vessels or small vessels close to the nerve, haemostasis can be achieved by 3-mm titanium vascular clips.

Extraction of the Lobe and Resection

At this point in time the lobe is completely freed. The endoscope and the retractors can be removed and the upper portion of the gland rotated and pulled out using conventional forceps. A gentle traction over the lobe allows the complete exteriorization of the gland. The lobe is freed from the trachea by ligating the small vessels and dissecting the Berry ligament. The isthmus is then dissected from the trachea and divided. After completely exposing the trachea, the lobe is finally removed. Drainage is not necessary. The midline is then approached by a single stitch; platysma is closed by a subcuticular suture and a cyanoachrilate sealant is used for the skin (Fig. 35.6).

35.3.4.2 MIVAP Operative Technique

The access to the operative field is same described in step 1 for MIVAT. In case of re-do surgery, a lateral access instead of the standard midline access is possible. This avoids entering fibrous tissue where recognition of anatomical planes and structures such as the recurrent nerve may be difficult. The incision is made just medially to the sternocleidomastoid muscle and the same blunt dissection is performed until the thyroid space is well-exposed.

The exploration first starts on the side in which the adenoma is supposed to be on the basis of the preoperative imaging, but bilateral exploration can be achieved through the central incision. The endoscopic magnification allows very easy identification of the relevant neck structures like the recurrent laryngeal nerve. Once the adenoma is located it is dissected without disrupting the capsule performing a cautious blunt dissection by means of the above described spatulas. The pedicle of the gland which is well visible under optical magnification (Fig. 35.7), is then clipped: the use of small disposable vascular clips is strongly suggested (2 mm) because of the relatively small operative field. Washing and cleaning of the operative field can be simply achieved in absence of trocars. Water can be injected directly with a syringe; its aspiration is facilitated by the use of the spatula-shaped aspirator. Smoke and fluids can be sucked without introducing extra instruments into the incision.

The adenoma is then retrieved through the skin incision. No drainage is necessary but we strongly advocate not to close tightly the midline so to better evaluate early bleedings. Skin is generally closed only by means of a skin sealant (Dermabond®) after a subcuticular running suture has been performed in order to approach the two edges of the incision. In the meanwhile the surgeon is waiting for the result of Quick intraoperative intact parathyroid hormone assay (qPTHa). The completeness of the surgical resection of all hyperfunctioning parathyroid tissue is confirmed by a decrease of more than 50 % in qPTHa values compared to the highest pre-excision level. Measurements are obtained when

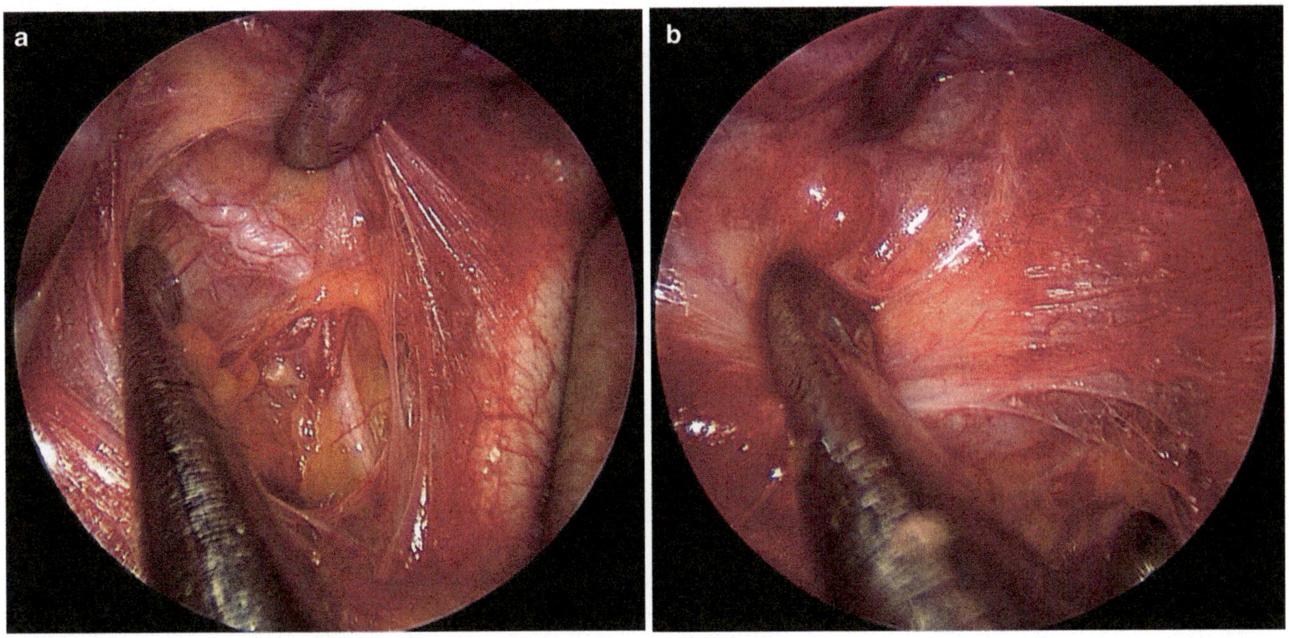

Fig. 35.5 Recurrent nerve (a) and parathyroid glands (b) dissected from the thyroid

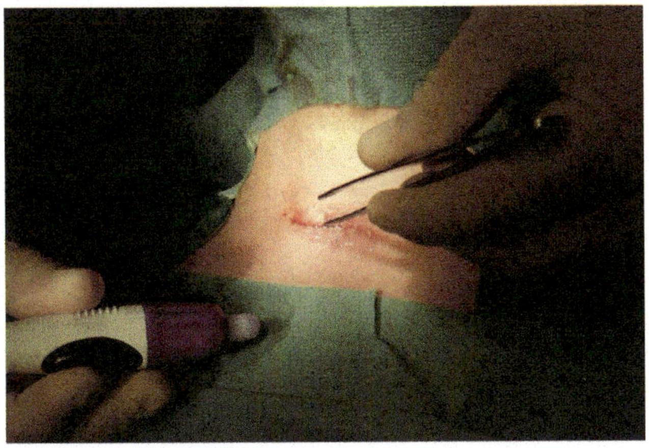

Fig. 35.6 Cyanoachrilate sealant used for closing the skin

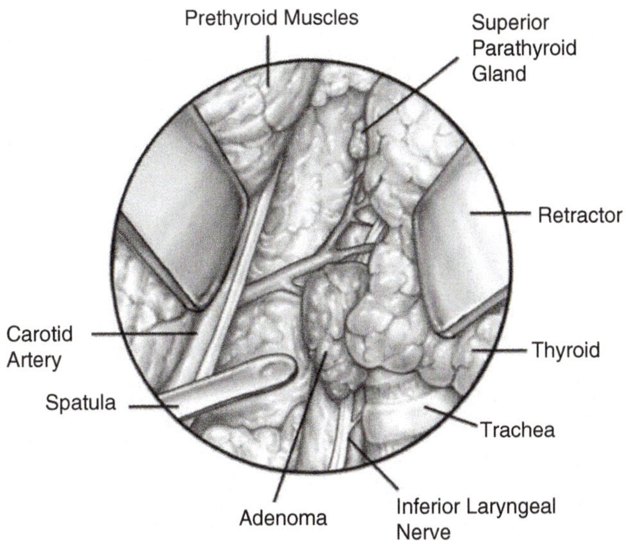

Fig. 35.7 Pedicle of the gland well visible under optical magnification

anesthesia is induced, when the adenoma is visualized and 5 and 10 min after the adenoma is removed.

35.3.5 Postoperative Care

After surgery, patients undergoing MIVAP and MIVAT require strict observation during the first 5–10 h on the ward. Dysfonia, airway obstruction, and neck swelling must be carefully checked. No drain is left, so careful surveillance for postoperative hematomas is required during the immediate postoperative period. Postoperative bleeding risk is very low, especially after MIVAP, and dramatically decreases after 5 h, especially using the harmonic scalpel. In fact, one of the major advantages when using the Harmonic Scalpel, is represented by the fact that the postoperative hemorrhage occurs immediately or at least after few hours.

In case of postoperative hematoma, if compressive symptoms and airway obstruction are present, re-intervention and immediate hematoma evacuation is strongly required.

Patients can start oral intake since the evening on the operative day, and will be discharged the day after. Patients

Table 35.3 Management of postoperative hypocalcemia

Management of hypocalcemia following thyroidectomy on the first postoperative day	
Acute symptomatic	Calcium gluconate IV
Asymptomatic calcium ≤7.5[a] mg/dL	Calcium (3 g) + vitamin D (0.5 μg) per os daily
Asymptomatic calcium 7.5–7.9 mg/dL	Calcium (1.5 g) per os daily

[a]Normal range: 8–10 mg/dL

undergoing MIVAP could be discharged the same day, especially if surgery has been performed under local anesthesia, when allowed by the national health care system.

On the first and second postoperative day serum calcium must be checked, in order to control hypoparathyroidism by substitutive therapy, as described in Table 35.3.

Wound care is not really necessary after MIVAP and MIVAP, because of the glue covering the skin and postoperative pain will be controlled by means of both iv or oral analgesics.

Voice impairments and subjective or objective dysfonia require immediate postoperative vocal cord check by and ENT doctor. In case of normal postoperative course, vocal cord check can be delayed after 3 months.

References

1. Miccoli P, Materazzi G. Minimally invasive video assisted thyroidectomy (MIVAT). Surg Clin North Am. 2004;84:735–41.
2. Miccoli P, Elisei R, Materazzi G, Capezzone M, Galleri D, Pacini F, Berti P, Pinchera A. Minimally Invasive Video Assisted Thyroidectomy for Papillary Carcinoma: a prospective study about its completeness. Surgery. 2002;132:1070–4.
3. Miccoli P, Pinchera A, Materazzi G, Biagini A, Berti P, Faviana P, Molinaro E, Viola D, Elisei R. Surgical treatment of low- and intermediate-risk papillary thyroid cancer with minimally invasive video-assisted thyroidectomy. J Clin Endocrinol Metab. 2009; 94(5):1618–22.
4. Lombardi CP, Raffaelli M, Traini E, De Crea C, Corsello SM, Bellantone R. Video-assisted minimally invasive parathyroidectomy: benefits and long-term results. World J Surg. 2009;33(11): 2266–81.
5. Miccoli P, Elisei R, Donatini G, Materazzi G, Berti P. Video-assisted central compartment lymphadenectomy in a patient with a positive RET oncogene: initial experience. Surg Endosc. 2007;21(1):120–3.

Part XIV

Adrenal

Laparoscopic Transperitoneal Adrenalectomy

36

Luigi Boni, Stefano Rausei, Matteo Di Giuseppe, Elisa Cassinotti, and Gianlorenzo Dionigi

36.1 Introduction

First described by Gagner et al. and Higashihara et al. in 1992 laparoscopic adrenalectomy is now considered the gold standard treatment for removal of adrenal masses. Reduction in post-operative stay, wound related complications, pain and faster return to normal activities in comparison to standard open technique represent the main benefits of the minimally invasive approach.

36.2 Indications

Current indications for laparoscopic transperitoneal approach to the adrenal glands are removal of benign functioning and non-functioning tumors of the adrenal gland <12-cm.

In detail, about 80 % of minimally invasive procedures are performed for endocrine cause of hypertension such as unilateral aldosteronoma, Cushing's syndrome and pheochromocytoma without any preoperative evidence of local invasion or metastases. Other less common indications include adrenal cyst, metasteses, myelolipoma, primary adrenocortical neoplasm, androgen-secreting tumors, adrenal hemorrhage, ganglioneururoma, adrenal tuberculosis and primary hydatid cyst. Bilateral laparoscopic transperitoneal approach has been used in the treatment of Cushing's syndrome that includes refractory Cushing's disease, ectopic adrenocorticotrophic hormone (ACTH) production, bilateral ACTH-secreting adenomas, and bilateral pheochromocytomas.

L. Boni, MD, FACS (✉) • S. Rausei, MD • M. Di Giuseppe, MD
E. Cassinotti, MD, PhD • G. Dionigi, MD, FACS
Minimally Invasive Surgery Research Center, University of Insubria, Azienda Ospedaliero Universitaria, Fondazione Macchi, Varese, Italy
e-mail: luigi.boni@uninsubria.it

36.3 Contraindications

Contraindications for laparoscopic transperitoneal approach are *relative* and include the uncooperative patient, uncorrectable coagulation defects, severe congestive heart failure, respiratory insufficiency, hemodynamic instability resulting from a ruptured adrenal gland, pregnancy, associate bowel obstruction and inability to perform the procedure safely with minimally invasive techniques.

As for pregnancy, first-trimester surgery risks teratogenesis and miscarriage while during the third-trimester surgery might cause preterm labor and premature delivery, as well as difficulties related to poor visualization. The second trimester is safest, with less risk for preterm labor but, if possible, elective surgery should be postponed until few months after delivery.

As usual cardiac diseases and cardiopulmonary obstructive diseases (COPD) are nowadays considered only relative contra-indications to laparoscopic surgery but in those cases the used of low-pressure pneumoperitoneum is recommended.

The elderly and morbidly obese patients have increased risk for complications with general anesthesia and a careful preoperative assessment is recommended. Special care should be taken in obese patients for the prevention of deep vein thrombosis using compression stockings, low-dose heparin, early post-operative ambulation.

Laparoscopic transperitoneal approach may also be challenging in case of previous abdominal open procedure and it might require modification of the usual trocar insertion site. In case of severe adhesion the minimally invasive retroperitoneal or the standard open approach should be considered.

The only *absolute* contraindications for laparoscopic transperitoneal approach include benign tumors greater than 12 cm (because of the increased incidence of malignancy at this size and technical limitations of extraction), tumors with gross local invasion, adrenocortical carcinomas, and metastatic pheochromocytomas.

H.J. Bonjer (ed.), *Surgical Principles of Minimally Invasive Procedures*, DOI 10.1007/978-3-319-43196-3_36

36.4 Advantages & Disadvantages

The main advantages of the laparoscopic adrenalectomy over open surgery are the same as those describe for other minimal access procedures: smaller incisions, better visualization of the operative field, possibility to easily explore the entire peritoneal cavity, shorter postoperative length of stay, less postoperative pain, decreased analgesics usage and improved patient satisfaction.

The disadvantages are that it is more technically demanding in terms of equipment, costs and the experience of the surgeon, bilateral adrenalectomy cannot be performed without repositioning the patient and that it is not recommended for the treatment of malignant neoplasm. Furthermore, drawbacks of this technique are the fact that frequency of adrenal tumours is relatively low, a minority of patients qualify for this approach as the volume of the adrenal masses to be removed often exceeds the possibilities of endoscopic surgery. Moreover, the learning curve is quite long for the surgeon and the availability of surgeons experienced both in endocrine and in endoscopic surgery is still low. De facto, it is difficult, outside high volume speciality centres, for practicing surgeons and residents in training to develop enough experience to become proficient with this technique, especially in more difficult cases.

36.5 Alternative Treatment Options

Alternative minimally invasive treatment options for adrenal tumor include retroperitoneoscopic approach, single port access adrenalectomy (both anterior and posterior), hand-assisted, robotic assisted surgery, and imaging-guided percutaneous ablation (by means of radiofrequency, microware, etc.).

36.6 Preoperative Work-Up

Adrenal lesions are characterized by size, growth, imaging characteristics, and functional status and these criteria are useful to determine whether an adrenal tumor is likely to be malignant or if it should be resected based on its functional status.

Abdominal ultrasound (US) represents an easy tool for the first diagnostic step: in case of a suspicion of adrenal lesion, the US finding needs an implementation by computer tomography (CT) scan. Adrenal lesions are initially assessed without contrast agent to measure their attenuation value since almost 70 % of benign cortical adenomas will contain sufficient intracellular lipid to significantly lower the attenuation value: if the attenuation value is high, immediate and delayed scans are performed following administration of contrast for the calculation of contrast agent washout. In general, adenomas will have greater washout than a nonadenomatous lesion; this technique has a sensitivity of 98 % and a specifity of 92 % in differentiating an adenoma from other adrenal tumours. Furthermore, using a multidetector CT, it is now possible to obtain image reconstructions of the adrenal glands in any plane: this has demonstrated helpful in determining whether a large mass is of renal or adrenal origin and also for detecting possible invasion of surrounding structures.

When CT evaluation is unsatisfactory, magnetic resonance images (MRI) might be useful due to its great contrast resolution and its high accuracy to distinguish normal and pathological tissues, as well as cyst, oedema, necrosis, haemorrhage, vascular and cellular density.

MRI does not involve the use of ionising radiation and relies on the difference in resonance frequencies of protons in water and intracytoplasmic lipid.

Radiological criteria to be considered in case of adrenal lesion are: size, morphology, CT density, MRI signal characteristics as well as enhancement after administration of contrast agents.

In order to evaluate the functional status of adrenal lesion together with its morphologic assessment, both US National Institutes of Health and American Association of Endocrine Surgeons guidelines suggest a set of preoperative functional studies.

The hormonal pattern evaluation includes an overnight dexamethasone suppression test (for subclinical Cushing's syndrome), the ratio of plasma aldosterone concentration to plasma renin activity (for aldosteronoma) and plasma fractionated metanephrines or 24-h total urinary fractionated metanephrines (for pheochromocytoma).

Only in very few cases, when radiology associated with hormonal tests is not able to identify the nature of adrenal mass functional imaging such as PET-CT and SPECT could be useful since they provide both anatomical and functional information, indeed ^{18}F-FDG-PET exploits the increased metabolism of glucose in malignant lesions and it has a high specificity for the detection of malignant adrenal lesions although there have been reports of FDG uptake also in benign lesions, such as adrenal adenomas and myelolipomas.

The accuracy of the current imaging techniques in characterizing adrenal incidentalomas greatly reduces the need for adrenal fine needle biopsy (FNB).

The use of FNB is now limited for distinguishing an adrenal metastasis from an extra-adrenal malignancy and, although the complication rate is less than 3 %, it must not be performed before having excluded the possibility of a pheochromocytoma. Furthermore the risk of a diffusion of cancer cells along the needle track also should be considered.

Nevertheless even after a thorough workup, many adrenal lesions lack a definitive diagnosis and it remains difficult to identify patients with functioning tumor preoperatively and to avoid the unnecessary resection of non-functioning mass so, to date, the decision whether to remove an adrenal lesion depends on the results of the aforementioned diagnostic work-up.

36.7 General Operative Settings

Patients are usually put on "nil by mouth" 12 h before the operation, once in the operating theatre, they will be placed on the operating table above a "bean-bag" that will be later used to keep the lateral position required for the procedure.

Foley bladder catheter is inserted in a sterile manner and, once oral-tracheal anaesthesia is completed, temporary oro-gastric tube should be placed in order to empty the stomach both to prevent aspiration and to facilitate dissection especially in case of left adrenalectomy.

Venous Central line is usually not required while an arterial line might be useful for continuous blood pressure monitoring especially in case of feocromocytomas.

36.8 Instrumentation

Instruments required for trans-peritoneal laparoscopic adrenalectomy are:

- Laparoscopic ancillary equipment including:
  - *30° 5/10 mm scope*
  - *High definition camera*
  - *CO2 insufflator*
  - *Light source*
- High frequency generator
- Ultrasonic generator and hand piece
- Ancillary laparoscopic instrumentations including:
  - *10 and 5 mm trocar*
  - *Atraumatic forceps*
  - *"Right angle" dissector*
  - *Hook*
  - *Scissors*
  - *Suction and irrigation device*
  - *Atraumatic liver laparoscopic retractor*
  - *Medium/large and large 5/10 mm clip applier*
- Retrieval endoscopic bag

36.9 Surgical Technique for Right Adrenalectomy

36.9.1 Positioning of the Patient

Once oral-tracheal anaesthesia is completed, the patient is gently rotated on his left site with an angle between 80° and 90°, the table should be split at the level of the left flank in order to increase the space between the costal margin and the iliac spine.

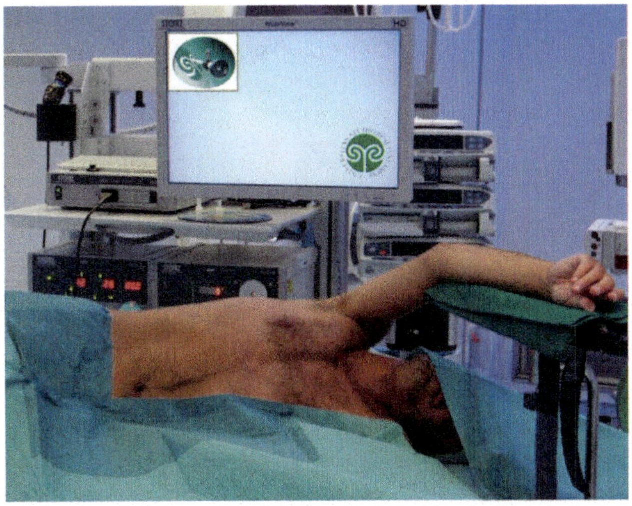

Fig. 36.1 Positioning of patient for transperitoneal adrenalectomy

The right harm should be fixed above patient's head using an arch and special care should be taken for positioning the left shoulder correctly in order to avoid accidental damage, a soft pillow is usually placed between patient's knees to prevent pressure sores (Fig. 36.1).

At this point the "bean bag" can be vacuum and patient fixed in the final position, during the procedure the operating table could be adjusted by tilting it on the left or right side so gravity can be used to achieve a better exposure.

The patient is then prepped with iodine or alcohol based solution from half of the chest to the sovra-pubic abdominal area, sterile drapes are then placed and secured.

The main monitor or the laparoscopic tower is placed on the right side of the bed towards patient's shoulder and adjusted according to surgeon's preferences.

The operating surgeon, the camera holder as well as the assistant stand on the left side, while the scrub nurse is usually on the lower right part of the bed watching and accessory monitor.

36.9.2 Pneumoperitoneum and Trocar Placements

The pneumoperitoneum can be induced either using a Veres needle or an "open" technique.

The Veres needle can be carefully placed in the elevated right flank around the middle point between the iliac and the umbilical scar, the pneumoperitoneum is induced up to 12 mmHg of intra abdominal pressure and the first 10 or 5 mm (depending on the diameter of the optic) trocar is introduced at the level of the middle right clavicle line just under the right costal margin (Fig. 36.2). Using this "closed" technique care should be taken not to damage accidentally the

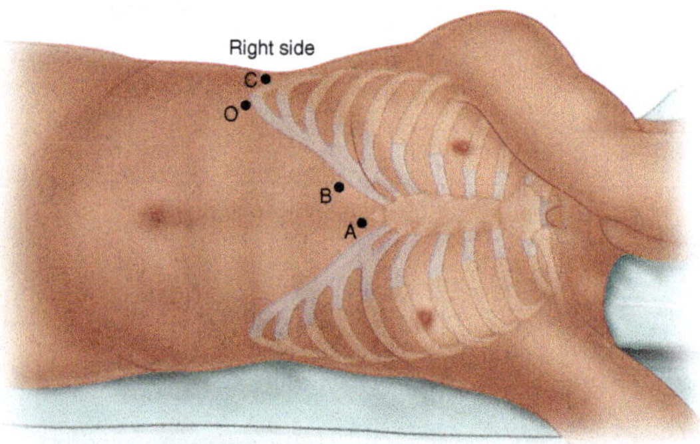

Fig. 36.2 Position of the trocar for right adrenalectomy (*O*: optic, *A*: liver retractor, *B*: surgeon's right hand, *C*: surgeon's left hand)

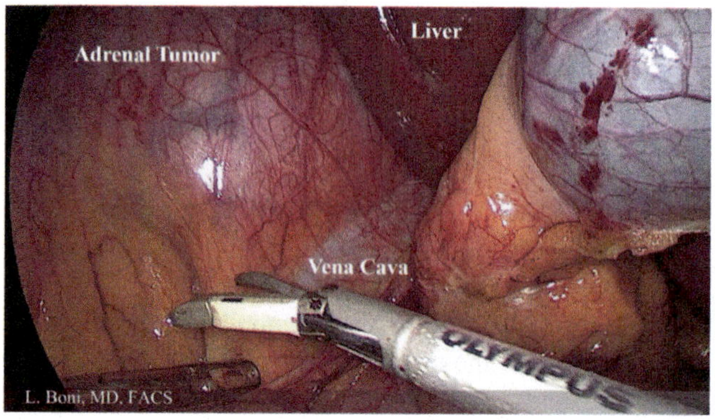

Fig. 36.3 Operative field after retraction of the right lobe of the liver

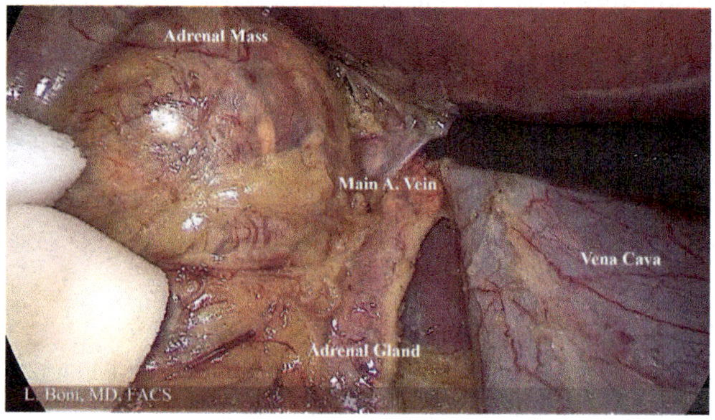

Fig. 36.4 Exposure of the main adrenal vein

right lobe of the liver: an "optic trocar" can also be used for entering the abdominal cavity.

As alternative, the pneumoperitoneum can be induced using an "open" technique with the Hasson's trocar inserted "under vision" in the same position as described above: nevertheless once the abdominal cavity is distended the position of such trocar is lowered resulting in a non optimal ergonomic setting.

Three further ports are required and can be introduced under direct vision (Fig. 36.2):

- One 5 or 10 mm trocar at the level of the midline will be inserted just on the right side of the xifoid and will be used by the assistant to introduce the atraumatic retractor and lift the right lobe of the liver. The diameter of the trocar will be chosen according to the size of retractor (Fig. 36.2).
- One 5 or 10 mm trocar on the level of the anterior clavicle line just under the right costal margin and will be used by the surgeon right hand to perform most of the dissection, so the size of the trocar will depend by the size of the dissection instruments used for the procedure (Fig. 36.2).
- Finally usually a 5 mm trocar is placed on the lateral clavicle line once again the costal margin and will be mainly used for the introduction of a retracting instrument during the procedure (Fig. 36.2).

36.9.3 Surgical Steps

Once the trocar are placed the right lobe of the liver is gently lifted using an atraumatic retractor introduced through the midline trocar, this will give access to the right adrenal area. In some cases adhesion between the liver and the transverse colon or the Gerota's fascia might be encountered and divided.

Once the right lobe of the liver is elevated the inferior vena cava (IVC) and the second and third part of the duodenum are exposed (Fig. 36.3).

Using the harmonic scalpel or the hook attached to low voltage monopolar electrocautery, partial mobilization of the duodenum is carried out in order to achieve a good exposure of the vena cava up to the level of the right renal vein.

At this point the IVC should be gently separated upwards from the right kidney by means of blunt and low voltage electric dissection. During this part of the procedure the left hand of the surgeon should gently push downward on renal parenchyma to facilitate the dissection of the IVC.

The main adrenal vein will be easily identified once the dissection of the IVC is completed up to the diaphragm (Fig. 36.4). The right adrenal vein is the only the main vessel that has to be dissected during right adrenalectomy but it is usually quite short and sometime it enter the IVC on its posterior wall.

The dissection of the main adrenal vein should be carried out with care using a "right angle" instrument (Fig. 36.4) or the hook, avoiding any accidental damage of the vein or the IVC that will result in significant bleeding difficult to be controlled.

Once the main adrenal vein is fully freed by the surrounding structures it should be secured between clips (Fig. 36.5) and divided with laparoscopic scissors.

At this point the procedures carries on with the mobilization of the adrenal gland from the Gerota's fascia using the harmonic scalpel: this part of the operation does not present significant difficulties but care should be taken in not accidentally enter the gland that could results in bleeding as well as tumour's cells spillage.

Once the dissection of the gland is completed the specimen can be introduced into a laparoscopic bag (Fig. 36.6) and extracted through one of the incisions that sometime have to be enlarged according to the size of the gland.

The surgical field must be carefully checked for bleeding and all the trocars removed under vision; surgical drain is usually not required but, if needed, it should placed through the lateral incision just under the right lobe of the liver.

Any fascia defects larger than 10 mm should be closed using re-absorbable suture.

36.10 Surgical Technique for Left Adrenalectomy

36.10.1 Positioning of the Patient

For left adrenalectomy the patients is placed in a mirrored position as for the right, the monitor is placed on the left while the surgical team stand on the right side (Fig. 36.7). The pneumoperitoneum is induced as described above either with the Veres needle or "open technique".

The first 10 or 5 mm trocar (depending from the diameter of the optic) is introduced at the level of the middle left clavicle line just under the costal margin (Fig. 36.8), at this point used direct vision 2 more 10 or 5 mm (depending from the size of the instruments) trocars are inserted at the level of the anterior and posterior left clavicle line respectively. Occasionally a 4th trocar can be added laterally in order to achieve a better exposure in case of large masses or obese patients.

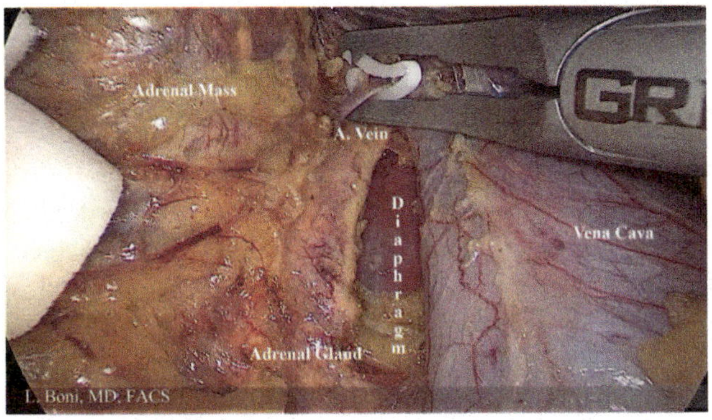

Fig. 36.5 Clipping of the main adrenal vein

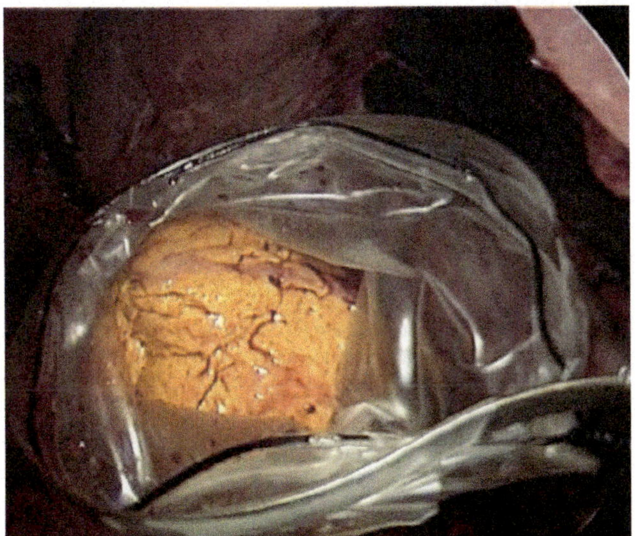

Fig. 36.6 Introduction of the adrenal gland into a bag

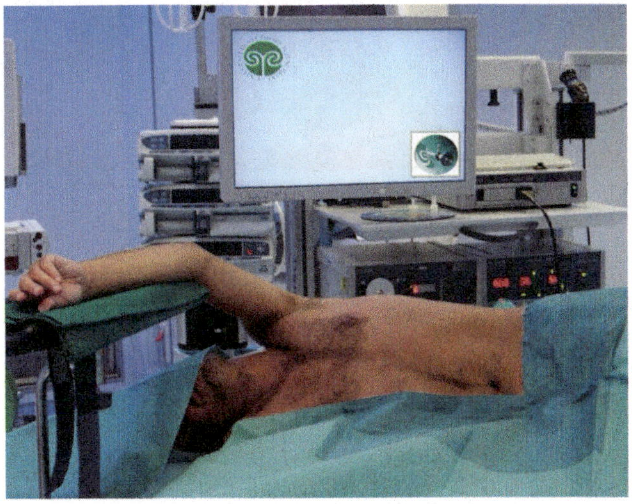

Fig. 36.7 Position of the patient for left adrenalectomy

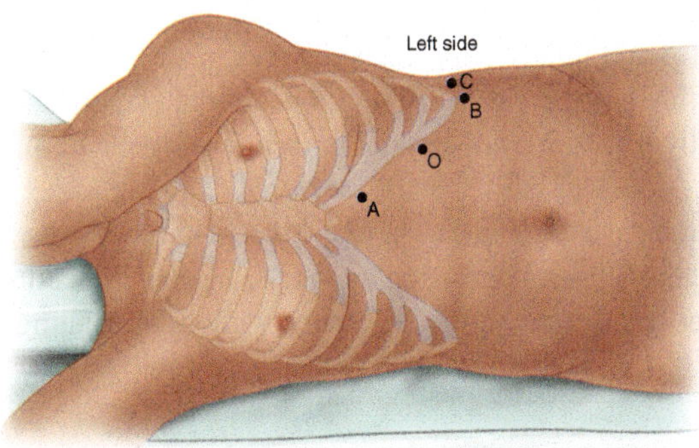

Fig. 36.8 Position of the trocar for left adrenalectomy (*O*: optic, *A*: surgeon's left hand, *B*: surgeon's right hand, *C*: optional trocar for retraction)

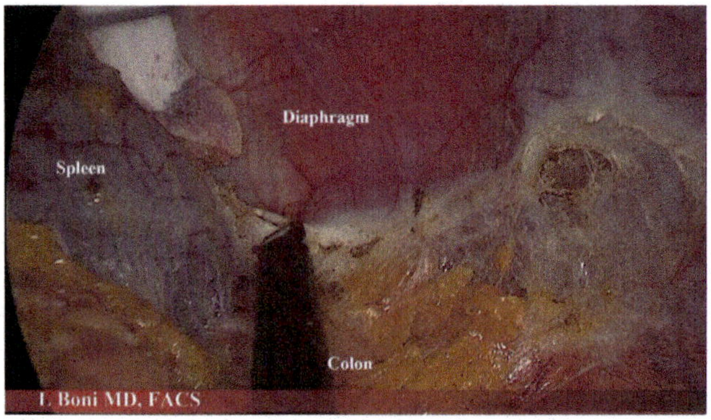

Fig. 36.9 Mobilization of the spleen and splenic flexure

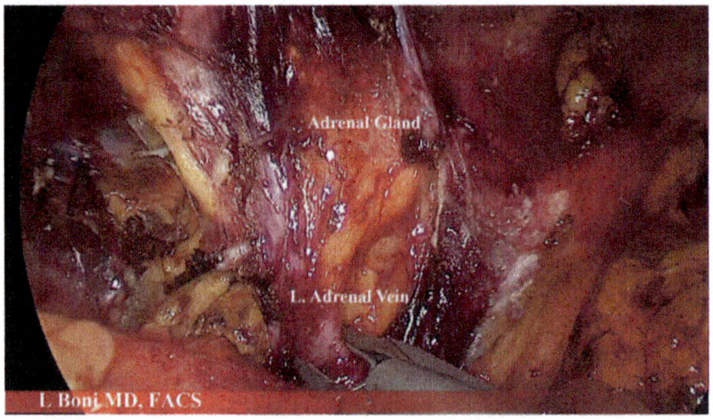

Fig. 36.10 Clipping and division of the main left adrenal vein

The procedure starts with a full mobilization of the splenic flexure by means of low voltage monopolar or ultrasonic dissection. Once the colon is mobilized further mobilization of the spleen should be carried out dividing the spleno-colic, spleno-renal and spleno-diaphragmatic ligaments in order to access to the retroperitoneal space (Fig. 36.9).

Dissection between the Gerota's fascia and the transverse mesocolon should be carried out in order to expose the left renal vein followed by the main adrenal vein, that usually run almost orthogonally to it (Fig. 36.10). Once identified the adrenal vein can be gently dissected from the surrounding structures using the hook and an atraumatic "right angle" dissector and finally clipped and divided.

At this point the dissection of the adrenal gland is started medially dividing small arterial branches using the harmonic shears (Fig. 36.11).

Leaving so fatty tissue around the gland will allow to apply gentle lateral retraction that facilitates the dissection of both posterior and superior aspect without damaging the parenchyma resulting in annoying bleeding. During the mobilization of the upper pole of the adrenal, the left phrenic vein should be dissected, clipped and divided.

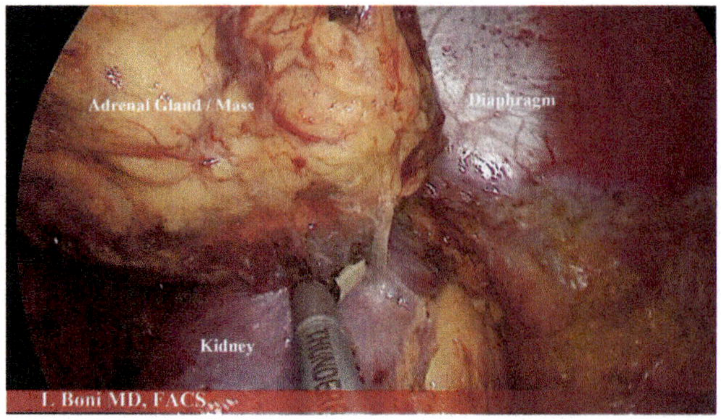

Fig. 36.11 Mobilization of the left adrenal gland with harmonic scalpel

Once the dissection of the gland is completed an endoscopic bag can be introduced and the specimen removed from one of the trocar site.

36.11 Post-operative Care

The bladder catheter is removed at the end of the procedure and the patient is allowed to free liquid diet 4 h after surgery and usually return to solid diet within 24 h. When a surgical drain is left in place, it is usually removed after 24 h according to the post-operative course.

Deep vein thrombosis prophylaxis is recommended with light weight heparin up to 15 days after surgery and patients are usually discharged 24–36 h after the procedure.

References

1. Gagner M, Lacroix A, Bolté E. Laparoscopic adrenalectomy in Cushing's syndrome and pheochromocytoma. N Engl J Med. 1992;327(14):1033.
2. Gumbs AA, Gagner M. Laparoscopic adrenalectomy. Best Pract Res Clin Endocrinol Metab. 2006;20(3):483–99.
3. Young Jr WF. Clinical practice. The incidentally discovered adrenal mass. N Engl J Med. 2007;356(6):601–10.
4. Caoili EM, Korobkin M, Francis IR, et al. Adrenal masses: characterization with combined enhanced and delayed enhanced CT. Radiology. 2002;222:629–33.
5. NIH state-of-the-science statement on management of the clinically inapparent adrenal mass ("incidentaloma"). NIH Consens State Sci Statements. 2002;19:1–25

Retroperitoneal Adrenalectomy

37

H. Jaap Bonjer and M. Walz

37.1 Selection of Patients

A multidisciplinary approach involving surgery, anaesthesiology, endocrinology, nuclear medicine, radiology and pathology is strongly recommended to manage patients with adrenal disease. Assessing hormonal activity of adrenal lesions and high resolution imaging are essential steps to determine whether surgical removal is necessary. Hormonally active adrenal tumors and non-functional adrenal lesions greater than 4 cm in diameter merit removal. In the latter group, it is important to identify any signs of malignancy. In patients with adrenal suspicious pathology, open surgery is advocated because these adrenal malignancies tend to be very fragile predisposing to tumor spill during laparoscopic manipulation.

Patients with adrenal tumors smaller than 6 cm in diameter and devoid of previous (peri) renal surgery are good candidates for retroperitoneal surgery. Approaching the adrenal gland retroperitoneally avoids interference with intraperitoneal adhesions and obviates the necessity to mobilize the right lobe of the liver in right adrenalectomy and to mobilize the spleen in left adrenalectomy. The retroperitoneal approach can be performed with the patient in lateral decubitus position and in prone position [1, 2]. The latter offers advantages in patients with bilateral adrenal disease because both adrenalectomies can be done without turning the patient unlike the lateral approach.

H.J. Bonjer, MD, PhD, FRCSC (✉)
Department of Surgery, VU University Medical Center, Amsterdam, The Netherlands
e-mail: j.bonjer@vumc.nl

M. Walz (✉)
Department of Surgery, Center of Minimally Invasive Surgery, Kliniken Essen-Mitte, Amsterdam, The Netherlands
e-mail: mkwalz@kliniken-essen-mitte.de

37.2 Retroperitoneal Adrenalectomy with the Patient in Lateral Decubitus

The patient is place in full lateral decubitus position on a bean bag with the lumbar space between the iliac crest and the tip of the tenth rib at the crack of the table. The table is broken maximally to expose this lumbar space fully. The skin in this area should be tout indicating proper positioning. The bean bag is deflated and care should be taken to pad it down to avoid interference with movements of the laparoscopic instruments. The arm on the affected side is supported in an arm rest. Pressure points such as the knee and ankle are carefully padded. The screens are placed at the top of the bed. The surgeon stands on the back side of the patient and the first assistant on the opposite side.

The first incision of 1.5 cm is made in the mid axillary line just below the tip of the tenth rib (Fig. 37.1). The fascia is incised and with forceps or the index finger the muscles are passed in between the fibers. The fascia transversalis is

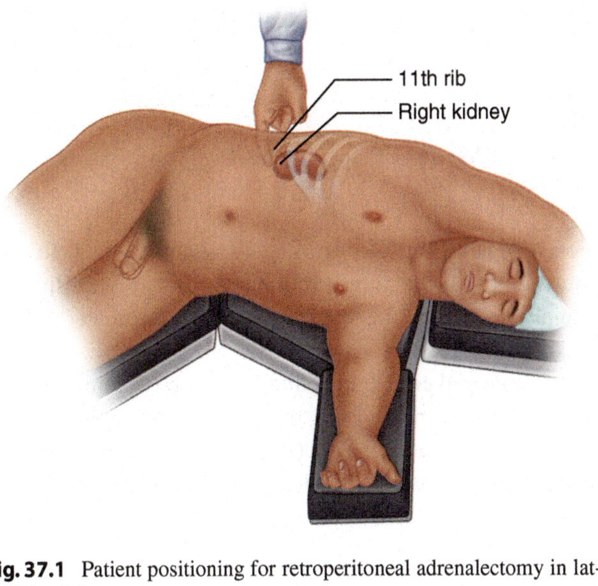

Fig. 37.1 Patient positioning for retroperitoneal adrenalectomy in lateral decubitus

H.J. Bonjer (ed.), *Surgical Principles of Minimally Invasive Procedures*, DOI 10.1007/978-3-319-43196-3_37

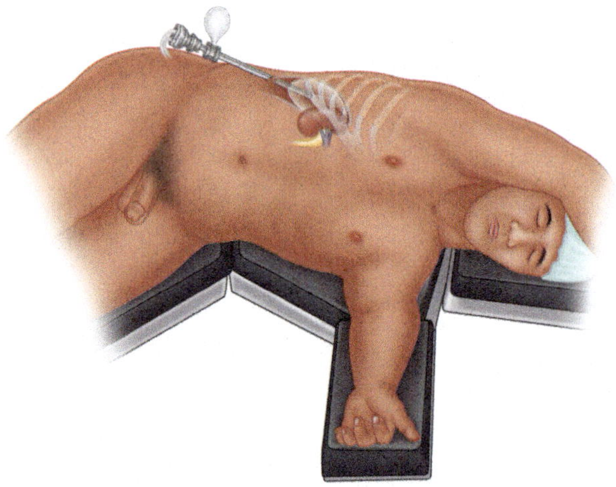

Fig. 37.2 Creating of the retroperitoneal space with a spacemaker

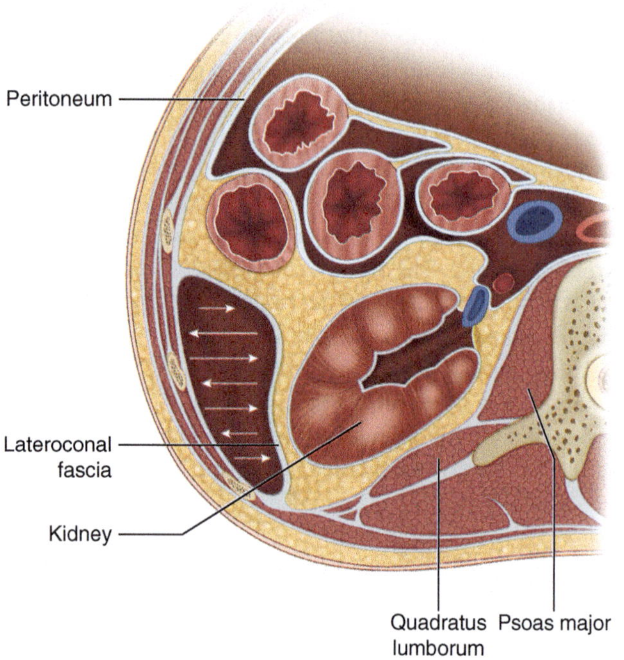

Fig. 37.3 Retroperitoneal space (*horizontal arrows*) that is created with the spacemaker

opened and then the retroperitoneal space is reached. To confirm this, the index finger should be inserted and directed cranially to palpate the inside of the ribs. The lower pole of the kidney can also be palpated.

A spacemaker is introduced, aimed cranially and inflated under direct vision by placing a 0° endoscope in the shaft of the spacemaker (Fig. 37.2). The first structure to be identified is the quadratus lumborum muscle. The boundaries of the retroperitoneal space created by balloon dissection is shown in Fig. 37.3. For proper orientation it is helpful to push down on the abdominal wall to correct the horizon of the endoscopic image for any undue rotation of the scope. In the first part of the dissection with few anatomic landmarks, malrotation of the endoscopic image can occur easily. The balloon of the spacemaker is inflated approximately 20 times but less in patients with Cushing's syndrome or disease considering the frailty of the tissues in these patients. After deflation of the spacemaker, a Hasson's trocar is placed and the retroperitoneal space is insufflated to a pressure between 15 and 20 mmHg. A 0° scope used mostly throughout the entire procedure but particularly in the initial phase when the working space is small. Orientation in small spaces appears to be more difficult when using angled endoscopes.

The second trocar is placed posteriorly just beneath the ribs. A 5 mm port is placed under direct vision. Care should be taken not to insert this port too cranially to avoid entering the pleural cavity. Through this posterior trocar a dissecting forceps with cautery or a 5 mm sealing device to mobilize the peritoneum from the anterior abdominal wall (Fig. 37.4). This should proceed until sufficient space is created to place a third and fourth trocar with sufficient distance in between. A 10 mm trocar is placed anteriorly to the optics' trocar and another 5 mm trocar is placed medial from the 10 mm trocar (Fig. 37.5). At insertion, these trocars should be aimed at a point where the adrenal gland is expected.

The next step of the procedure is opening the lateroconal fascia which extends between the peritoneum and the quadratus lumborum muscle (Fig. 37.6). This fascia is translucent and can be opened easily with scissors in a craniocaudal fashion about 2 cm from the muscle to avoid perforation of the peritoneum. When this occurs, the working space becomes smaller but is rarely interfering with progression of the procedure.

After opening the lateroconal fascia, the kidney needs to be identified and serves as anatomical guidance. The upper pole of the kidney is freed from peri-renal fat which can be quite adherent in some patients (Fig. 37.7). It is important to stay close on the kidney to avoid injury of the pancreatic tail on the left or right lobe of the liver on the right. During dissection of the upper pole the typical golden yellow colored adrenal tissue will become visible. Through the most medial trocar, the kidney is pushed posteriorly and caudally with an atraumatic instrument. The adrenal gland should not be grasped because the adrenal tissue is fragile. Indirect retraction is preferable. The anterior plan of the adrenal gland is avascular and can be readily exposed. The inferior adrenal vessels are taken down and dissection proceeds in a lateral to medial fashion. Care should be taken to preserve upper branches of the renal artery which are the origin of the inferior adrenal arteries.

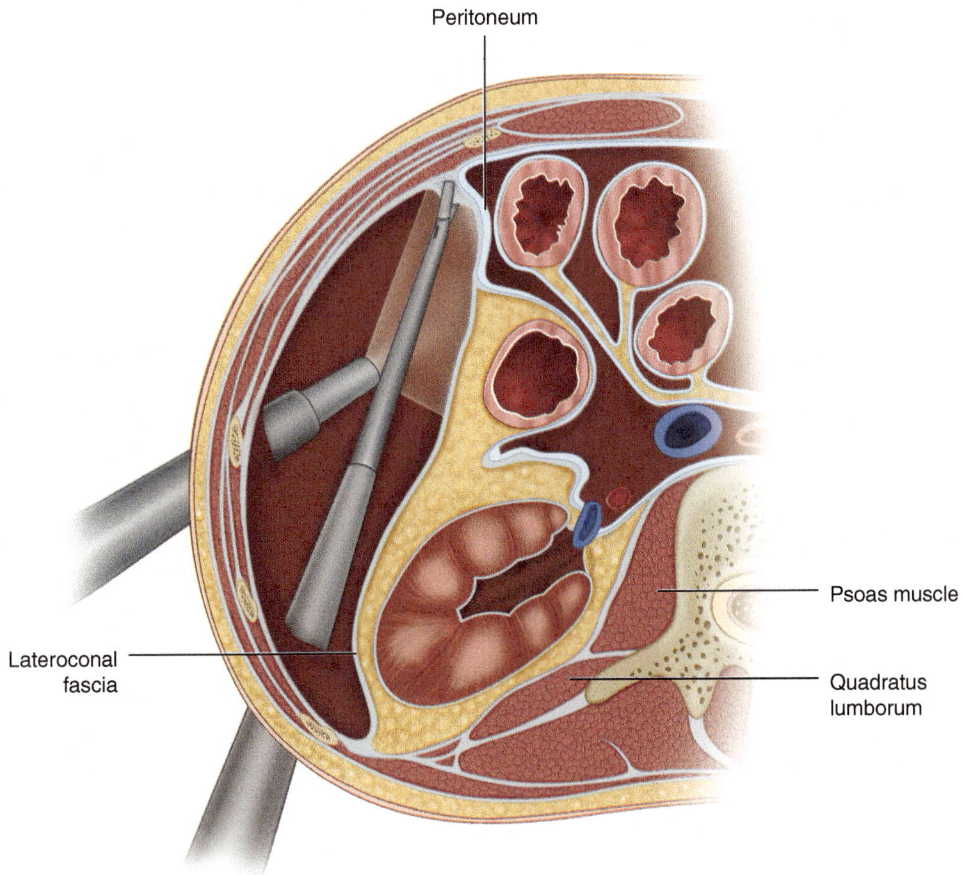

Fig. 37.4 Mobilization of the peritoneal sac

On the right side the caval vein will be identified and followed cranially while taking down medial arterial vessels coming from the aorta passing posteriorly to the aorta. Ultimately the short adrenal vein is exposed. Gentle lateral retraction of the adrenal gland is mandatory to prevent lacerating the adrenal vein. Once the adrenal vein has been ligated and cut, the adrenal will 'give' and only the superior arterial vessels arising from the phrenic artery. In case of a very short vein allowing limited length for placing clips, two clips on the caval side suffice and a clip on the adrenal side of the vein can be left out because the back bleeding is minimal (Fig. 37.8).

On the left side, the sequence of dissection is similar to the right. However, during dissection of the inferior aspect of the adrenal gland the adrenal vein draining into the left renal vein and is ligated and transected. The adrenal vein on the left is much longer than on the right and, hence, leaves more margin for clip placement. Within 2 cm from the adrenal tissue, a diaphragmatic vein drains into the adrenal vein. This vein can be left intact when all clips are placed distally from

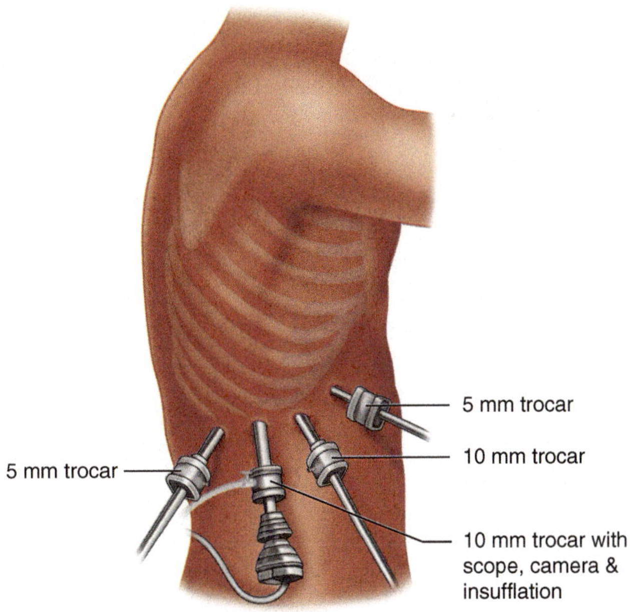

Fig. 37.5 Placement of trocars for retroperitoneal adrenalectomy

Fig. 37.6 Opening the lateroconal fascia

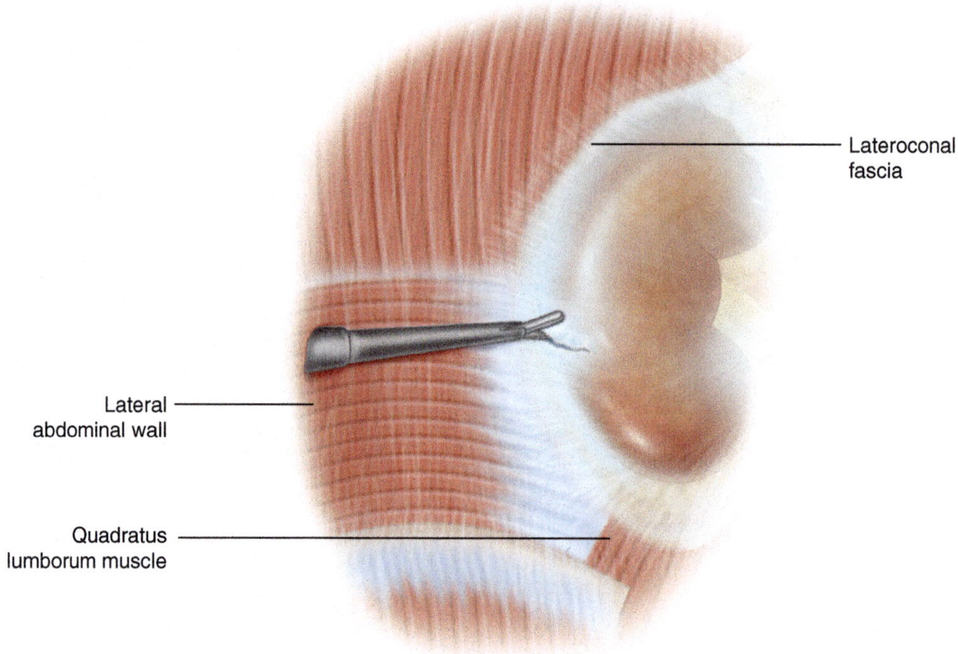

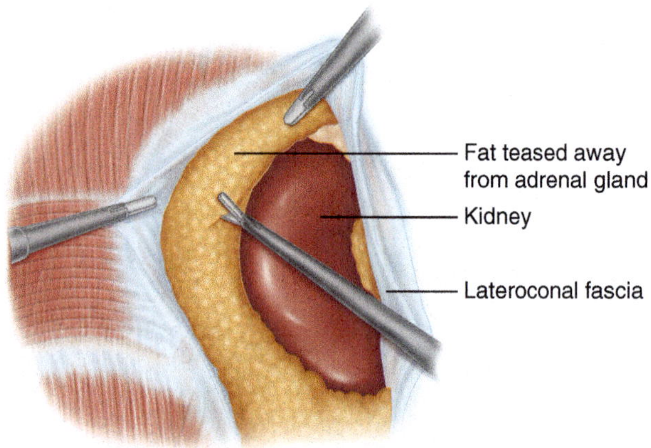

Fig. 37.7 Freeing up the superior pole of the kidney

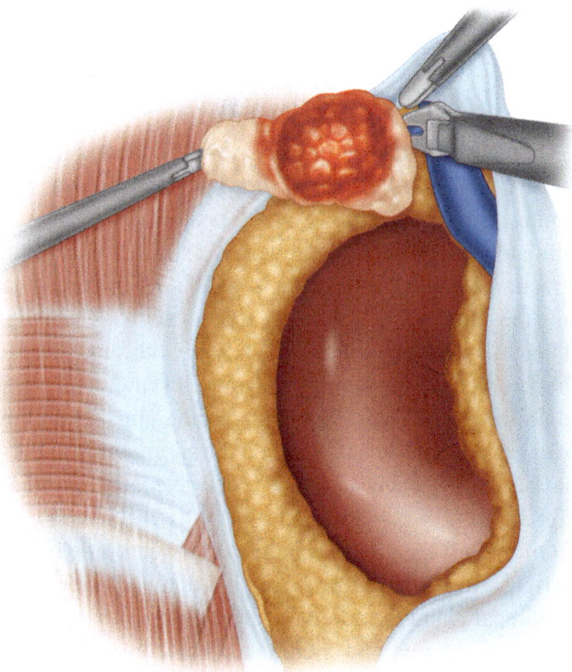

Fig. 37.8 Clipping the right adrenal vein

the junction between the diaphragmatic vein and the renal vein. Otherwise, the diaphragmatic vein needs to be cut and ligated. After transaction of the adrenal vein, medial dissection follows with taking down of the medial adrenal arteries arising from the aorta. Finally, the cranial part of the adrenal is dissected and superior adrenal arteries coming from the phrenic artery are taken down.

Once the adrenal gland has been freed completely, it is placed in a bag and extract through the incision of the Hasson's trocar because this is the largest incision. The scope is placed in the other 10 mm trocar during extraction. Lowering the insufflation pressure at the end of the procedure is advisable to identify any bleeding from venules. Drainage of the operative space is not necessary.

37.3 Troubleshooting

Perforation of the peritoneal sac reduces the working space rendering the procedures in some patients more difficult. The mobilisation of the peritoneum to create space for placement of the third and fourth trocar needs to take place flush on the muscles of the abdominal wall but posteriorly to the transversalis fascia. To get the right angle of dissection, the surgeon has to bow down by flexing the knees to get into the right plane. External manual pressure on the anterior abdominal wall helps as well.

Failure to identify the adrenal gland is another problem of this procedure. Some surgeons have advocated using laparoscopic ultrasonography and this may certainly prove helpful. However, the secret to finding the adrenal gland is meticulous dissection of the upper pole of the kidney. This will always reveal the inferior margin of the adrenal gland.

Bleeding from the adrenal gland or its arterial branches is relatively common in patients with phaeochromocytomas. Bleeding from small adrenal arteries can be managed by inserting a sponge and compression for several minutes. Bleeding from adrenal tissue is more difficult to control because cauterizing or sealing adrenal tissue is not very effective. Indirect retraction and suction will allow sufficient exposure for further dissection of the adrenal gland. The 5 mm suction device is a helpful atraumatic instrument to indirectly retract the adrenal gland and evacuate blood or water vapour when ultrasonic dissection is used.

Bleeding from the adrenal vein is the most challenging situation, particularly on the right side, requiring compression with sponges and suction to identify the exact site of the bleeding. In some instances application of clips partly on the caval vein is sufficient. If this is not possible, a laparoscopic Satinsky vessel clamp can be placed on the caval vein followed by laparoscopic oversewing of the laceration of the vessel. If vascular control can not be readily accomplished, conversion to lumbotomy is necessary.

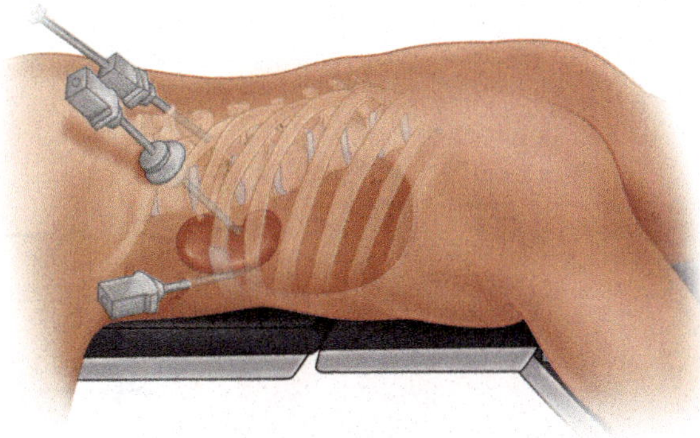

Fig. 37.9 Placement of trocars in retroperitoneal adrenalectomy in prone position

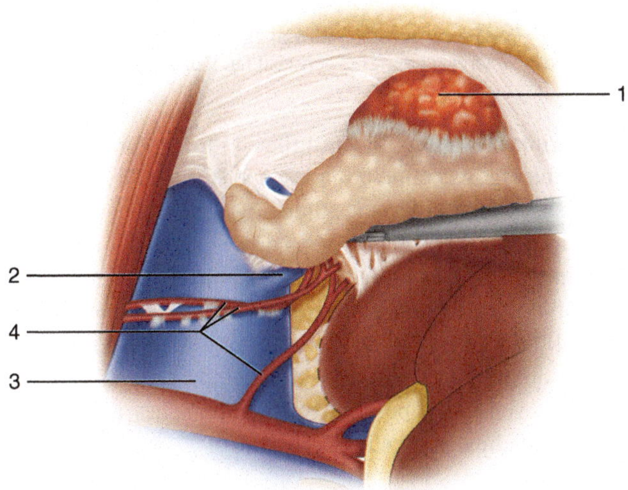

Fig. 37.10 Posterior view of the right adrenal gland. *1* adrenal tumor, *2* right adrenal vein, *3* vena cava, *4* inferior adrenal artery

37.4 Retroperitoneal Adrenalectomy with the Patient in Prone Position

The procedure is performed under general anesthesia with the patient in prone position. The patient is lying on a rectangular support with central space for the anterior abdominal wall. A cental venous line and arterial line are inserted. The first incision is made 1.5 cm transversally just below the tip of the twelfth rib. The retroperitoneal space is entered by a combination of blunt and sharp dissection. Either a space maker or finger dissection can used to create a small retroperitoneal working space subsequently two trocars are inserted four to five cm laterally and medially to the first incision (Fig. 37.9). This is done without visual control. The

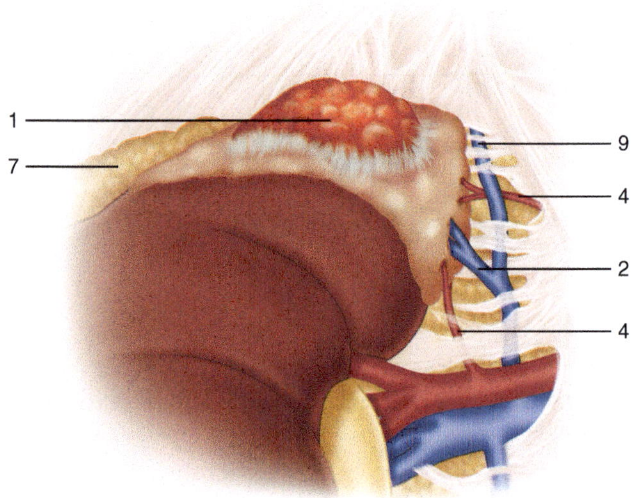

Fig. 37.11 Posterior view of the adrenal gland. *1* adrenal tumor, *2* left adrenal vein, *4* adrenal arteries, *7* perirenal fat, *9* diaphragmatic vein

retroperitoneal space is insufflated to a pressure of 12–25 mmHg. A 5 mm 30° endoscope is used. Dissection is commenced laterally to the adrenal which tends to be relatively avascular. The dissection is carried cranially up to the diaphragm. Care is taken to only manipulate the adrenal gland bluntly and delicately to prevent tearing the fragile adrenal tissue. Dissection proceeds along the medial border of the adrenal gland. On the right side, the adrenal arteries cross the vena cava posteriorly these branches are ligated either with clips or a sealing device.

The short right adrenal vein runs posterolaterally and is secured with clips and cut or transected with a sealing device (Fig. 37.10). Dissection is completed and the adrenal gland is placed in an extraction bag.

On the left side, the lateral side of the adrenal gland is freed up first. On the medial side, the inferior and medial adrenal artery are encountered and taken down (Fig. 37.11). A branch of the diaphragmatic vein drains into the left adrenal vein. When the adrenal vein is transected on the adrenal side of the junction between the diaphragmatic branch and the adrenal vein, the diaphragmatic vein can be left intact. After transection of the vein, mobilization of the cranial part of the adrenal gland is completed by taking down the cranial adrenal artery.

In patients with bilateral adrenal disease such as MEN-IIa syndrome, unilateral partial adrenalectomy van be performed to preserve corticosteroid producing adrenal cortex. In these cases, the adrenal gland is only dissected cranially and laterally to preserve the blood supply of the adrenal gland. After identification, the adrenal tumor is dissected with a margin of 0.5–1 cm of normal tissue. Transection the adrenal tissue is done either with electrosurgery or sealing devices.

References

1. Bonjer HJ, Sorm V, Berends FJ, Kazemier G, Steyerberg EW, de Herder WW, Bruining HA. Endoscopic retroperitoneal adrenalectomy: lessons learned from 111 consecutive cases. Ann Surg. 2000;232:796–803.
2. Walz MK, Peitgen K, Walz MV, et al. Posterior retroperitoneoscopic adrenalectomy: lessons learned within five years. World J Surg. 2001;25:728–34.

Part XV

Innovative Minimally Invasive Techniques

NOTES and Hybrid NOTES Procedures in Clinical Practice

38

K.H. Fuchs, W. Breithaupt, G. Varga, and T. Schulz

38.1 Introduction

Natural orifice transluminal endoscopic surgery (NOTES) has emerged in the early 2000 as a logic development of ideas originating from interventional endoscopists and gastroenterologists as well as surgeons. After the initial hype of ideas and fantasies the concept of NOTES has become a clinical reality [1, 2]. The principle of minimal access surgery is the reduction of access-size and access-trauma aiming for a shorter patient recovery, improved postoperative well-being, better cosmesis, less inhibiting postoperative restrictions in order to get the patient quickly back to full physical and psychologic abilities, and possibly an improved long term outcome. The latter could be achieved by less wound infections and less incisional hernias over time. The advantage of this concept of minimal access surgery over conventional open surgery has been clearly shown in the past decades. It must be emphasized that the improvements in patient care 20 years ago with the advent of minimal access surgery were not only caused by the reduction of abdominal incisions, but also caused by conceptional changes that came along with re-thinking perioperative care [3].

The concept of NOTES reduces the access trauma further by using a natural orifice as an access route to the intraabdominal cavity [2, 4]. Minimizing access trauma at the abdominal or thoracic wall could possibly lead to less postoperative pain, improved and quicker recovery from surgery, less postoperative complications, less wound infection and less longterm problems such as hernias.

K.H. Fuchs, PhD (✉) W. Breithaupt • G. Varga • T. Schulz
Department of Surgery, Agaplesion Markus-Krankenhaus, Frankfurt, Germany
e-mail: Karl-Hermann.Fuchs@fdk.info

38.2 Basic Considerations in NOTES and Hybrid-NOTES Procedures

Some very important issues have to be kept in mind, when a NOTES procedure is planned. Table 38.1 summarizes the list of challenges and important topics of the initial NOSCAR meeting and white paper [1]. The initial thoughts and fears characterize the chosen topics of peritoneal access, gastric closure, infection, suturing in anastomosis special orientation, platforms and new technology, complications, intraperitoneal events and education and training.

The danger of infection has been overestimated in the beginning of NOTES research. The infection rate was kept low by limiting contamination. This can be accomplished by desinfection of the pharynx, esophagus and stomach, and bowel, as well as an adequate antibiotic prophylaxis, which is routine practice in gastrointestinal surgery. A number of studies on clinical experience showed that the desinfection of flexible endoscopes to be used in the mediastinum or abdominal cavity seems to be sufficient in limiting contamination and thus preventing infection. Today, infectious complications in NOTES procedures are in most series in an acceptable low range below 3 % [5–7].

Several access routes via natural orifices were evaluated in the past years and peritoneal access was trained [4]. The transvaginal route is most frequently used, since the clini-

Table 38.1 Important challenges and questions, established by the NOSCAR group during their initial working meeting and publication [1, 2]

Peritoneal access
Gastric closure
Prevention of infections
Suturing and anastomotic devices
Maintaining spatial orientation
Development of a multitasking platform
Management of intraperitoneal complications and hemorrhage
Physiologic untoward events caused by NOTES
Training

H.J. Bonjer (ed.), *Surgical Principles of Minimally Invasive Procedures*, DOI 10.1007/978-3-319-43196-3_38

cal experience in gynecology is 100 years old. The transesophageal and transanal/transcolonic were initially considered the most dangerous approaches, since infections were thought to play a role, but it is established in clinical practice today. The transgastric route was initially thought to be the most important. Currently, experimental and clinical experience showed, that there is a place for all these routes for different indications and procedures. In the meantime also several closure techniques have been established quite successfully for the different approaches. In 2012, the transesophageal, the transgastric, the transvaginal and the transcolonic-transanal approaches are well established in clinical practice.

The principle of Hybrid techniques have overcome some of the limitations that inhibited the clinical breakthrough of NOTES techniques. In Hybrid procedures, transabdominal trocards are used in limited number and limited size in order to fascilitate, assist and/or enable the maneuvers through the natural orifice via graspers for better retraction, exposure and/or delivery of rigid energy devices. Despite the fact, that transabdominal instruments will somewhat limit the possible positive effects of NOTES, Hybrid procedures increase patient safety by fascilitating the use of experienced and safe laparoscopic techniques.

Organisational and legal as well as ethical requirements may vary between countries but also between different institutions. The evaluation of the protocol to introduce a new innovative technique should be performed by an independent committee such as the IRB, the ethical committee or a similar body. It is important to fulfill these requirements, when introducing such a potential dangerous procedure in order to create more safety for all involved; the patient, the responsible endoscopist, the hospital and the method. Notes has great potential, if performed safely [8].

38.3 The Transvaginal Access

The transvaginal route is established in operative gynecology since a century. In addition, transvaginal endoscopy or culdoscopy has also been performed many decades ago. The advantage of the transvaginal access is the possibility to use rigid laparoscopic instruments, which surgeons are familiar with.

The concept of Hybrid transvaginal cholecystectomy is comprehensible to surgeons and can be quickly introduced with a steep learning curve in clinical practice [9–11]. In addition to cholecystectomy, also transvaginal appendectomy and colon resections were introduced into clinical practice with remarkable safety record [9].

Discussions focused on possible side effects of postoperative dyspareunia. However, the transvaginal technique has a good safety record and is well established.

Several working groups recommended that transvaginal NOTES procedures should be performed initially in cooperation with gynaecologists, until surgeons have gained enough experience to perform this technique safely [9, 11]. Usually 10–15 procedures are advised under guidances. A perioperative antibiotic prophylaxis with cephalosporin should be given and a preoperative gynaecologic examination is advised.

Contraindications for transvaginal access are rectovaginal endometriosis, pregnancy and malignomas of the cervix and vagina. Previous gynaecologic operations can cause severe adhesions. Therefore it is advisable to use extra precautions such as a preliminary capnoperitoneum and intraperitoneal visual control, when penetrating the vagina. It is advised to perform a suture closing of the access route of the posterial vagina wall. Also a gynaecologic postoperative check could be advised. Regarding indications and contraindication one should consult the available literature on cholecystitis and cholecystolithiasis.

38.3.1 Operative Technique of Transvaginal Cholecystectomy

A prophylaxis with antibiotics such as cephalosporines should be administered prior to surgery. The patient is brought in a lithotomy and Trendelenburg position. As with many Hybrid techniques, primary abdominal access is performed via a safe standard laparoscopic approach with establishment of a capnoperitoneum and a transumbilical camera trocard, preferably of 5 mm. This allows for a safe introduction of a larger access via the vagina with several trocards and/or instruments. For a cholecystectomy a larger trocard (10–12 mm) is inserted transvaginallly as well as a seperate long grasper, which reaches into the subphrenic region of the right upper quadrant in order to lift the liver and gallbladder for adequate exposure of the important anatomic structures. Then the cameraposition is changed to the transvaginal main trocard for visualisation of the right upper quadrant. The energy device is brought into the abdominal cavity via the umbilical 5 mm trocard and the dissection of the gallbladder can be started.

The dissection of the gallbladder follows the rules of the traditional laparoscopic dissection with starting at the Callot's triangle and evaluated the "critical view" after completion of the preparation. For safe closure of the cystic duct, either ligatures, 5 mm clips via the umbilical port or 10 mm clips vis the transvaginal port are necessary. Once the gallbladder is free, it can be retrieved with or without a bag, using the large port in the vagina, while the camera is changed into the transumbilical position. At the end of the procedure the vagina is closed with sutures under direct vision from the outside. This allows for a very safe closure with a minimal risk for problems.

A similar approach is used for transvaginal colon resections [12, 13].

38.4 The Transesophagel Access

The transesophageal route, used in peroral endoscopic myotomy (POEM) is also evaluated for mediastinal work. Currently, several clinical indications are evaluated for the POEM techniques such as Achalasia, Diffuse Esophageal Spasm and other spastic motility disorders and in the near future mediastinal explorations.

Patients with Achalasia, an esophageal motility disorder, present usually with occasional to persistent dysphagia and/or retrosternal pain and burning. The major clinical problem is intermittent obstruction of the esophageal passage of food and/or fluids, which forces the patient to see a doctor. The underlying disease is a functional disorder, which involves the lower esophageal sphincter and its incomplete or lacking relaxation during swallowing, an aperistalsis of the esophageal body and an increased tone of the lower esohageal sphincter.

The therapeutic spectrum of this disorder consists of medical therapy, endoscopic balloon dilatation, endoscopic Botox-injection, open or laparoscopic Cardia-myotomy and most recently transesophageal endoscopic Myotomy, introduced by H. Inoue as POEM (peroral endoscopic myotomy) [14]. POEM is now introduced in clinical practice in dedicated centers around the world [15–17].

38.4.1 Requirements for Establishing POEM

The most important requirement is a well experienced team in interventional flexible endoscopy [14]. The endoscopist as well as the assisting staff should have experience in advanced therapeutic endoscopic techniques and hemostasis to handle all necessary endoscopic instruments such as injection-needles, needle-knife, triangle-knife, coagulation-graspers and endoscopic clip handling and closures. During the POEM-procedure, there is a certain time–pressure, since gas-insufflation in the submucosal tunnel is necessary for visualisation, which increases the risk with time for extensive mediastinal, retroperioneal and subcutaneous emphysema. The prevention of this problem needs quick and safe operative steps with the available flexible endoscopic techniques.

In addition advanced surgical and especially laparoscopic skills and experience as well as surgical knowledge about esophageal disease must be available in case of conversion and/or consultation. Our team has performed extensive experimental training in submucosal tunnelling and other NOTES-procedures, before introducing this technique into clinical practice.

The necessary equipment consists of the modern endoscopic and laparoscopic technology such as high-resolution video endoscopes and laparoscopes, flexible endoscopic instruments as well as energy sources to provide spray coagulation technique, which is essential for a safe submucosal dissection.

For the introduction of this new technique, patients with Achalasia should be selected without prior endoscopic nor surgical treatment in order to find optimal tissue conditions in the esophageal wall. The patients should be able to understand the procedure well and should also be able to understand the possible risk of complications with such a new technique as well as the possible advantages and disadvantages. The investigators, who initially published their experience, emphasized the importance of informing the patient sufficiently. In Europe the requirements in the different countries may vary remarkable regarding informed consent and IRB approval.

38.4.2 The Operative Technique of POEM

Prior to the operation the patient must be npo for 8 h. In the 3 days before the procedure the Achalasia patient is asked to eat only semisolid food and have much fluid to prevent food obstruction in the esophagus above the cardia.

The procedures is performed in our institution in general anesthesia. The patient is brought in a supine position and the abdomen is free for inspection and palpation during the procedure to check the possible presence of a capnoperitoneum. In this case, a Veres-needle is brought in under sterile conditions to release the CO2-gas from the abdominal cavity. The infection-contamination issue is addressed by discontinuing all antisecretory drugs of the patient 1 week prior to the operation in order to keep the intragastric environment as acidic as possible to reduce bacterial growth. Also antibiotic prophylaxis (Ciprofloxacin and Metronidazole) is given intraveneously. After the operation daily high dosage Protonpumpinhibitors are administered for better healing of the esophagotomy.

Prior to the actual procedure, the upper Gastrointestinal tract is checked with an endoscope to remove all fluid and/or food, which can be quite often present in Achalasia patients. The esophageal, pharyngeal and gastric lumen is rinsed and cleared completely. Then it is rinsed extensively with chlorhexidine.

Then the patient is covered with sterile drapes up to the mouth. Then a gastroscope is introduced into the esophagus, attached to a CO2-insufflator. A transparent cap is attached on the tip of the scope for better exposure of the sites. Initially the important esophageal landmarks are measured such as the distal end of the cardia, the narrowing of the Cardia in the distal esophagus, representing the upper end of the pathologic non-relaxing high-pressure zone. The myotomy should start a few cm above the latter area. Thus, the starting-point of the myotomy is determined. As a consequence, the point of the esophagotomy will then be about 5 cm above the starting-point of the myotomy, if one aims for a safe tunnel distance of 5 cm. Usually this entrance or esophagotomy will between 28 and 32 cm from the teeth.

After the measurement, a 5–10 ml depot of blue-stained saline and suprarenin will be injected in the submucosal area. This will lift the mucosa from the muscular layer and the following incision of the mucosa with a Triangle-Tip-knife will create the entrance into the tunnel. Further careful alternating application of injection of blue-stained saline, spray-coagulation and moderate pushing of the endoscope will complete a tunnel down to the area below the cardia. This steps should be performed with extreme care and caution in order to prevent damage to the mucosa, which is the only intact layer towards the mediastium, once the myotomy is completed.

It is important to remove the endoscope from the tunnel several times to double-check the correct direction of the tunnel within the esophageal circumference as well as the advancement of the tunnel towards and below the cardia. A final check should include an endoscopic view during intragastric inversion to confirm the blue-stained gastric mucosa at the end of the tunnel below the cardia.

Then the endoscope is repositioned in the tunnel at the starting point of the myotomy and the myotomy is advanced distally with the Triangle-Tip-knife, possibly severing only the circular layer of the muscle and leaving the longitudinal muscle fibers intact.

At the end of the procedure, the extent of the myotomy is checked, all fluids are sucked out of the tunnel and the esophagotomy is closed by adaptation of the esophageal mucosa and clip closure.

In Europe, so far only a few centers with large experience in esophageal disease, laparoscopy and especially advanced interventional endoscopy have started to introduce this POEM-technique in their clinical practice. Initial success and low complications rates are quite promising and show a great future perspective for this technique.

38.5 The Transgastric Access

The transgastric route, initially thought to be ideal way to enter the abdomen, has been tested for several indications such as peritoneal exploration, appendectomy, cholecystectomy, ovarian tube ligation, small bowel tumor resection and gastric tumor resection [1, 2, 4, 7]. Despite a tremendous effort of many teams to establish appendectomy, cholecystectomy and staging peritoneoscopy in clinical practice, the latter indications are currently not well established for the transgastric technique in a clinical practice. Reasons for this might be the technical limitations of flexible endoscopy in the abdominal cavity. As a consequence, the transgastric route and associated techniques are currently used for full thickness gastric wall resections with increasing success specially in the Asian countries because of the higher number of cases. In Europe few studies have been performed with cholecystectomy, staging peritoneoscopy and appendectomy [4, 7]. Transgastric cholecystectomy is quite time consuming and seems to be technically very demanding compared to the transvaginal cholecystectomy, which has proved to be successful. Transgastric Appendectomy is under trial evaluation.

38.5.1 Operative Technique of Transgastric Procedure

There are several methods to get access to the peritoneal cavity by transagstric approach. A first decision is made, whether to use as safety back-up a visual control via a umbilical port for a laparoscope. Another way is the PEG-technique to enter the peritoneum without laparoscopic help by first introducing a wire-connection between gastric lumen and the abdominal wall to make sure that no interposition is possible between stomach and abdominal wall. Then the wire can be released and used dilatate the transgastric penetration for the passage into the abdominal cavity.

An alternative is the penetration of the gastric wall with the needle-knife gastrotomy by the flexible endoscope under laparoscopic guidance to use the appropriate location at the anterior gastric wall.

The patient is prepared with an overnight fast and antibiotic prophylaxis with cephalosporine usually an hour before the operation. The patient is brought in a supine position and for safety reasons a regular pneumoperitoneum is established with all safety regulations after which a 5 mm port is entered and an optic with attached camera is introduced into the peritoneal cavity A regular size endoscope is used to pass the esophagus and enter the gastric lumen. All fluids are removed by suction and an optimal spot is chosen under both flexible endoscopic and laparoscopic guidance. Then a needle-knife is used to perform a direct gastrotomy. Then via a guidewire the endoscope is passed into the peritoneal cavity and can be explored, depending on the clinical indication.

Closure of the gastromy can be performed with the over-the-scope-clip or by using miniinstruments by the usual laparoscopic suture technique.

38.6 The Transanal and Transcolonic Access

The transanal- transcolonic technique was initially considered problematic because of the infection issue and the bacterial load of the colon. A large clinical experience existed for transanal endoscopic procedures, created as Transanal Endoscopic Microsurgery (TEM) bei Gerhard Buess in the early 1980s [18]. The most important idea behind the transanal/transcolonic route is the use of the anastomotic site as the access into the peritoneal cavity [19–22]. As a consequence, since no additional opening in the gut is necessary, there is no additional risk of the access site infection and complications other than the risk of the anastomosis. With completion of the anastomosis, also the access via the natural orifice is closed.

The latter idea is improved by hybrid technology using transabdominal mini-laparoscopy and rigid small-size energy devices for safe dissection. These ideas led to the introduction of Transanal Hybrid Colon Resections, creating a compromise between the concept of NOTES (using access via natural orifice) and the experience in safe technique of mini-laparoscopic dissection to complete the resection of the bowel and performing the anastomosis. This made it possible to perform transanal-transcolonic colorectal resections in clinical practice.

Today, we can differentiate in the transanal approach using the principal of the original TEM technique to dissect the rectum and perform colorectal resections and rectal anastomosis, and secondly use the transanal access to pass deeper into the abdominal cavity and use a transcolonic approach at the anastomotic site to perform colon resections.

38.6.1 Technique of Transanal Hybrid Colon Resection

After establishing a capnoperitoneum via a Veres needle and after necessary safety-tests, a periumbilical port was introduced in the abdominal cavity. Two additional 5 mm ports were brought in the right lower quadrant for dissection of the colon and rectum. Via these ports also the dissection of the anastomotic site, all necessary hemostasis as well as an energy device were applied. The dissection of the mesentery was stepwise performed under careful laparoscopic control to ensure that the pelvic nerve plexus was not in danger and the dissection planes could be followed.

In case of sigmoid resection for prolaps surgery, the colon-lumen was clamped at the level of the descending segment and a sigmoidoscopy was performed to make sure that this bowel segment was clean, which was clarified by rinsing of the rectum and colon. After removal of the scope, bougies of the sizes 25, 28 and 33 were introduced into the anus, rectum and sigmoid colon. A careful bougienage of the rectum facilitates the following maneuvers. The next step was the transanal introduction of a Transanal Endoscopic Applicator, which allows for safe introduction of endoscopes, linear staplers, grasping devices and specimen removal. Then the anvil of a 28 mm circular stapler was introduced into the rectum with a special grasper and maneuvered more proximal up to the descending colon to the future anastomotic site.

This was followed by an incision of the colon – usually the distal sigmoid – at the distal anastomotic site. Here, a transanally introduced linear stapler could exit the colon into the abdominal cavity and was used to transsect the proximal end of the sigmoid segment, which needed to be removed for shortening of the colon. Via the transanal positioned Applicator, the application, removal and change of stapling cartridges was technically rather easy to be performed. At the proximal colon stump, the intraluminal anvil was grasped through the bowel wall and stabilized. The central pin of the anvil was penetrated through the bowel wall at the stapled line to be available for later anastomosis. The penetration of the pin was facilitated by performing a small hole at the stapled line with the ultrasound cutting device.

Once the sigmoid segment was resected and free of detachments, a grasper was advanced via the Trananal Endoscopic Applicator to reach for the specimen in the abdomen. Then the specimen was pulled through the luminal opening at the distal rectosigmoid stump, via the rectal lumen and transanally to the outside.

After removal of the specimen transanally, a pursestring suture was placed at the distal rectosigmoid stump in order to complete the anastomosis with the circular stapling device. A circular stapler was inserted transanally and advanced to the distal rectosigmoid opening, carrying the purse-string suture. The central pin was opened and the purse-string suture was tied down around the central pin. Furthermore, the anvil was connected to the stapler, followed by approximating and firing the device in the usual manner under laparoscopic visual control. Thus the actual anastomosis could be performed under the same optimal conditions, that laparoscopic surgery can provide.

In case of a rectal prolaps, a rectopexy was added in the usual technique with non-absorbable sutures between peritoneal, pararectal tissue and the sacral bone at the promontorium using the 5 mm ports, straight needles and miniinstruments.

In case of slow transit constipation, subtotal colon resection was performed by dissection and severing of the complete colon mesentery with the 5 mm Energy- device usually via two 5 mm ports, occasionally added by another 3 mm grasper without trocard for assisting and better exposure. The ileum as well as the sigmoid colon was transsected via a transanal linear stapler. Then the complete colon was removed transanally. The anvil was advanced transanally to the distal ileum and inserted into to lumen, followed by penetration of the central pin through the antimesenteric ileal wall for later anastomosis. The ileum was closed via a transanal linear stapler. The tissue remnant was removed transanally. The ileosigmoidostomy was performed similar as described above.

After control of hemostasis, inspection of the anastomosis, leak test with air and water as well as placement of a drainage, the procedure was finished by removal of the three ports.

38.7 Training NOTES and Hybrid NOTES Techniques

Since NOTES procedures require both capabilities in interventional endoscopy and advanced laparoscopic surgery, many speculations emerged regarding the future role of surgeons and gastroenterologists or endoscopists performing these procedures. With increasing experimental and clinical experience, it became clear that NOTES procedures and Hybrid NOTES procedures depending on their nature, require a long training phase and usually a large background of clinical and technical experience, necessary to perform NOTES procedures safely in the abdominal [2, 4, 7, 23].

There is no doubt that these new techniques should be trained in the preclinical setting and extensive experimental work is needed, before taking these techniques to the patient. Interventional endoscopy and advanced laparoscopy must be well established prior to involving NOTES techniques. The prerequisites for clinical introduction of an innovative procedure such as NOTES procedures in clinical practice have been outlined in detail by EAES consensus recommendations [8].

References

1. Rattner D, Kalloo AN, ASGE/SAGES working Group. White Paper on Natural Orifice translumenal endoscopic surgery. Surg Endosc. 2006;20(2):329–33.
2. Rattner D, Hawes R, Schwaitzberg S, Kochman M, Swanstrom L. The second SAGES/ASGE white paper on natural orifice translumenal endoscopic surgery: 5 years of progress. Surg Endosc. 2011;25:2441–8.
3. Kehlet H, Whilmore DW. Evidence-based surgical care and the evolution of fast-track surgery. Ann Surg. 2008;248:189–98.
4. Fuchs KH, Meining A, Von Renteln D, Fernandez-Esparrach G, Breithaupt W, Zornig C, Lacy A. The Euro-NOTES Status Paper – from the concept to clinical practice. Surg Endosc. 2013;27(5):1456–67.
5. Narula VK, Happel LC, Volt K, Bergmann S, Roland JC, Dettore R, Renton DB, Reavis KM, Needleman BJ, Mikami DJ, Ellison EC, Melvin WS, Hazey JW. Transgastric endoscopic peritoneoscopy does not require decontamination of the stomach in humans. Surg Endosc. 2009;12(6):1331–6.
6. Nau P, Ellison EC, Muscarella Jr P, Mikami D, Narula VK, Needleman B, Melvon WS, Hazey JW. A review of 130 humans enrolled in transgastric NOTES protocols at a single institution. Surg Endosc. 2011;25(4):1004–11.
7. Meining A, Feussner H, Swain P, Yang GZ, Lehmann K, Zorron R, Meisner S, Ponsky J, Martiny H, Reddy N, Armengol-Miro JR, Fockens P, Fingerhut A, Costamagna G. Natural-orifice transluminal endoscopic surgery (NOTES) in Europe: summary of the working group reports of the Euro-NOTES meeting 2010. Endoscopy. 2011;43(2):140–3.
8. Neugebauer EA, Becker M, Buess GF, Cuschieri A, Dauben HP, Fingerhut A, Fuchs KH, Habermalz B, Lantsberg L, Morino M, Reiter-Theil S, Soskuty G, Wayand W, Welsch T. EAES recommendations on methodology of innovation management in endoscopic surgery. Surg Endosc. 2010;24(7):1594–615.
9. Lehmann KS, Ritz JP, Wibmer A, Gellert K, Zornig K, Burghardt J, Büsing M, Runkel N, Kohlhaw K, Albrecht R, Kirchner TG, Arlt G, Mall JW, Butters M, Bulian DR, Bretschneider J, Holmer C, Buhr HJ. The German registry for natural orifice translumenal endoscopic surgery: report of the first 551 patients. Ann Surg. 2010;252(2):263–70.
10. Zorron R, Palanivelu C, Galvão Neto MP, Ramos A, Salinas G, Burghardt J, DeCarli L, Henrique Sousa L, Forgione A, Pugliese R, Branco AJ, Balashanmugan TS, Boza C, Corcione F, D'Avila Avila F, Arturo Gómez N, Galvão Ribeiro PA, Martins S, Filgueiras M, Gellert K, Wood Branco A, Kondo W, Inacio Sanseverino J, de Sousa JA, Saavedra L, Ramírez E, Campos J, Sivakumar K, Rajan PS, Jategaonkar PA, Ranagrajan M, Parthasarathi R, Senthilnathan P, Prasad M, Cuccurullo D, Müller V. International multicenter trial on clinical natural orifice surgery-NOTES IMTN study: preliminary results of 362 patients. Surg Innov. 2010;17(2):142–58.
11. Zornig C, Siemssen L, Emmermann A, Alm M, von Waldenfels HA, Felixmüller C, Mofid H. NOTES cholecystectomy: matched pair analysis comparing the transvaginal hybrid and conventional laparoscopic techniques in a series of 216 patients. Surg Endosc. 2011;25(6):1822–6.
12. Lacy AM, Delgado S, Rojas OA, Almenara R, Blasi A, Llach J. MA-NOS radical sigmoidectomy: report of a transvaginal resection in the human. Surg Endosc. 2008;22(7):1717–23.
13. Tarantino L, Linke GR, Lange J, Siercks I, Warschkow R, Zerz A. Transvaginal rigid-hybrid natural orifice transluminal endoscopic surgery technique for anterior resection treatment of diverticulitis: a feasibility study. Surg Endosc. 2011;25(9):3034–42.
14. Inoue H, Minami H, Kobayashi Y, et al. Peroral endoscopic myotopmy (POEM) for esophageal achalasia. Endoscopy. 2010;42:265–71.
15. von Renteln D, Inoue H, Minami H, Werner YB, Pace A, Kersten JF, Much CC, Schachschal G, Mann O, Keller J, Fuchs KH, Rösch T. Peroral endoscopic myotomy for the treatment of achalasia: a prospective single center study. Am J Gastroenterol. 2012;107(3):411–7.
16. Ren Z, Zhong Y, Zhou P, Xu M, Cai M, Li L, Shi Q, Yao L. Perioperative management and treatment for complications during and after peroral endoscopic myotomy (POEM) for esophageal achalasia (EA) (data from 119 cases). Surg Endosc. 2012;26(11):3267–72.
17. Eleftheriadis N, Inoue H, Ikeda H, Onimaru M, Yoshida A, Hosoya T, Maselli R, Kudo SE. Training in peroral endoscopic myotomy (POEM) for esophageal achalasia. Ther Clin Risk Manag. 2012;8:329–42.
18. Buess G, Mentges B, Manncke K, Starlinger M. Technique and results of transanal endoscopic microsurgery in early rectal cancer. Am J Surg. 1992;163:63–9.

19. Sylla P, Rattner DW, Delgado S, Lacy AM. NOTES transanal rectal cancer resection using transanal endoscopic microsurgery and laparoscopic assistance. Surg Endosc. 2010;24(5):1205–10.
20. Lacy AM, Adelsdorfer C, Delgado S, Sylla P, Rattner D. Minilaparoscopy-assisted transrectal low anterior resection (LAR): a preliminary study. Surg Endosc. 2013;27(1):339–46.
21. Telem DA, Berger DL, Bordeianou LG, Rattner D, Sylla P. Update on transanal NOTES for rectal cancer: transitioning to human trials. Minim Invasive Surg. 2012;2012:287613.
22. Fuchs KH, Breithaupt W, Varga G, Schulz T, Reinisch A, Josipovic N. Transanal Hybrid Colon resection – from laparoscopy to NOTES. Surg Endosc. 2012;27(3):746–52.
23. Fuchs KH, Breithaupt W, Kuhl HJ, Schulz T, Dignaß A. Experience with a training program for transgastric procedures in NOTES. Surg Endosc. 2010;24:601–9.

Single Incision Laparoscopy

39

Helmut G. Weiss, Jan Schirnhofer, Eberhard Brunner, Katharina Pimpl, Christof Mittermair, Christian Obrist, and Michael Weiss

39.1 Introduction

In the last decades general surgery has undergone a change from open to laparoscopic surgery to reduce morbidity, shorten hospital stay and accelerate recovery. Nowadays, both simple as well as complicated procedures in benign and malignant diseases are performed endoscopically. This has led to development of new instrumentation and standardization.

The quest for even less invasive procedures led to further reducment of the surgical trauma by minimizing the size and number of trocar incisions, with the ultimate goal to omit any visible scar in the abdominal wall. One of these attempts is Single Incision Laparoscopy (SIL), which is generally carried out through a single incision hidden in the umbilicus.

Although the first steps in laparoscopy have been developed in the eighteenth century through one single umbilical incision, technical limitations mandated the use of multiple trocars to perform minimal invasive surgery other than solely diagnostic laparoscopy. Almost 200 years later gynecologists recycled the transumbilical single incision approach for laparoscopic tubal ligation [1]. Recent advantages in instrumentation provided the opportunity to reuse the SIL concept in technically more demanding procedures. The field was pioneered with the first SIL hysterectomy [2] and SIL appendectomy in 1991 [3]. General surgeons cautiously adopted the SIL technique by developing either extraumbilical one-trocar techniques [4] or stepwise reducing the incisions for appendicectomy by means of transumbilical laparoscopic assisted techniques [5]. The first report on SIL cholecystectomy is attributed to Paganini in 1995 [6], but first published by Navarra in 1997 [7].

H.G. Weiss, MD, MSc, FEBS (✉) • J. Schirnhofer, MD
E. Brunner, MD • K. Pimpl, MD • C. Mittermair, MD
C. Obrist, MD • M. Weiss, CM
General Surgery Department, Saint John of God Hospital, Salzburg, Austria
e-mail: helmut.weiss@bbsalz.at

Due to the slow penetration of new inventions within the medical society it lasted another 10 years to introduce SIL in daily surgical routine. Beside the contemplative reluctance of surgeons evaluating safety and feasibility, there was another main factor supporting the advancement of SIL. Namely the scientific realization of the opportunity to perform surgery without any scar utilizing the mouth, vagina or anus as the entrance to the surgical field - natural orifice transluminal endoscopic surgery (NOTES). This new methodology immediately attracted patients who stated that they would prefer NOTES over standard laparoscopy if the risks associated with the two approaches were similar [8]. This was a first express of patients request for unmaimed cosmesis beside other negative effects of surgical scars apart from the proven risks of pain, bleeding, infection or hernia.

However, the concept of NOTES has several disadvantages and limitations with the currently available instruments, including abdominal spillage of gastric, urinary, or colonic contents, the necessity of many special instruments, difficulties in maintaining the spatial orientation, difficult tasks of viscerotomy closure with the additional risk for leakage from gastrotomy or colotomy. Since there are so many obstacles in the development of NOTES it is still in its early developmental stages. NOTES has to be evaluated thoroughly in experimental models before it is introduced into clinical routine.

However, it has stimulated a revived interest in SIL. SIL represents an attractive alternative to both, conventional laparoscopy and NOTES, by hiding the scar in the depth of the umbilicus. And in addition, it can be performed with standard laparoscopic instruments and according to well known strategic surgical steps. Thereby, surgical safety and outcomes remain unaffected. Also, conversion from a single-port surgery to multi-port conventional laparoscopy can be performed immediately on demand.

H.J. Bonjer (ed.), *Surgical Principles of Minimally Invasive Procedures*, DOI 10.1007/978-3-319-43196-3_39

39.2 Terminology

SIL initially was described using many synonyms, some of which were trademarks others more intuitive link the transumbilical approach to natural orifice concept.

Table 39.1 lists the most commonly used synonyms of SIL.

Table 39.1 Most commonly used synonyms of Single Incision Laparoscopy

Synonyms for single incision laparoscopy
Single incision laparoscopic surgery, SILS™
Laparo-endoscopic single-site surgery, LESS (U-LESS)
Embryonic NOTES, E-NOTES
Transumbilical endoscopic surgery, TUES
Single port access (SPA) surgery
Single port laparoscopy (SPL)
Single-access-site (SAS) laparoscopic surgery
Single-site-access (SSA) laparoscopic surgery
Single site umbilical laparoscopy (SSUL)
One port umbilical surgery, OPUS
Natural orifice trans-umbilical surgery, NOTUS
Trans-umbilical laparoscopic assisted, TULA
Single incision pediatric endosurgical techniques (SIPES)
Hybrid procedures (on the way to NOTES)

39.3 Indications–Contraindications

For surgeons having passed the learning curve indications for the SIL approach are basically the same as for conventional laparoscopy. With regard to the expected outcome preexisting scars or planned redo-surgery other than SIL contest at least the cosmetic benefit. Contraindications are similar to those given for conventional laparoscopy, namely, generalized peritonitis or patients at a high operative risk. Due to the relation between height of patients and length of instruments small children are not optimal candidates for SIL.

Table 39.2 shows the number of patients with regard to the defined SIL procedures operated at our department from August 2008 to August 2013 (Table 39.2).

Table 39.2 Most commonly used synonyms of Single Incision Laparoscopy

Transumbilical SIL procedures	Number
Cholecystectomies	756
Inguinal hernia repairs	508
Colorectal resections	362
Appendectomies	253
Liver resections	32
Small bowel resections	28
Fundoplications	21
Gastric resections	20
Pancreas resections	9
Adrenalectomies	9
Others	94
Total	2092

39.4 Technique and Instrumentation

The entrance at the umbilicus is variable. Most surgeons prefer cutting vertically in the groove of the navel to hide the scar [9]. For larger incisions the cut initially juts out the navel at the lower margin. At the end of the procedure a virtually scarless aspect can be achieved by incorporation of the incision within the restored umbilical crease using a intracutaneous running suture that combines a linear with an purse-string closure (Fig. 39.1).

Others advocate to cut at the upper margin of the umbilicus with a slight lengthening to both sides resulting in a omega-shaped line [10]. In the standing position this scar is hardly detectable after surgery.

The length of the skin incision depends on both, the number and size of trocars and the diameter of any specimen that have to be retrieved. The positive correlation between length of incision and risk for wound complications has been scientifically proven [11] for incisions longer than four centimeters in open surgery. Presumably, for SIL and conventional laparoscopy a similar correlation exists although available data can not convincingly identify a threshold. In our experience the better ability to perform a fascial closure under direct vision after SIL might outweigh the risk of a longer incision compared to conventional laparoscopy.

The prevalence of fascial gaps or preexisting umbilical hernia is about 40% in our patient population. By using the transumbilical approach these defects are detected more accurately and can be closed simultaneously during the SIL procedure. Closure of umbilical hernia with non-absorbable sutures or mesh augmentation is generally recommended. Use of absorbable single stitches or running sutures in cases other than preexisting hernia is under debate. Skin closure can be preferentially performed with subcuticular sutures or glue (Fig. 39.2).

Initially SIL was performed with an optical trocar to minimize the approach. Limitations in surgical performance mandated the use of additional trocars. Therefore, additional trocars were used low profile through separated fascial incisions. Later on, single-port devices enclosing three to four working channels or a gel cap were developed to bring three or more instruments through one fascial incision (Fig. 39.3).

It is of paramount importance for SIL that sufficient sealing of the pneumoperitoneum is facilitated. These port devices increase the procedural costs but reduce the risk for wound complications significantly [9]. In order to reduce procedural costs hand-made ports are developed that com-

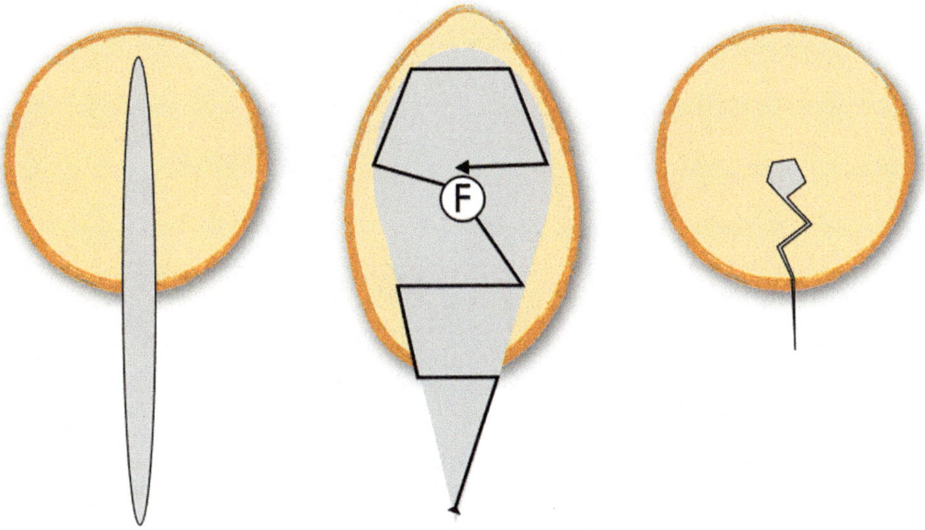

Fig. 39.1 Closure of incision that jut out the navel at the lower margin: a running suture combines a linear with an purse-string type closure. *F* depicts the deep fascial stitch whereas all other stitches are intracutaneous

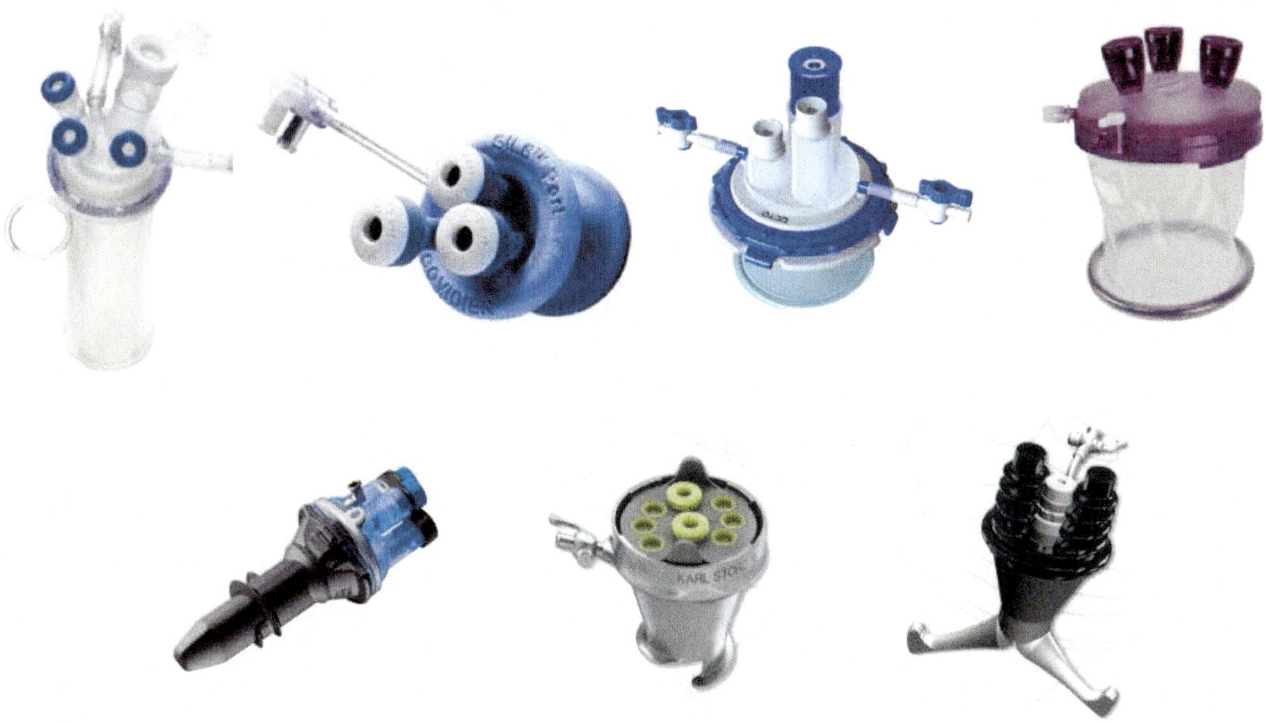

Fig. 39.2 An assortment of frequently used single port devices: Disposable and reusable systems are shown in the *upper* and *lower panel*, respectively

bine an Alexis wound protecting foil with a sterile surgical glove where the fingertips serve as points of access, yet maintain an airtight seal for insufflation. As an alternative, reusable SIL ports are available that are cost effective with a break-even in procedural costs after 15–20 procedures compared to conventional laparoscopy.

The technical challenges encountered with single-port surgery are the fight of instruments inside and outside the body since surgical movements have to be deflected at a single fulcrum in the umbilicus. As a consequence specific tricks are mandatory to restore triangulation during the manipulations:

First, crossing the instruments leads to a virtual exchange of the right and left side, meaning that the instrument that is deployed with the right hand is positioned at the left side of the operative field and vice versa (Fig. 39.4).

In this situation the use of at least one articulating or bended instrument reestablishes triangulation and prevents

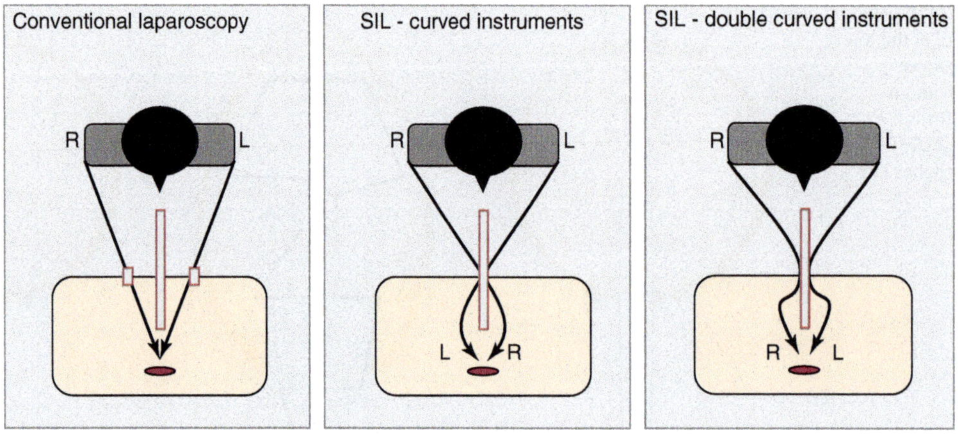

Fig. 39.3 Compared to conventional laparoscopy (*left*) crossing the instruments to reestablish triangulation leads to a virtual exchange of the right and left hand side using single bent instruments (*middle*). Thereby the working path is slightly longer than the direct route. Double curved instruments allow for instrument guidance as effectively delivered (*right*)

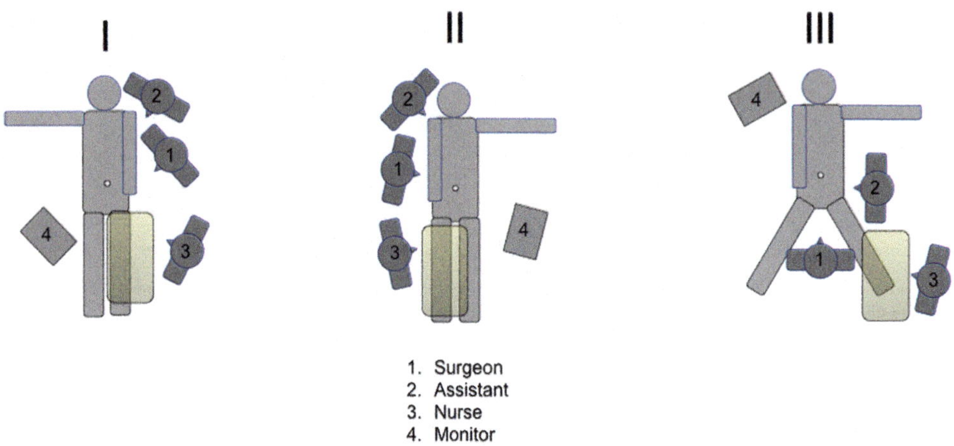

Fig. 39.4 *I* OR setting for SIL-AE, right side TAPP/TEP, SIL right hemicolectomy. *II*: OR setting for left side SIL-TAPP/TEP, SIL left hemicolectomy, SIL rectal resection, SIL pancreas resection. *III*: OR setting for SIL-CHE, SIL gastric and esophageal procedures, SIL liver resection

clashing of the hands outside. Furthermore use of longer graspers helps to reach the target via the longer curved way. Handling with pre-bent instruments seems easier when starting with SIL. However, articulating instruments with rotating tips enable more degrees of freedom for complex movements in advanced procedures. The bended or articulating instrument should always be used in the supporting hand whereas the straight instrument is in the operating hand to facilitate dissection, sealing, clipping or suturing.

Second, double-curved instruments have been developed to allow instrument guidance for both hands. This benefit is attenuated by the fact that almost all movements with the instruments are no longer in a linear axis.

Third, retracting devices, suspending sutures or magnetic anchoring are available to expose the dissection field. Thereby it is possible to substitute working instruments and to exclusively use straight tools throughout the procedure with little clashing outside.

Fourth, the most sophisticated devices for SIL are operative platforms, such as the disposable SPIDER™ (Single Port Instrument Delivery Extended Reach, TransEnterix, DACH Medical) device or the da Vinci Single-Site™ Instrumentation robot (Intuitive Surgical, Inc). These systems offer all possible degrees of freedom for dissection or retraction. The SPIDER™ delivers two flexible instruments as graspers, hooks or scissors together with a five millimeter camera and an additional straight trocar through a four channel shaft. The da Vinci SI robot additionally offers stereoscopic vision and subtle guidance of instruments. At present, high costs and longer operation times due to laborious installation impede wide acceptance of this robotic platform, at least for non-advanced procedures.

Cameras that are recommended for SIL should be extralong to prevent collision of hands outside. Getting the light cable out of the field is advantageous and can be achieved by a right-angle connector or an end-on light source. It seems insignificant to take a straight, 30° or 45° optic or a laparoscope with a flexible tip. For the benefit of a better amount of light it is advisable to use a 10 mm instead of a 5 mm laparoscope for complex procedures.

39.5 Procedures–Operating Room–Technique Step by Step

In the new area of SIL a variety of basic and advanced surgical procedures are described. The setting in the theatre is depicted in Fig. 39.5.

As most of the procedures are carried out with at least one straight instrument our preferred standard of delivery through the single port device is shown in.

39.5.1 SIL Appendicectomy (SIL-AE)

In 1991 Pelosi described the first successful SIL-AE [3]. This approach has the potential to offer the same benefits commonly associated with laparoscopic surgery in terms of recovery and pain with, perhaps, an even better cosmetic result. It is regarded the easiest of the surgical standard SIL procedures with the shortest learning curve [12]. However, for beginners the SIL technique limits the surgeon's working angles and has the potential to be a more technically demanding approach with potentially increase of operation time. This may jeopardize acceptance and patience of the operative team during acute surgery which is carried out commonly outside office hours.

The patient is placed in the supine position with the left arm alongside the body. The surgeon and assistant stand on the left side of the patient, with the monitor placed on the patient's right side. An umbilical incision of about 15 mm is performed. A SIL port is inserted, pneumoperitoneum is reached and the abdominal cavity is inspected with a 5 mm 30° laparoscope.

Then the operating table is tilted to a 30° Trendelenburg position associated with a left tilt to allow adequate exposition of the right lower quadrant of the abdominal cavity. The mesoappendix is divided as usual. Transection is performed sharply after placing an absorbable loop (Endoloop; Ethicon Endosurgery) or by using an intestinal load of an endostapler. The appendix is slowly retrieved through an appropriate channel of the port device without squeezing or contact with the abdominal wall. Bulky, inflamed, vulnerable or perforated specimen are removed in a bag to prevent wound complications.

Data of randomized controlled studies, comparative studies and meta-analyses revealed that in SIL-AE compared to the conventional laparoscopic appendectomie operative time is longer

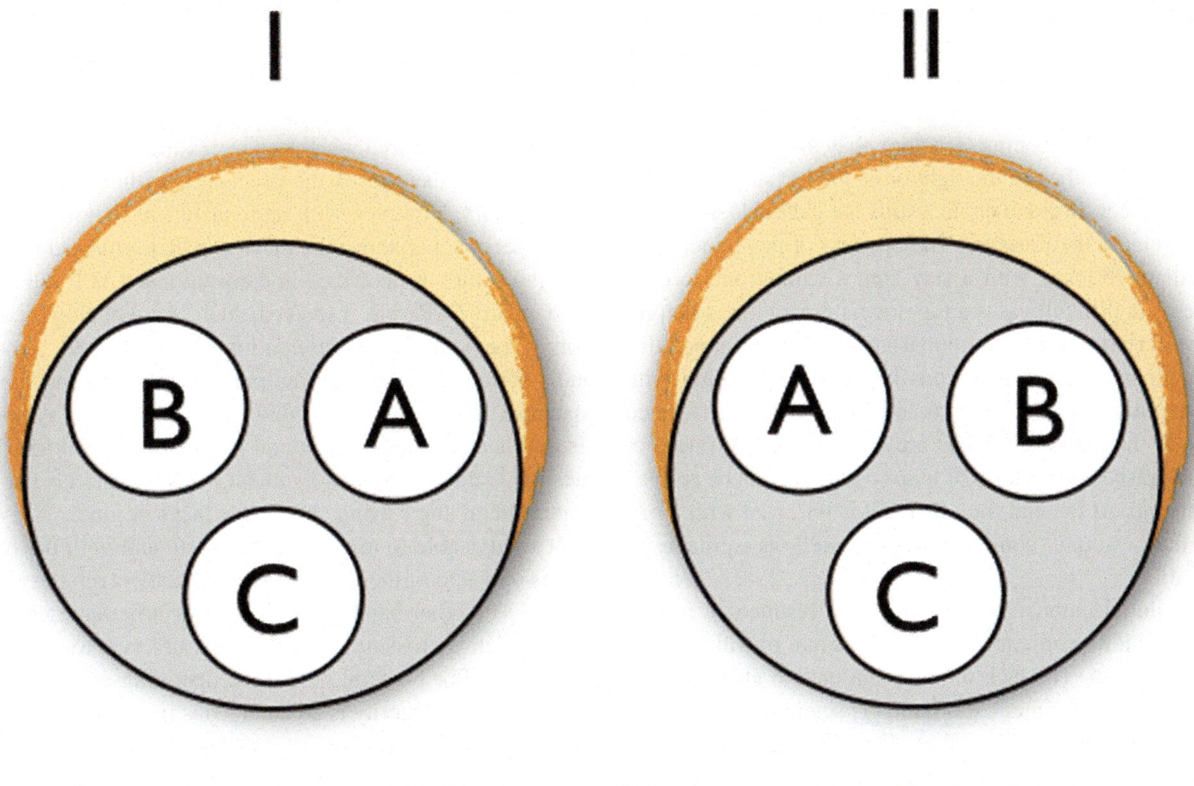

Fig. 39.5 *I* Trocar position of camera (C), operating (A) and supporting (B) instruments to reach targets left to the optical axis (e.g., SIL-CHE, left side SIL-TAPP/TEP, SIL-CR). *II*: Trocar position for right side SIL-TAPP/TEP, SIL-AE

in children and obese and therefore results in greater costs. In contrast, less pain and faster recovery is reported in cases with perforation when operated by means of SIL [13–17]. However, these small differences are likely of marginal clinical relevance. SIL-AE did not increase the rate of complications and therefore is a valuable alternative to conventional laparoscopic appendectomy with the benefit of better cosmetic satisfaction.

39.5.2 SIL Cholecystectomy (SIL-CHE)

As mentioned above the first official presentation of SIL-CHE by Paganini and Navarra dates back almost 20 years. A variety of different techniques is described so far, of which some obviously ignore the rules of safety by compromising the standard dissection in the triangle of Callot. However, more or less sophisticated variations have been published using sutures, wires, endohooks, SPIDER™, robotics etc. All of those showed safety and feasibility for SIL-CHE at least in non-acute cases.

In brief, the patient, surgeon, assistant and monitor are exactly positioned according to multiport laparoscopy. After a two centimeter incision through the folds of the umbilicus a single port device is inserted. Thereafter, the operating table is tilted to a 30° Anti-Trendelenburg position associated with a slight left side rotation to allow adequate exposition of the right upper quadrant of the abdominal cavity. The fundus of the gallbladder is retracted by use of either a stay suture, endoscopic retractors (Endograb, TPEA Lifter, AFS Medical Austria) or an additional extra-long grasper (DACH Medical, Austria). During dissection of the triangle optical view can be optimized by placing a suture that allows pulling the infundibulum either on the right or on the left side according to a puppeteer. In acute cholecystitis the gallbladder is emptied to release the pressure. The opening of this puncture is immediately closed with a stay suture without any consequences. In difficult cases a top down preparation is helpful as it would be used in conventional laparoscopy. Intraoperative cholangiography, a rendez-vous bile duct exploration with intraoperative ERCP/EPT or stone removal can be performed easily in this approach. Clips are available with straight or curved graspers. Any form of loops or sutures can be applied on demand. At the end the specimen is retrieved with a bag to protect wound complications as well as spillage of content.

The initial enthusiasm for SIL-CHE resulted in a high number of low profile feasibility studies that provoked justified skepticism. The lack of sufficient data to clearly prove any inferiority or benefit still hampers scientific conclusion. The current evidence shows that SIL-CHE offers a safe alternative to conventional cholecystectomy with a comparable profile in intra- and postoperative complications [18–20]. The need for a longer operating time is balanced by a trend towards lower postoperative pain and improved patient satisfaction.

39.5.3 SIL Inguinal Hernia Repair (SIL-TAPP, SIL-TEP)

Inguinal hernia repair is one of the most commonly performed surgical procedures worldwide. Laparoscopic techniques, including transabdominal preperitoneal (TAPP) and totally extraperitoneal (TEP) inguinal hernia repair, have resulted in reduced postoperative pain, faster recovery, and low recurrence rates. Both methods can be performed through a single skin incision with safe and feasible outcome [21–23].

SIL-TAPP is carried out with the patient in the supine position arms along side the body. The surgeon and the assistant are both standing at the contralateral side of the hernia. A two centimeter incision is performed intraumbilically and the pneumoperitoneum is installed after insertion of a single port device. Dissection of the groin region requires substantial shear stress at the fulcrum. Three isolated trocars mostly result in gas leakage and unstable pneumoperitoneum. This is why we strongly recommend to use a single port system for SIL-TAPP rather than three isolated trocars via separate fascial incisions. For dissection and reposition of the hernia the table is tilted head down. For simplicity a slight modification in peritoneal incision and preparation of the peritoneal flap is commonly used: the incision line is not directed towards the inner ring of the inguinal channel but at a some centimeters higher level. Thereby only a dorsal peritoneal flap is prepared which can be readjusted by re-absorbable tacks at the end of the procedure without the risk of nerval injury. However, with more technical training closure of the peritoneum above the mesh can be performed using a running suture as described in conventional TAPP. All steps of standard TAPP are respected, such as meticulous reduction of the hernial sac, preservation of the epigastric vessels and vas deferens, defining the pubic symphysis and finally placing a 15–12 cm mesh medially across the pubic symphysis and laterally up to the lateral end of iliopubic tract. The mesh is fixed to Cooper's ligament medially and also at the upper-lateral angle using absorbable tacks or glue.

It is advisable to use a straight instrument with the hand that is opposite of the hernia side to directly reach the target region. The other hand guides a bent or articulating instrument which is crossing the path of the first one to allow triangulation. For bilateral hernia the operating team changes the side. Ambidexterity is advantageous in this case.

The SIL-TEP technique is performed as follows:

The patient is placed in the supine position with the surgeon and assistant standing opposite of the site of the hernia.

A single curvilinear skin incision at the lower margin of the umbilical crease is performed on average two to three centimeter in length. Dissection of subcutaneous tissue to the anterior sheet of the rectus muscle is performed. The anterior sheet is incised for another two centimeter in a curved path to get access to the preperitoneal space which is preformed with a blunt 5 mm dissector underneath the rectus muscle. A single port device is placed to allow insufflation without further balloon dilator. A 30° laparoscope and two five millimeter instruments–one of which is articulating–are delivered through the channels. The use of three independent trocars all adjacent to each other with a distance of about one centimeter has been shown to sometimes fail in sealing the gas and are therefore not recommended by us. Dissection, reposition, and mesh placement are carried out in the same way as in conventional laparoscopy. The technical challenge for the camera man is during the accurate dissection lateral to the semilunar line. As in conventional TEP mesh fixation is not done routinely. No drain is inserted at the end of the procedure. Gas is stepwise released under vision to reposition the peritoneal sac onto the mesh without kinking it.

Both techniques, SIL-TAPP and SIL-TEP, are regarded technically advanced procedures. This is why the penetration rate of these techniques among surgeons is not as high as the rate for SIL-CHE or SIL colon resections. The benefit of the invisible scar is counterbalanced by longer operating time, the demand for higher technical skills and higher procedural costs if disposable instruments are used.

Good comparative scientific studies comparing SIL-TAPP and SIL-TEP with conventional TAPP and TEP are warranted to identify one method having the edge over the other.

39.5.4 SIL Colorectal Resection (SIL-CR)

SIL in general is best suited for a subset of patients who require specimen extraction or stoma creation. Therefore it is convincing to apply the SIL approach to colorectal surgery.

Since 2008 [21, 24, 25] various SIL techniques have been described for resection of the right, transverse or left colon, as well as rectal resections.

When performing SIL-CR two alternative approaches other than the transumbilical route can be considered: The "classical" site at the umbilicus has the advantage of an easy access to all parts of the colorectal frame. But, in cases requiring a protective ileostomy or Hartmann's procedure the entire operation can be carried out via the proposed stoma site at the right or left lower quadrant. A valid alternative might be through a Pfannenstiel incision with the aim to reduce any wound complication risk in the midline.

SIL-CR transvaginal and transrectal instrument delivery or specimen extraction extends the surgical options. Both intracorporeal and extracorporeal anastomosis are as feasible as in conventional laparoscopy.

With the experience of more than 350 SIL-CR we standardized the technique as described briefly:

39.5.5 Ileocolic Resection and Right Hemicolectomy

The patient is prepared supine and secured to the table as for any laparoscopic procedure. Surgeon and assistant are standing on the left side of the patient. Split-leg extenders can be beneficial for the scrub nurse for better assistance while watching the operation. The table is tilted with the left-side down and in Trendelenburg position. A three to five centimeter transumbilical incision is adequate depending on the size of the specimen or a prevalent hernia. Adhesions near the incision can often be taken down sharply through the incision with adequate retraction and lighting. Achieving an adequate view of the anatomy while being able to work untroubled is one of the more challenging aspects of SIL-CR.

Dissection, vessel sealing and intestinal transection follow the oncologic principles of complete mesocolic excision of open and conventional laparoscopic surgery. Traction and countertraction is mandatory and can be established with an additional straight instrument guided by the assistant or by using a lifting device or suspending suture.

Ligating, stapling, clipping or sealing the ileocolic artery and branches of the superior mesenteric veins is at the discretion of the surgeon.

Visualization and dissection of the hepatic flexure is alleviated by moving the table to the reverse Trendelenburg position and, with a bowel grasper, sweep the right colon medially and anteriorly, which will display the hepatocolic attachments in reference to the duodenum. After transection the specimen is retrieved in a tearproof bag to protect the peritoneum from any bacterial or tumor cell contamination through the spillage of squeezed fluid.

39.5.6 Left Colectomy, Low Anterior Resection, Total Colectomy, and Proctocolectomy with Ileal Pouch-Anal Anastomosis

The patient is prepared and stabilized to a split-leg extender table with the operating team on the right side. A three to five centimeter incision is made either in the planned stoma site or the umbilicus. A single port device in combination with a wound protector is strongly recommended to reduce the risk for wound complications. The challenge to drive the camera is acceptable if learning can occur in a laboratory setting. A technique for providing sufficient retraction and triangulation is using an increased table angulation and gravity to tent the mesentery over the articulated instrument while dissecting with the other. Again, ambidexterity substantially saves time and enhances performance. All steps of SIL dissection, vessel ligation, bowel transection and anastomosis entirely follow the standards of conventional laparoscopy.

When below the peritoneal reflection, visualization can be difficult. A floppy uterus can be retracted anteriorly using a (temporarily transcutaneous) suture. Clips can also be used to tack a floppy ovary or fallopian tube above the broad ligament. To get further separation between the vagina and the rectum, a probe can be placed into the vagina for anterior retraction or into the rectum for posterior retraction. Both retraction methods can be utilized to create more operating space in the deep narrow pelvis.

Placing the stapler in an anterior-to-posterior fashion might be easier to fit the rectum within the stapler jaws. The proximal and distal transected colon specimen is wrapped in a bag and extracted through the wound protector. Thereafter the proximal colon segment is advanced externally to place the anvil. Reaching at least two centimeter past the symphysis is sufficient to ensure appropriate length for any anastomosis.

39.5.7 Ileostomy and Colostomy Creation

Stoma creation is definitely one of the under-appreciated benefits of SIL, particularly in the re-do patient. SIL requires only an incision at the stoma site which will be used to free adhesions and establish pneumoperitoneum under direct vision. The bowel should be marked to ensure proximal versus distal orientation. It is essential not to twist the segment to maintain mesenteric orientation during extraction.

Randomized controlled trials between SIL and conventional CR indicate a comparable outcome which favors SIL-CR in terms of shorter hospital stay and a trend to less pain. Therefore SIL-CR might serve as a safe alternative to the conventional approach in a selected group of non-obese patients [26–28].

Furthermore, SIL has been shown to be feasible in fundoplication, gastric resection, metabolic surgery (Gastric banding, gastric sleeve resection, gastric RY-bypass, mini-gastric-bypass, biliopancreatic diversion), liver, pancreas, spleen resections, adrenalectomies, in small bowel obstruction and some other advanced procedures with optimal outcome.

39.6 How to Start–Learning Curve

The SILS approach is technically more challenging than conventional laparoscopy. For novices this difference in performance is flattened within some procedures. Moreover, learning to carry out SIL appears to result in better skills that improve abilities to carry out both SIL and LC, whereas training in LC fails to have the same effect [29]. The same is true for experienced laparoscopic surgeons. During SIL, performance scores drop and frustration, effort, and mental and physical demands are all increased. Training is paramount to prevent an obstacle race during the first SIL procedures. Proctoring might be helpful for surgeons to get SIL skills in their repertoire [12]. Last but not least parameters, such as limited time, loss of patience, wrong patient selection, inappropriate instruments, and substantial air leak might end up in frustration and dishonor the SIL approach. It has been published that operating times generally are brought in line after 10–25 SIL cases.

A surgeon who offers SIL has the responsibility to inform his patients by fully explaining the procedure, mentioning any lack of safety profile, offering alternative traditional methods and giving the patients enough decision time. As SIL is still not a common standard, thorough documentation in a prospective database is recommended to pass external audits.

Conclusion

The tendency towards either limiting the number of abdominal incisions or eliminating them completely represents the ultimate goal for surgeons in their quest to perform SIL as the 'minimized' surgery aiming to avoid any visible scars.

Improving surgical skills, overcoming commercial temptation and pressure and focus on the clinical outcome will allow to conduct more valid studies to proof any benefit of SIL other than cosmesis.

Literature

1. Siegler AM. An instrument to aid tubal sterilization by laparoscopy. Fertil Steril. 1972;23(5):367–8.
2. Pelosi MA, Pelosi 3rd MA. Laparoscopic hysterectomy with bilateral salpingo-oophorectomy using a single umbilical puncture. N J Med. 1991;88(10):721–6.
3. Wolenski M, Markus E, Pelosi MA. Laparoscopic appendectomy incidental to gynecologic procedures. Todays OR Nurse. 1991;13(12):12–8.
4. Inoue H, Takeshita K, Endo M. Single-port laparoscopy assisted appendectomy under local pneumoperitoneum condition. Surg Endosc. 1994;8(6):714–6.
5. Kala Z, Hanke I, Neumann C. A modified technic in laparoscopy-assisted appendectomy–a transumbilical approach through a single port. Rozhl Chir. 1996;75(1):15–8.
6. Paganini A, Lomonto D, Navordino M. One port laparoscopic cholecystectomy in selected patients. Third International Congress on New Technology in Surgery. Luxemburg; 1995.
7. Navarra G, Pozza E, Occhionorelli S, Carcoforo P, Donini I. One-wound laparoscopic cholecystectomy. Br J Surg. 1997;84(5):695.
8. Varadarajulu S, Tamhane A, Drelichman ER. Patient perception of natural orifice transluminal endoscopic surgery as a technique for cholecystectomy. Gastrointest Endosc. 2008;67(6):854–60.

9. Weiss HG, Brunner W, Biebl MO, Schirnhofer J, Pimpl K, Mittermair C, Obrist C, Brunner E, Hell T. Wound complications in 1145 consecutive transumbilical single-incision laparoscopic procedures. Ann Surg. 2014;259(1):89–95.
10. Huang CK, Tsai JC, Lo CH, Houng JY, Chen YS, Chi SC, Lee PH. Preliminary surgical results of single-incision transumbilical laparoscopic bariatric surgery. Obes Surg. 2011;21(3):391–6.
11. Laurent C, Leblanc F, Bretagnol F, Capdepont M, Rullier E. Long-term wound advantages of the laparoscopic approach in rectal cancer. Br J Surg. 2008;95(7):903–8.
12. Ahmed I, Ciancio F, Ferrara V, Jorgensen LN, Mann O, Morales-Conde S, Paraskeva P, Vestweber B, Weiss H. Current status of single-incision laparoscopic surgery: European experts' views. Surg Laparosc Endosc Percutan Tech. 2012;22(3):194–9.
13. Cai YL, Xiong XZ, Wu SJ, Cheng Y, Lu J, Zhang J, Lin YX, Cheng NS. Single-incision laparoscopic appendectomy vs conventional laparoscopic appendectomy: systematic review and meta-analysis. World J Gastroenterol. 2013;19(31):5165–73.
14. Li P, Chen ZH, Li QG, Qiao T, Tian YY, Wang DR. Safety and efficacy of single-incision laparoscopic surgery for appendectomies: a meta-analysis. World J Gastroenterol. 2013;19(25):4072–82.
15. Gao J, Li P, Li Q, Tang D, Wang DR. Comparison between single-incision and conventional three-port laparoscopic appendectomy: a meta-analysis from eight RCTs. Int J Colorectal Dis. 2013;28(10):1319–27.
16. Frutos MD, Abrisqueta J, Lujan J, Abellan I, Parrilla P. Randomized prospective study to compare laparoscopic appendectomy versus umbilical single-incision appendectomy. Ann Surg. 2013;257(3):413–8.
17. Kye BH, Lee J, Kim W, Kim D, Lee D. Comparative study between single-incision and three-port laparoscopic appendectomy: a prospective randomized trial. J Laparoendosc Adv Surg Tech A. 2013;23(5):431–6.
18. Hao L, Liu M, Zhu H, Li Z. Single-incision versus conventional laparoscopic cholecystectomy in patients with uncomplicated gallbladder disease: a meta-analysis. Surg Laparosc Endosc Percutan Tech. 2012;22(6):487–97.
19. Wu XS, Shi LB, Gu J, Dong P, Lu JH, Li ML, Mu JS, Wu WG, Yang JH, Ding QC, Zhang L, Liu YB. Single-incision laparoscopic cholecystectomy versus multi-incision laparoscopic cholecystectomy: a meta-analysis of randomized clinical trials. J Laparoendosc Adv Surg Tech A. 2013;23(3):183–91.
20. Trastulli S, Cirocchi R, Desiderio J, Guarino S, Santoro A, Parisi A, Noya G, Boselli C. Systematic review and meta-analysis of randomized clinical trials comparing single-incision versus conventional laparoscopic cholecystectomy. Br J Surg. 2013;100(2):191–208.
21. Brunner W, Schirnhofer J, Waldstein-Wartenberg N, Frass R, Pimpl K, Weiss H. New: single-incision transumbilical laparoscopic surgery. Eur Surg. 2009;41:98–103.
22. Cugura JF, Kirac I, Kulis T, Janković J, Beslin MB. First case of single incision laparoscopic surgery for totally extraperitoneal inguinal hernia repair. Acta Clin Croat. 2008;47(4):249–52.
23. Kroh M, Rosenblatt S. Single-port, laparoscopic cholecystectomy and inguinal hernia repair: first clinical report of a new device. J Laparoendosc Adv Surg Tech A. 2009;19(2):215–7.
24. Remzi FH, Kirat HT, Kaouk JH, Geisler DP. Single-port laparoscopy in colorectal surgery. Colorectal Dis. 2008;10(8):823–6.
25. Bucher P, Pugin F, Morel P. Single port access laparoscopic right hemicolectomy. Int J Colorectal Dis. 2008;23(10):1013–6.
26. Huscher CG, Mingoli A, Sgarzini G, Mereu A, Binda B, Brachini G, Trombetta S. Standard laparoscopic versus single-incision laparoscopic colectomy for cancer: early results of a randomized prospective study. Am J Surg. 2012;204(1):115–20.
27. Egi H, Hattori M, Hinoi T, Takakura Y, Kawaguchi Y, Shimomura M, Tokunaga M, Adachi T, Urushihara T, Itamoto T, Ohdan H. Single-port laparoscopic colectomy versus conventional laparoscopic colectomy for colon cancer: a comparison of surgical results. World J Surg Oncol. 2012;10:61.
28. Fung AK, Aly EH. Systematic review of single-incision laparoscopic colonic surgery. Br J Surg. 2012;99(10):1353–64.
29. Kwasnicki RM, Aggarwal R, Lewis TM, Purkayastha S, Darzi A, Paraskeva PA. A comparison of skill acquisition and transfer in single incision and multi-port laparoscopic surgery. J Surg Educ. 2013;70(2):172–9.

Robotic Surgery

40

Ivo A.M.J. Broeders

40.1 Introduction

Telesurgery was initially explored to enable battlefield care from a remote location. A prototype called the Green manipulator was developed in the eighties by the National Air and Space Administration (NASA) and the Stanford Research Institute (SRI). The research team involved developed a four-degrees of freedom robotic system that enabled manipulation of surgical instruments over distance using cables for data transfer. The company Intuitive Surgical Inc commercialized this prototype (Fig. 40.1). By that time Computer Motion Inc. has already launched their Easop robotic arm for voice controlled steering of rigid endoscopes. They expanded their concept to the Zeus robotic telemanipulator, a remote surgery system that held three separate arms. Intuitive Surgical inc. acquired this company and is the sole provider of commercially available robotic systems for endoscopic surgery from 1998 up to 2016.

Their da Vinci® system was launched to enable minimally invasive cardiac bypass surgery. Nevertheless, the CE mark was acquired by presenting data on safety in endoscopic surgical procedures such as cholecystectomy and fundoplication for reflux disease.

Robotic cardiac surgery didn't reach the assumed market potential but widespread introduction followed a few years later when urologists started using the da Vinci® system at large scale for radical prostatectomy. This led to interest among gynaecologists and ENT specialists. General surgeons used the system from start at limited scale. Robotics started to gain popularity when larger studies on low anterior resection appeared in 2008 and on.

Up to now 1.8 million procedures have been performed worldwide with surgical robotics and over 3000 systems are installed (old numbers or put in reference with date stated).

Ivo A.M.J. Broeders
Department of Surgery, Meander Medical Centre,
Amersfoort, The Netherlands
e-mail: iamj.broeders@meandermc.nl

The key element of telemanipulation is the introduction of dedicated computer technology between the surgeon and the surgical instruments. This enables surgical support, advanced imaging and the use of dedicated computer -steered tools. The inherent drawbacks of endoscopic surgery are dealt with by reversing the tip response of the instruments, and by introducing scaling to lower the fulcrum effect. Two degrees of freedom are added to the instrument tip to enable refined and complex dissection and suturing tasks (add: the instrument are wristed and the tip can turn 360° and therefore can perform precise tasks in small defined areas such as the pelvis).

The surgeon also steers the camera by pressing a foot paddle, which leads to blocking of the instrument arms and control of the camera arm by the joysticks. The endoscope is completely stable during surgery, and a high level 3-D view is provided by a 12 mm optic (and in the latest version the Xi model a 8,5 mm optic) with two optical channels. The two separate images are fused in the workstation to deliver the true 3-D image.

The surgeon controls three arms, to operate with two and assist with one. Usually one extra assistant trocar is placed, and surgery is preferably performed with one dedicated OR nurse only. The surgeon can adapt the position of the chair, the arm- and head rests to work in an ergonomically favourable position.

A drawback is the complete absence of haptic feedback in combination with loss of direct contact with the instruments. This is of less importance in refined work, but is an issue to deal with in case larger forces are exerted. Telemanipulation surgery separates the surgeon from the tableside team, which inherently leads to loss of direct control within the sterile field. Also, there are substantial differences between the surgeon and the OR nurse in vision, horizon dependency, instrument handling and body position. This demands extensive collaboration between the team members and clear communication with a feedback check system.

Robot-assisted surgery usually increases direct surgical costs and requires intensive training by both surgeon and OR

H.J. Bonjer (ed.), *Surgical Principles of Minimally Invasive Procedures*, DOI 10.1007/978-3-319-43196-3_40

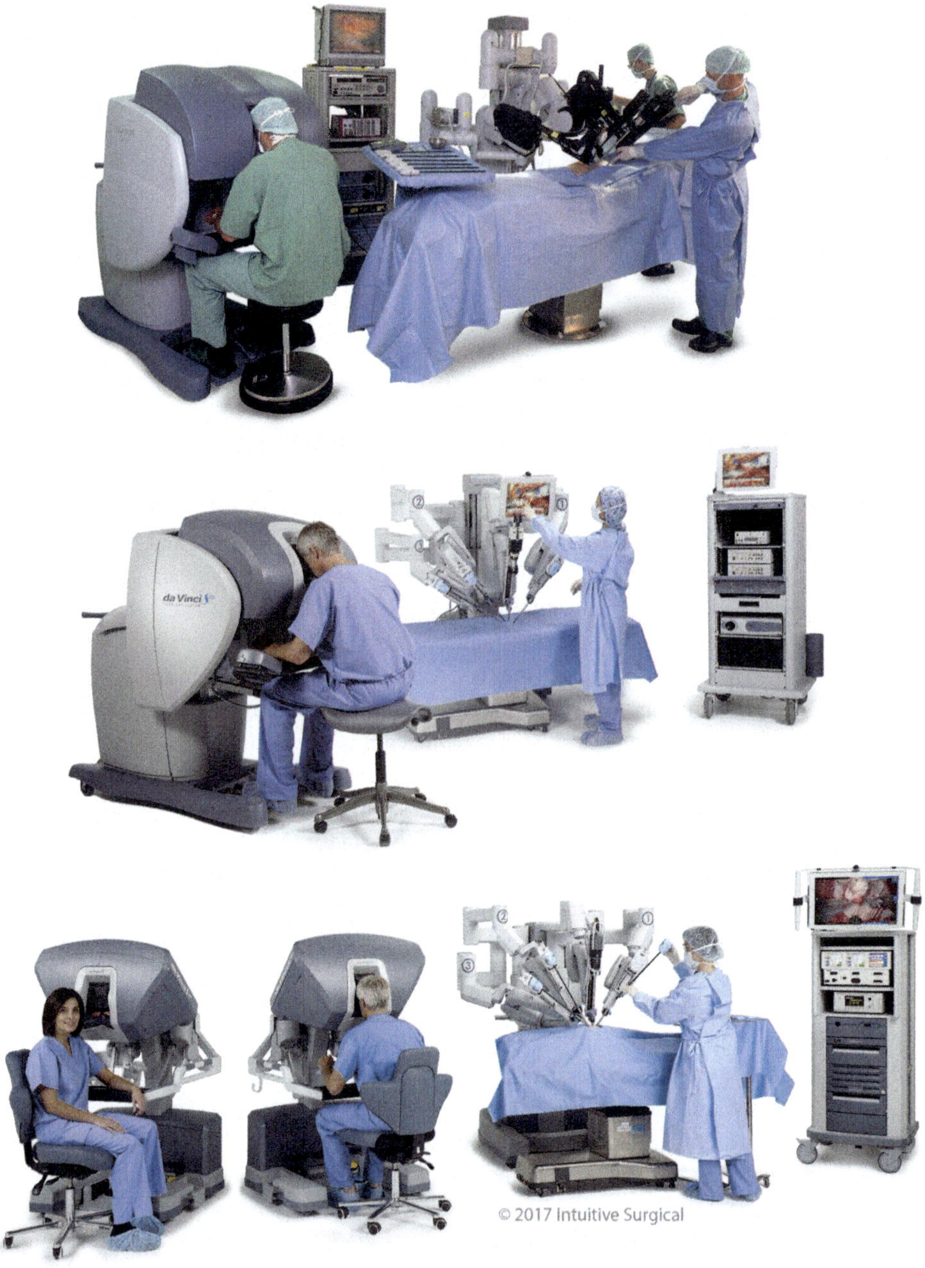

Fig. 40.1 Development of robotic surgical (da Vinci) system through the years (Permission for reproduction: ©2017 Intuitive Surgical, Inc.)

nurses. It puts demands on OR space, time management and anaesthesia.

Users of the current robotic systems should therefore aim at complex endoscopic surgery, from a technical and financial perspective. One should however realize that computer aided surgery is not just about surgical performance. telemanipulation systems open the way to a new era in surgery, were virtual reality, big data analysis and artifical intelligence will be incorporated to bring surgery to the next level. Competing systems will bring new economic models, which surgeons get the opportunity to stay in line with revolutionary concepts in digital healthcare.

40.2 Indications

There is abundant ex-vivo evidence on superiority of robotics systems when performing complex surgical tasks [1–7]. Articles on clinical use of robotic systems in endoscopic surgery are also abundant, but high quality comparative- or randomized studies are scarce. A large international randomised prospective trial on robot versus laparoscopical rectum surgery (the Rolarr trial) did only show a lower conversion rate after robotic rectum surgery for a specific group of obese and male patients (ref abstract ESCP Barcelona sept 2015).

Experienced teams will drape a robotic system while preparing the patient and dock in five minutes, and time required for instrument changes is comparable to standard endoscopic surgery. The initial time loss will not be compensated in routine surgery, such as cholecystectomy, fundoplication or uncomplicated right-hemicolectomy. This type of laparoscopic procedures also allow reasonable to good ergonomics for the surgeon, so no clear benefit for robot use with the currently available systems. Additionally, trocar size in robotics is bigger; the camera port measures 12 mm (or 8.5 in the latest Xi version), and the working ports 8.5 mm. In routine procedures, the added value in imaging, dissection and ergonomics will therefore not compensate for time loss, trocar size and costs. Apart from this, it will be difficult to demonstrate superiority of robotic surgery on standard parameters, such as blood loss, postoperative complications and length of stay when comparing the technique to standard endoscopic techniques. One should therefore seek for procedures that are technically demanding or ergonomically unfavourable. Optimal visualisation, dissection and tissue reconstruction in combination with a good working position should increased results in long term functional outcome and should enable experienced surgeons to perform these procedures routinely for many years without the physical complaints related to standard endoscopic surgery.

Oesophageal- and lung cancer are the primary targets in thoracic general surgery. The precise dissection enables extensive lymph node dissection in difficult areas such as the aorto-pulmonary window [8]. The assisting arm and the stable, surgeon-controlled camera are of particular value in the transhiatal approach.

Robotics have been used in anti-reflux surgery, but there are hardly studies focusing on long term outcome, and early results are comparable [9–11]. Excellent results have been published on the use in myotomy in achalasia and the system is of value in the repair of giant hiatal hernia's and redo surgery for reflux and para-esophageal hernia [12]. The suturing support or robotic systems can be of particular value in pancreatic and liver resection and biliary reconstruction, the repair of visceral aneurysms and pelvic floor reconstruction [13, 14].

Rectal cancer is a main focus at this point of time. Robotics may support the surgeon in optimal dissection in the right plane while avoiding nerve damage.

A number of comparative studies have been published, and meta–analysis suggests comparable outcome, but lower conversion rates in the robotic group [15]. These studies on early results are subject to many confounders. The Rolarr trial compared both laparoscopic as robot technique in a multicentre randomized setup with conversion as primary end point. This study showed a lower conversion rate after robotic rectum surgery for a specific subgroup of patients (male and obes) (ref abstract ESCP Barcelona sept 2015).

Robotics surgery provides surgical support by eletromechanical instrument and camera manipulation, but the computer-based setup also offers extensive additional gain in perioperative diagnostics and additional onlay imaging. This may prove to be a main benefit in the upcoming years. Examples are near infrared technology with fluorescence imaging. This will be used for tissue discrimination, sentinel node detection and analysis of colorectal vascularisation in prevention of anastomotic dehiscence. Computer aided stapling allows pressure measurement within the stapler beak to ensure the application of the correct stapler height.

40.3 The Business Case for Robotics

Robotic surgery adds costs to treatment. In-hospital cost recovery is difficult when comparing robotic surgery to standard endoscopic surgery, because one cannot expect much difference in OR time, hospital stay and complications. Optimal exploitation of robotic systems is therefore most desirable.

Cost consists of fixed annual expenses and procedure related costs. Annual expenses include the depreciation of the 1.8 million system expenses of a period of maximally 8 years, and a 10 % annual burden of this amount for full service and software upgrades. This leads to about 400 K euro fixed annual system costs. Procedure related costs consist of sterile drapes and the use of (semi) disposable instruments. These costs average 1500 euro's per procedure and depend on the type and number of instrument used.

When using the system for 100 procedures annually, robotics add 5500 euro's to patient hospital costs, but this amount lowers to 2300 euro's when using the system 500 times per year. It is therefore most important to build a realistic business case, based on the number of complex endoscopic procedures that are performed in the hospital in the past years. Most hospitals will require a multidisciplinary robotic surgery program to reach the numbers needed to bring costs in an acceptable range. A multidisciplinary team of medical specialists, OR staff, OR planners and hospital board is therefore advisable to prepare acquisition of a robotic system and allow cost-efficient use from start.

40.4 Preparation and Training

Robotic surgery requires dedicated training because of inherent differences with standard endoscopic surgery. Surgeons and OR nurses need to understand the technical details of the console and robot to enable efficient and safe use. Also team and communication training should be part of the training program.

Training starts with building knowledge on technical details. These comprise connection, cable management and startup, ergonomic settings of the console, and moving and storing of the console and robot. OR nurses will subsequently focus on draping the arms while surgeons work on technical details of instrument- and camera settings, and on understanding all steering capacities with graspers and pedals. Learning how to connect the robot to the trocars is a team effort.

Currently, the selling company guides preparation and training. The program includes site visits to understand the general concepts, followed by dedicated team training of surgeons and OR nurses. This training includes learning technical knowhow as mentioned, followed by (procedure specific) surgery on a pig- or human model. Company trainers and medical proctors guide the initial procedures.

The USA project Fundamentals of Robotic Surgery has realized a training curriculum with the objective to "create and develop a validated multispecialty, technical skills competency based curriculum for surgeons to safely and efficiently perform basic robotic-assisted surgery" (see www.frsurgery.org) (https://www.nicholsoncenter.com/sites/default/files/research/Fundamentals%20of%20Robotic%20Surgery.pdf). This program aims to deliver an obligatory and independent training course for residents and registered surgeons who intend to start robotic surgery, comparable to the Fundamentals of Laparoscopic Surgery program. Meanwhile, numerous joint initiatives and dedicated training centres offer specialism-dedicated courses to practice basic and advanced robotics surgery skills.

Basic skills can also be trained using simulators (Fig. 40.2). The company Mimic offers a table top simula-

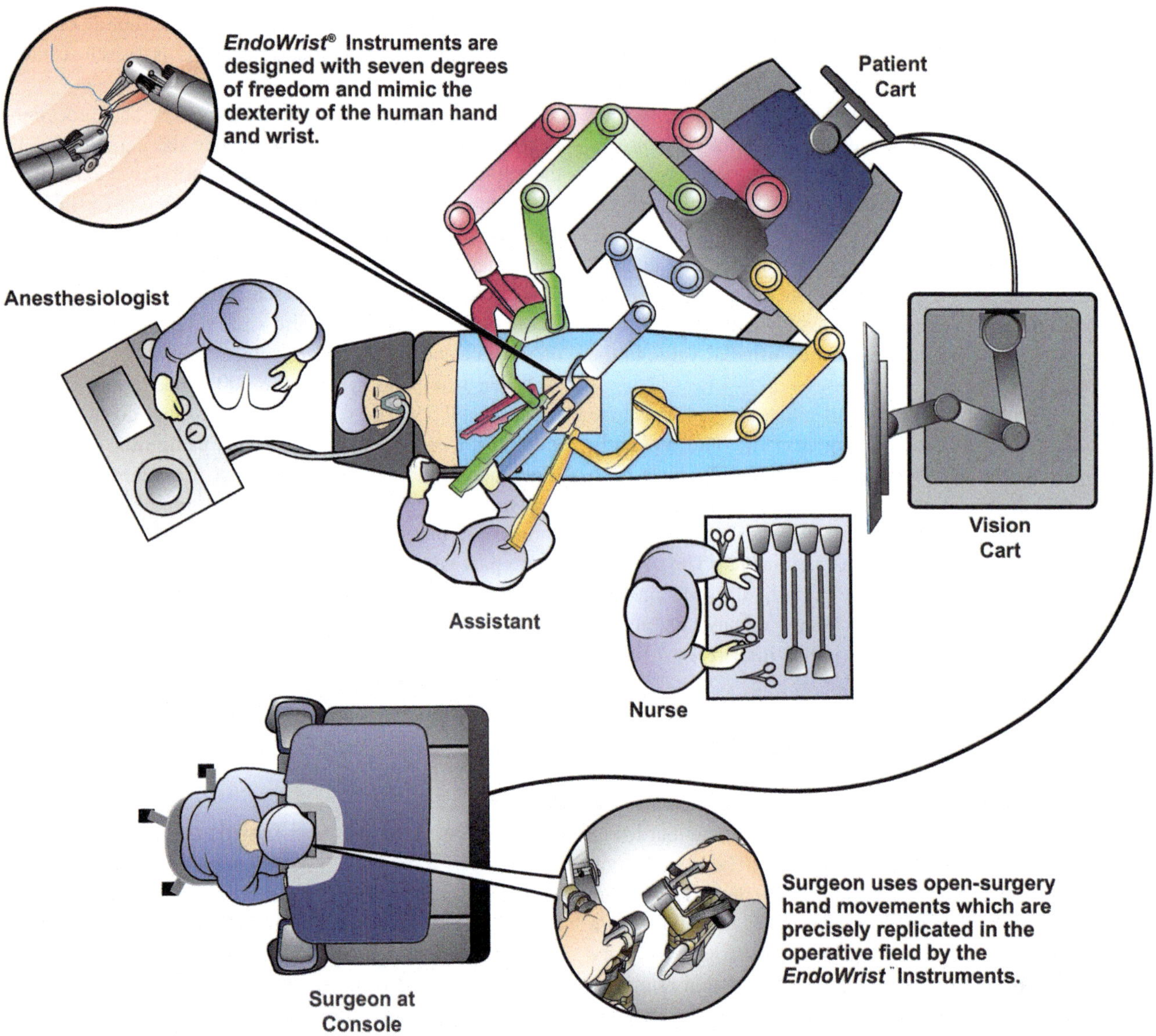

Fig. 40.2 An example of an OR set-up with robot system (Permission for reproduction: ©2017 Intuitive Surgical, Inc.)

tion device that teaches basic instrument and camera manipulation with a number abstract drills and a scoring system comparable to endoscopic surgery trainers, that also allows table side OR technicians to train robot skills together with the surgeon. Intuitive Surgical also offers the software of this trainer in a hardware setup that is mounted on the robotic console. This allows training in the actual surgical environment.

Surgeons who start with robotic surgery should be familiar with all details, risks and pitfalls of endoscopic surgery and the pneumoperitoneum. Moderate to extensive experience in more complex endoscopic surgical procedures is desirable. The actual clinical use should start with straightforward procedures that are completely familiar to the surgeon and the complete OR team. Such procedures include e.g., cholecystectomy or uncomplicated ileocecal resection. Step-up to more complex procedures is usually appropriate after some ten cases. It is essential to operate at least weekly to develop the skills needed to deal with the complex setup and delicate technology and to minimize time loss during start-up.

40.5 Efficient and Safe Use of Robotic Systems

Robotic surgery is a team effort. Both console surgeons and table side OR nurses or surgeons should understand the differences in appreciation of the surgical scenario and ergonomics. Surgeons should be aware of the risks of abrupt arm movements for table-side staff, who usually assist though a port in between two robotic arms. Console surgeons should also be aware of the loss of haptic feedback and the large forces that can be embedded on tissue with the instruments, both in- and outside their field of view. They should also create a high level of awareness on endoscopic surgery related issues such as gas leakage of heat damage by optics, because they are no longer in direct touch with the patient. Robotic arms may deliver pressure damage to body parts such as the upper or iliac crest in small pelvis surgery, or direct damage to the patient face of chest by the large camera head. Additionally, the high definition 3-D view usually allows visualisation from a larger distance to the target, and the console surgeon is less horizon dependent, because there is no direct contact with instruments and patient and the surgeon's field of view is completely limited to the operating field due to the design of the head rest. A gyroscope is projected in the upper border of the screen to show the amount of rotation and to allow correction.

Good and direct contact between console surgeon and table-side team is essential because of these differences in appreciation of the surgical procedure. This implies that the console should be positioned in such a way that direct eye contact is guaranteed when the surgeon lifts the head from the head rest. Verbal communication is supported by a microphone and speaker system.

The procedure starts with correct placement of trocars. Robotic surgery is less forgiving in this aspect. Ideally, the central column of the robot is in line with the target and the camera port. The latest generation robotic system allows docking from the side, which allows better access to the head or perineum during surgery. Trocars should ideally be placed 8–10 cm apart, and not in each others working line towards the target in order to avoid contact between the robotic arms during surgery. The assistant port is usually positioned between the camera port and the left- or right surgical port. The ports should not be to close to the target to avoid large exterior excursions of the arms due to the fulcrum effect. All team members should check for unwanted contact of the moving parts of the arms with the patient's head or body.

The OR table is placed in the correct position before connection to the robot. In case of pelvic surgery, legs are positioned as low as possible to allow connection of the arms in Trendelenburg position. Downward tilting of leg rests should be avoided after draping to avoid excess strain in the groin. In case of upper abdomen surgery, the patient's head should be relatively close to the table top-end, otherwise robotic arm length may run short.

The robot is not connected to the OR table, so a change in table position will put unwanted force on trocars and may lead to trocar displacement or damage. Good access to the target area should therefore be guaranteed before connection. Excessive Trendelenburg is to be avoided in pelvic surgery. One can remove the small bowel from the smaller pelvis in 30–40° Trendelenburg, and then reduce table tilt as long as the small bowel stays beyond the promotorium. Good and continuing muscle relaxation is requested to maximize working space and to avoid patient straining or couching, which may lead to trocar displacement. In case table positioning during surgery appears necessary, release buttons on all four robotic arms need to be activated to allow save table movement. The XI system form Intuitive Surgical can be conneted digitally to a dedicated OR table, which allows OR table movement with the robot connected to the patient.

In case of emergency conversion, table-side team members remove instruments and remove arms one by one, by pressing the release button with one hand and pulling the trocar with the other. Such a manoeuvre can be completed within 30 s. In the time out procedure before starting the procedure, an item can be added to discuss emergency conversion shortly as to whom drives the robot cart away, who is in charge of opening the laparotomy sets etc. It can also be considered to leave trocars and pneumoperitoneum to gain faster access to the abdomen in emergency setting, according to surgeons preference.

Success of robotic surgery depends on knowledge of the essentials endoscopic surgery and robotic technology. Teamplay is crucial and trocar positioning and coupling of the robot is best performed in joint effort by both console surgeon and tableside team. Good preparation and repetitive use of robotic systems will allow safe and time-efficient use and will deliver maximal proficiency of robots as a most useful companion in complex endoscopic surgery.

References

1. Stefanidis D, Wang F, Korndorffer Jr JR, Dunne JB, Scott DJ. Robotic assistance improves intracorporeal suturing performance and safety in the operating room while decreasing operator workload. Surg Endosc. 2010;24:377–8.
2. Chandra V, Nehra D, Parent R, Woo R, Reyes R, Hernandez-Boussard T, Dutta SA. Comparison of laparoscopic and robotic assisted suturing performance by experts and novices. Surgery. 2010;147:830–9.
3. Van der Schatte Olivier RH, Van't Hullenaar CD, Ruurda JP, Broeders IA. Ergonomics, user comfort, and performance in standard and robot-assisted laparoscopic surgery. Surg Endosc. 2009;23:1365–71.
4. Ruurda JP, Broeders IA, Pulles B, Kappelhof FM, van der Werken C. Manual robot assisted endoscopic suturing: time-action analysis in an experimental mode. Surg Endosc. 2004;18:1249–52.
5. Ruurda JP, Wisselink W, Cuesta MA, Verhagen HJ, Broeders IA. Robot-assisted versus standard videoscopic aortic replacement. A comparative study in pigs. Eur J Vasc Endovasc Surg. 2004;27: 501–6.
6. Narula VK, Watson WC, Davis SS, Hinshaw K, Needleman BJ, Mikami DJ, Hazey JW, Winston JH, Muscarella P, Rubin M, Patel V, Melvin WS. A computerized analysis of robotic versus laparoscopic task performance. Surg Endosc. 2007;21:2258–61.
7. Hubens G, Coveliers H, Balliu L, Ruppert M, Vaneerdeweg W. A performance study comparing manual and robotically assisted laparoscopic surgery using the da Vinci system. Surg Endosc. 2003;17:1595–9.
8. van der Sluis PC, Ruurda JP, van der Horst S, Verhage RJ, Besselink MG, Prins MJ, Haverkamp L, Schippers C, Rinkes IH, Joore HC, Ten Kate FJ, Koffijberg H, Kroese CC, van Leeuwen MS, Lolkema MP, Reerink O, Schipper ME, Steenhagen E, Vleggaar FP, Voest EE, Siersema PD, van Hillegersberg R. Robot-assisted minimally invasive thoraco-laparoscopic esophagectomy versus open transthoracic esophagectomy for resectable esophageal cancer, a randomized controlled trial (ROBOT trial). Trials. 2012;13:230.
9. Wang Z, Zheng Q, Jin Z. Meta-analysis of robot-assisted versus conventional laparoscopic Nissen fundoplication for gastro-oesophageal reflux disease. ANZ J Surg. 2012;82:112–7.
10. Mi J, Kang Y, Chen X, Wang B, Wang Z. Whether robot-assisted laparoscopic fundoplication is better for gastroesophageal reflux disease in adults: a systematic review and meta-analysis. Surg Endosc. 2010;24:1803–14.
11. Frazzoni M, Conigliaro R, Colli G, Melotti G. Conventional versus robot-assisted laparoscopic Nissen fundoplication: a comparison of postoperative acid reflux parameters. Surg Endosc. 2012;26: 1675–81.
12. Horgan S, Galvani C, Gorodner MV, Omelanczuck P, Elli F, Moser F, Durand L, Caracoche M, Nefa J, Bustos S, Donahue P, Ferraina P. Robotic-assisted Heller myotomy versus laparoscopic Heller myotomy for the treatment of esophageal achalasia: multicenter study. J Gastrointest Surg. 2005;9:1020–9.
13. Lai EC, Tang CN. Current status of robot-assisted laparoscopic pancreaticoduodenectomy and distal pancreatectomy: a comprehensive review. Asian J Endosc Surg. 2013;6:158–64.
14. Casciola L, Patriti A, Ceccarelli G, Bartoli A, Ceribelli C, Spaziani A. Robot-assisted parenchymal-sparing liver surgery including lesions located in the posterosuperior segments. Surg Endosc. 2011;25:3815–24.
15. Trastulli S, Farinella E, Cirocchi R, Cavaliere D, Avenia N, Sciannameo F, Gullà N, Noya G, Boselli C. Robotic resection compared with laparoscopic rectal resection for cancer: systematic review and meta-analysis of short-term outcome. Colorectal Dis. 2012;14:134–56.

Index

A

Abdominal cavity, 15, 26, 29, 34, 72, 80, 87, 91, 102, 164–166, 189–191, 194, 198, 228, 256, 267–271, 279, 280
Achalasia, 41–43, 45, 48, 269, 287
Acute abdomen, 71, 189
Adenoma, 231–232, 245, 246, 248, 249, 253, 254
Adhesiolysis, 34, 35, 37, 38, 183–186
Adhesions, 15, 27, 34–38, 51, 57, 64, 81, 84, 95, 103, 119, 122, 132, 136, 139, 140, 145, 146, 155, 158, 169, 178, 183–185, 189, 203, 208, 211, 215, 218, 221, 259, 268, 281, 282
Adrenalectomy, 159, 201, 253–264
Aldosteronoma, 253, 254
Appendicectomy, 275, 279–280
Appendicitis, 71, 183, 189–195

B

Bacterial infection, 167
Banding (gastric banding-GB), 87–92, 282
Bariatric, 77–85, 87–88, 92, 93, 98, 101, 105, 107–109, 115–122
Bile duct, 84, 111, 131, 132, 135, 136, 139, 141, 145–150, 161, 165, 280
Biliopancreatic, 78, 82–85, 87, 92, 94, 101, 105, 107–114, 118, 282
Bypass, 7, 78, 82–83, 87, 92–99, 101, 105, 107, 115, 120, 121, 282, 285

C

Cancer, 45, 53, 54, 58, 61–67, 99, 131, 139, 147, 161–163, 166, 183, 201–202, 207, 208, 215, 220, 227, 231, 232, 237, 238, 254, 287
Carcinoma, 53, 66
Cholecystectomy, 21, 27, 71, 84, 102, 110, 128, 131, 135, 139–143, 145, 146, 151, 163, 177, 180, 201, 268–269, 275, 280, 285, 287, 289
Cholecystitis, 139, 140, 143, 145, 146, 268, 280
Cholecystolithiasis, 139, 201, 268
Choledochotomy, 136, 149–151
Closed, 15–16, 26, 30, 33, 36, 66, 67, 82–85, 91, 94, 96–98, 105, 112–114, 148, 150, 151, 166, 168, 170, 171, 178, 183, 194, 200, 205, 221, 223, 229, 239, 248, 255, 257, 268, 270–272, 276, 280
Colectomy, 197–205, 207–212, 278, 281–282, 287
Colon cancer, 201, 207
Colorectal resection, 215, 271, 276, 281
Computer, 9, 42, 71, 254, 285–287
Cushing's syndrome, 253, 254, 260

D

Da Vinci, 278, 285
Diagnostic laparoscopy, 22, 68, 161, 189–195, 275
Disease, 7, 41, 42, 44, 47–51, 54, 62–64, 71, 78, 85, 88, 98, 101, 107, 108, 118, 125, 126, 132, 136, 139, 145, 161, 167, 175, 179, 183, 184, 189, 191, 197, 201–204, 207, 208, 215, 227, 245, 246, 253, 259, 260, 264, 269, 270, 275, 285
Disorder, 5, 17, 27, 41–45, 47, 48, 51, 77, 78, 88, 101, 107, 113, 145, 155, 167, 180, 189, 190, 192, 207, 269
Ductal calculi, 145–151
Duodenal switch (DS), 78, 82–85, 87, 101, 107–114, 117, 119, 121
Dysphagia, 41, 42, 48–50, 96, 104, 105, 117, 119, 269

E

Early and late subtypes, 167
Endoscopic, 3, 4, 7, 12, 21–27, 29, 34, 41, 42, 44, 54, 62, 64–66, 102, 110, 115, 145, 146, 150, 151, 156, 158, 168, 195, 197, 198, 231, 232, 235, 237, 238, 245–248, 254, 255, 258, 267–271, 280, 285–289
Ergonomics, 3–8, 11, 287, 289
Error, 3, 5, 9–12, 112, 220
Esophagus, 8, 41, 43–45, 47–51, 53–55, 58, 65–67, 80, 90, 97, 101–103, 115, 116, 246, 247, 267, 269, 270
Extraperitoneal, 21–26, 231, 238, 280

F

Failure, 42, 47, 48, 105, 107, 108, 115–119, 121, 131, 135, 146, 167, 179, 197, 215, 222, 226, 238, 253, 263
Femoral, 22, 24, 26–31

G

Gallbladder, 84, 102, 105, 114, 128, 129, 131, 132, 139–143, 146, 148, 149, 163, 192, 268, 280
Gallstones, 110, 145, 146
Gastric, 7, 43, 47, 54, 61–68, 71, 78, 87–99, 101, 107, 115, 155, 162, 176, 216, 267, 275
Gastroesophageal reflux disease (GERD), 45, 47–51, 78, 79, 102, 119, 121

H

Hemicolectomy, 202, 278, 281, 287
Hepatectomy, 125, 127–129
Hepatocellular carcinoma, 125, 131, 132
Hernia, 21–31, 33–38, 47, 73, 78, 88, 93, 105, 114, 143, 145, 183, 194, 197, 275, 287
Hernia repair, 5, 7, 8, 21–27, 29, 33–38, 186, 276, 280
Hiatus, 47, 49–51, 61, 80, 116, 119
High anterior, 215
Hybrid and open techniques, 15–16

H.J. Bonjer (ed.), *Surgical Principles of Minimally Invasive Procedures*, DOI 10.1007/978-3-319-43196-3

I

Inflammatory bowel disease (IBD), 101, 107, 108, 183, 197, 202, 207, 215, 227
Inguinal, 8, 21–31, 276, 280–281

L

Laparoscopic appendectomy, 189–195, 201, 280
Laparoscopic cholecystectomy, 9, 21, 27, 71, 139–143, 145, 151, 180, 201
Laparoscopic infracolic necrosectomy, 169–171
Laparoscopic ultrasound (LUS), 63, 132, 146, 147
Laparoscopy, 15, 22, 26, 33, 34, 37, 45, 54, 55, 62, 63, 68, 93, 94, 125, 126, 133, 143, 161, 176, 178, 180, 184, 189–195, 201, 205, 222, 238, 270, 272, 275–282
Liver cirrhosis, 108
Liver metastases (LM), 63, 131–133, 197
Local excision, 231, 232, 237
Low anterior, 185, 281–282

M

Mesh, 21–27, 29, 30, 33–38, 49, 50, 180, 225, 226, 276, 280, 281
Microwave ablation (MWA), 131–133, 135
Minimally invasive, 10–12, 15, 21, 41, 54, 55, 57, 68, 87, 125, 147, 161, 189, 197, 201, 246, 253, 254, 285
Minimally invasive esophagectomy (MIE), 53, 54, 58
Minimally invasive video assisted parathyroidectomy (MIVAP), 245–250
Minimally invasive video assisted thyroidectomy (MIVAT), 245–250
Motility, 41–45, 47, 88, 269

N

Natural orifice transluminal endoscopic surgery (NOTES), 195, 238, 267, 275

O

Obesity, 54, 77, 78, 85, 87, 88, 92, 101, 107, 145, 146, 201, 207, 215, 223
  surgery, 77, 88
Obstruction, 21, 30, 41, 42, 62, 64, 73, 85, 98, 117, 183–186, 191, 193, 197, 222, 249, 253, 269, 282
Operating room, 3–5, 8, 22, 27, 28, 34, 42, 56, 63, 71, 88–91, 93, 98, 99, 102, 109–110, 132–134, 161–166, 190, 202, 205, 227, 229, 239, 241, 246, 279–282
Options for surgical/endoscopic, 48, 62, 167–168

P

Pancreas, 55, 65, 95, 103, 111, 155–159, 161–165, 170, 176–180, 199, 204, 211, 221, 276, 278, 282
Pancreatectomy, 155–159
Pancreaticoduodenectomy, 161–166
Pancreatitis, 139, 145, 146, 155, 167–171
Parathyroid, 79, 245–250
Peptic, 62, 71–73
Perforation, 34, 35, 37–38, 42–45, 61, 71–73, 92, 105, 131, 143, 179, 185, 202, 222, 226, 233, 260, 263, 280
Peri-ampullar, 161
Pheochromocytoma, 253, 254
Polyps, 197, 237, 238
Proctocolectomy, 207, 281–282
Prolapse, 29, 30, 215, 225–229, 238

R

Radiological management, 254
Rectal cancer, 183, 202, 208, 215, 220, 231, 232, 237, 238, 287
Rectopexy, 225–229, 238, 271
Rectum, 185, 191, 202, 205, 207, 210, 212, 215–223, 231, 233, 237–239, 271, 282, 286
Reflux, 7, 41, 42, 44, 45, 47–51, 66, 79, 81, 88, 99, 101, 105, 108, 115, 116, 119, 201, 285, 287
Retroperitoneal, 29, 167, 178, 199, 204, 221, 253, 259–264
Revisional surgery, 122
Robotic, 11, 105, 254, 278, 280, 285–290
Roux-en-Y, 64, 66, 78, 82, 87, 93–97, 99, 115, 120, 121

S

Safety, 3, 7, 9–12, 16, 17, 38, 58, 66, 68, 106, 121, 129, 139, 141, 147, 201, 216, 222, 237, 268, 270, 271, 275, 280, 282, 285
Severe necrotizing acute pancreatitis, 167
Sigmoid, 41, 183, 191, 193, 201–205, 208, 210, 212, 217–219, 225–229, 271, 272
Sigmoidectomy, 201–205
Single incision laparoscopy (SIL), 275–282
Single port laparoscopy (SPL), 276
Sleeve, 78, 81–85, 87, 98, 99, 101–108, 110–112, 115, 118–121, 282
Spleen, 51, 55, 80, 82, 96, 103, 111, 155–159, 175–180, 204, 221, 222, 258, 259, 282
Splenectomy, 155, 158–159, 175–180, 201
Stomach, 41, 43, 44, 47–51, 54, 55, 61, 64–67, 73, 79–84, 88, 90–93, 95–97, 99, 102–105, 108, 109, 111, 112, 114, 115, 117–122, 131, 133, 155, 158, 162, 164–166, 176, 178, 179, 192, 197, 210, 255, 267, 270
Surgery, 3–8, 48–49, 87–88, 155–159, 175–180, 237, 285–290,
System approach, 3, 9, 10

T

Techniques, 11, 15–16, 21, 26, 33, 34, 36, 51, 57, 66, 73, 99, 125, 136, 139, 147, 155, 180, 183, 195, 197, 201, 218, 225, 238, 239, 253, 254, 268–270, 272, 275, 280, 281, 287
Telesurgery, 285
Theatre, 9–12, 217, 255, 279
Thoracic cavity, 15–17, 57
Total, 21–26, 41, 49, 53, 54, 62, 64, 67–68, 71, 84, 85, 104, 105, 108, 112, 122, 129, 135, 143, 168, 180, 185, 189, 194, 207–212, 215, 222, 231, 235, 238, 246, 254, 271, 276, 280–282
Totally extraperitoneal (TEP), 21–27, 278–281
Total mesorectal excision (TME), 210, 212, 215, 221, 222, 231, 232, 235, 237, 238
Transabdominal, 112, 268, 271, 280
Transabdominal preperitoneal (TAPP), 21, 27–31, 278–281
Transanal, 222, 231–235, 237–239, 268–272
Transanal endoscopic microsurgery (TEM), 231–235, 237, 239, 271
Transanal TME (taTME), 222
Transcolonic, 268, 271
Trans-cystic, 147, 149–150
Transesophageal, 268, 269
Transgastric, 268, 270, 271
Transperitoneal, 255
Transvaginal, 198, 199, 267–270, 281

U

Ulcer, 62, 71–73, 78, 88, 98, 101

V

Ventral, 3, 33–38, 73, 141, 225, 226, 238
Volvulus, 183, 197, 201, 202

Printed by Printforce, the Netherlands